DATE DUE

MAR 0 9 2005	
MAR 2 1 2005	
FEB 2 5 2008	
SEP 1 8 2008	
OCT 2 8 2013	
FEB 1 8 2016	

Cocaine Addiction

COCAINE ADDICTION

Theory, Research, and Treatment

JEROME J. PLATT

HARVARD UNIVERSITY PRESS

Cambridge, Massachusetts, and London, England 1997

Many of the designations used by manufacturers and sellers to distinguish their products are claimed as trademarks. Where those designations appear in this book and Harvard University Press was aware of a trademark claim, then the designations have been printed in initial capital letters (for example, Tylenol).

Library of Congress Cataloging-in-Publication Data

Platt, Jerome J.
    Cocaine addiction: theory, research, and treatment/Jerome J. Platt.
        p.   cm.
    Includes bibliographical references and index.
    ISBN 0-674-13632-2 (cloth: alk. paper)
    1. Cocaine habit.   I. Title
        [DNLM: 1. Cocaine.   2. Narcotic Dependence.   WM 280 P719c 1997]
    RC568.C6P53   1997
    616.86'47—dc21
    DNLM/DLC
    for Library of Congress   96-37435

To my wife, Kay, who graciously tolerated yet another volume
—thanks for morning coffee

romance with intoxicants were not insuperable. This feeling is supported by the evidence of the progress made which any reader of this book will come to appreciate. This book is clearly one of the rungs of a ladder we must climb to gain control over these problems and to minimize, or perhaps even abolish, their impact on our lives.

Edward C. Senay, M.D.

Contents

Preface

The problem of cocaine abuse and addiction is not a new one. Cocaine has been a public health problem since its introduction into the United States in the late nineteenth century. Initial failure to recognize the risks of cocaine use has resulted in periodic epidemics, interspersed with public forgetfulness concerning the risks of cocaine use, followed by a new love affair with the drug. Such has been the pattern of use in this country over the last century.

As yet, there is no "magic bullet" available for the treatment of this disorder, despite research on the problem over the last twenty years. Both laboratory and clinical scientists have been working intensively on the problem in this country and elsewhere, and have developed a large body of knowledge concerning the etiology, epidemiology, pharmacology, medical aspects, and psychology of cocaine abuse. This body of knowledge will likely contribute to the eventual development of effective treatments for cocaine abuse.

The primary purpose of this volume is to provide an overview of the present state of knowledge concerning cocaine abuse and addiction and its treatment. A second purpose is to provide some insight into the history of the problem, as well as an understanding of how cocaine achieves its effects and why these effects are so powerful. A third purpose is to provide a review of the strategies which have been employed in attempts to address the problem, and their current status. Finally, based on the material available, I have drawn conclusions and made some recommendations concerning what I believe are the implications for future research and policy making of the knowledge which is discussed.

This volume is certainly not meant to be, nor can it be, the final word on cocaine abuse and addiction. In fact, the very nature of the book publication process has no doubt resulted in some very recent findings not being included. Research, and with it increased understanding of the problem, will continue to accrue at a fast rate. Over the past twenty years, beginning in 1976, a parallel work on heroin addiction eventually resulted in three volumes on the subject. It is inevitable that periodic updates will be necessary with respect to cocaine as well. I hope that the development of increased understanding and efficacious treatment, which has evolved over the last two decades for heroin abuse and addiction, will also be the case for cocaine.

Finally, this volume is intended to serve as a review, as well as a means of access to the scientific and related literature on cocaine abuse and addiction and its treatment. While every effort has been made to report accurately the ideas, concepts, research findings, and opinions therein, the author cannot assume any responsibility for the validity, accuracy, or effectiveness in practice of the ideas, concepts, opinions, and data presented. This volume is not intended to serve as a treatment manual in actual clinical situations nor to substitute in any way for appropriate clinical training, experience, or supervision. Readers should consult the original sources for more detailed information concerning the ideas, findings, and interventions described, and should employ them only after appropriate consideration.

A number of persons have made important contributions to the completion of this volume. First, thanks are due to Mindy Widman for her major contributions throughout the preparation of this volume. In addition to her specific contributions to the preparation of Chapters 1 and 11, Dr. Widman oversaw the numerous tasks associated with managing over two thousand sources which were collected during the writing of this volume, and contributed in many ways, both major and minor, to the editing and proofreading of the final draft. Tobjörn Järbe, John DiGregorio, Stephen R. Max, Kay Platt, and of course Mindy Widman served as readers of the manuscript, and I hope that their incisive comments pointed me in the direction of greater precision—the blame for any lack of which must rest with me alone. And, of course, the yeomen of the book-writing process, Lee Sinclair and Stacey Chestnut, deserve my warmest thanks and appreciation for the countless numbers of trips to the library stacks, the seemingly endless searches for obscure articles and monographs in databases, and the management of the references. Their continued good cheer during this process still amazes me.

Cocaine Addiction

I

History, Use, and Pharmacology

1

The Problem of Cocaine Abuse and Addiction

I would rather have a life span of ten years with coca than one of ten million centuries without it.
—Paolo Mantegazza, 1859 (quoted in Owens, 1912, p. 329)

For William McKinley, Thomas Edison, and Sarah Bernhardt it deserved a written testimonial. For Pope Leo XIII it merited a medal. For Freud it resulted in "exhilaration and lasting euphoria" (Freud, 1884, reprinted 1984, p. 211). For Sherlock Holmes, it was "so transcendentally stimulating and clarifying to the mind that its secondary action is a matter of small moment" (Conan Doyle, 1888, reprinted 1967, p. 610). For the average late nineteenth-century American it was the "intellectual beverage and temperance drink" (Coca-Cola advertisement, as cited in Grinspoon and Bakalar, 1976, p. 28). For President William Howard Taft, in 1910 it was "Public Enemy No. 1" (Das, 1993, p. 298). In the 1970s it was a benign recreational drug (Musto, 1992; Reinarman and Levine, 1989). For America in the 1980s it had become (and remains to this day) a plague (Reinarman and Levine, 1989). Such have been the reactions to cocaine in its various forms and preparations, all of which have been developed from a native South American plant, *Erythroxylon coca*,[1] described in the dictionary as physically resembling tea.

A Brief History of *Erythroxylon coca*

When the Spaniards "discovered" Peru, they found the inhabitants continually chewing on a combination of leaves and ash which resulted, its users claimed, in increased strength and endurance. They were also fulfilling a religious rite. (Coca leaf chewing is still practiced in South America.) For the Incas, evidence of cocaine use has been found dating back between 2,500 and 5,000 years (Ray, 1978; Van Dyke and Byck, 1983).[2] Its use was likely initially reserved for the nobility or as part of religious ceremonies. By the time of the Spanish conquest, however, this exclusivity no longer existed, and coca acted as the commonly accepted medium of exchange (Johnston, 1853). Use, while constant, was in low doses (200–300 mg per day) as compared with the more than 2 grams of cocaine taken daily by high-dose users in the 1990s (Gold, 1992).

The Incan "Gift of the Gods" was viewed as idolatrous and as interfering with the process of conversion by the Spanish, who banned it (Van Dyke and Byck, 1983). Without coca, however, the Inca could not perform the heavy labor necessary to mine gold or work the fields (Freud, 1884; Kleber, 1988; Van Dyke and Byck, 1983). As a consequence of this new discovery, even the Catholic Church cultivated the plant (Spotts and Shontz, 1980). Leaves were distributed to workers three to four times daily during short rest breaks (Freud, 1884; Johnston, 1853). The properties of the plant in increasing endurance and combating hunger were noted and recorded very soon after the conquest, by priests and doctors alike (Freud, 1884). The euphoria and intoxication it produced were reported as the "Joyful Newes out of the New-found Worlde" (Monardes, 1569, translated by Frampton, 1596).

The use of coca, unlike many other substances found there, such as coffee and tobacco, was almost exclusively limited to the New World until the nineteenth century, largely because of the loss of potency of the leaves during transport (Van Dyke and Byck, 1983).

In 1847 von Tschudi, reporting on his travels in Peru, noted that "the moderate use of coca [was] not merely innoxious, but . . . may even be very conducive to health." As proof of this assertion, von Tschudi noted that there were numerous examples of long-lived natives who had chewed the leaves since boyhood and who "must in the course of their lives have chewed not less than 2,700 lb. of the leaf, and yet have retained perfect health" (von Tschudi, 1847, cited in Johnston, 1853). Johnston noted that the leaf possessed "two very remarkable properties not known to coexist in any other substance" (1853, p. 147): that is, it reduced the need for food and alleviated the respiratory effects of high altitude. Interest in the substance was also greatly increased by reports of the physiological and psychological versatility of coca published by Paolo Mantegazza in 1859 (Dowdeswell, 1876; Freud, 1884). Mantegazza recommended that the drug be used to assist digestion, stimulate the nervous system, increase muscular power, and induce tranquillity

(Dowdeswell, 1876). More scientific inquiry into the uses of coca leaf, however, found that "it has occasioned none of those subjective effects so fervidly described and ascribed to it by others—not the slightest excitement, nor even the feeling of buoyancy and exhilaration which is experienced from mountain air, or a draught of spring water. This examination was commenced in the expectation that the drug would prove important and interesting physiologically, and perhaps valuable as a therapeutic agent. This expectation has been disappointed" (Dowdeswell, 1876, p. 667).

Nevertheless, before 1870 Angelo Mariani, a French chemist, effectively introduced coca to the general public (Karch, 1993; Musto, 1992; Ray, 1978). Using imported coca leaves, he created coca lozenges and coca tea, but his most successful and wide-reaching product combined Bordeaux wine, a small amount of alkali, and 2 ounces of fresh coca leaf to create Vin Mariani or coca wine. His discovery made him one of the most respected and beloved manufacturers of the era. This "unequaled . . . tonic-stimulant for fatigued or overworked body and brain" (Vin Mariani advertisement, reproduced in Van Dyke and Byck, 1983, p. 5) was said to prevent "malaria, influenza and wasting diseases." Each 4-ounce glass contained 20 to 40 mg of coca, a dose similar to that received through chewing (Karch, 1993; Musto, 1992; Van Dyke and Byck, 1983; Verebey and Gold, 1988). The effects of coca wines, of which Mariani's was the best known, were widely praised by politicians, writers, composers, athletes, and even the clergy, including some who operated orphanages (Musto, 1992).

In the United States similar popular use of the drug was under way. In addition to more standard pharmaceutical preparations containing cocaine, Parke, Davis and Company produced coca cigarettes and cigars, coca cordial, and coca syrups (Das, 1993; Spotts and Shontz, 1980). In 1892 a formula for chocolate cocaine tablets appeared in *The Chemist and Druggist* (Musto, 1992). It was touted as a cure for catarrh, and patent medicines containing cocaine abounded, including Agnew's Powder, Anglo-American Catarrh Powder, and Ryno's Hay Fever and Catarrh Remedy (Gay et al., 1973).[3] It even became the official hay fever remedy of the American Hay Fever Association (Das, 1993). Cocaine content in these nostrums was usually low but could be highly variable. One of these drugs, Dr. Tucker's Asthma Specific, contained 420 mg of cocaine per ounce and was applied directly to the nasal mucosa, so that almost complete absorption was achieved (Karch, 1993).

In 1885 John Styth (sometimes reported as "Smith" or "Smyth") Pemberton, an Atlanta pharmacist, created a patent medicine he called

"French Wine Coca—Ideal Nerve and Tonic Stimulant." By 1886 the wine had been removed from the formula and caffeine substituted, thus creating the first batch of Coca Cola.[4] Asa Chandler, who acquired the original recipe from Pemberton, introduced the drink in 1888. It "was advertised to 'cure your headache' and 'relieve fatigue for only 5¢'" (Gay et al., 1973, p. 415). Each 6-ounce bottle contained approximately 4.5 mg of cocaine, and continued to do so until 1900, when the cocaine was removed from the formula and replaced with even higher levels of caffeine (Musto, 1992).[5] In addition to "Coke," Americans could also choose "Coca-Coke, Rocco Cola, Koca Nola, Nerv Ola, Wise Ola, and one simply called Dope" (Das, 1993, p. 297).

The popular use of the substance "helped prepare the way for the welcome for pure cocaine in the 1880s" (Musto, 1992, p. 8). In 1861 the isolation of its active ingredient by Niemann, who named it "cocaine,"[6] resulted in the establishment of practical and potent uses for the substance in Europe and North America (Van Dyke and Byck, 1983). In 1884 Carl Köller described the first practical use of cocaine as an ophthalmic anesthetic originally suggested by Schroff in 1862 and researched by von Anrep in 1880 (Köller, 1884). In *Über Coca* (1884) Freud reviewed the scientific literature available on cocaine at the time (approximately twenty studies). He also described his own experience with the use of the drug and recorded his observations about its use on patients (Freud, 1884). His description included the physiologic and mood-altering effects of the drug, as well as a series of recommendations for its use, including for stimulation, for digestive disorders, for wasting related to disease, for treatment of alcoholism and morphine addiction, for asthma, as an aphrodisiac, and as a local anesthetic—suggestions very similar to those made by Mantegazza in 1859.

As with Freud, physicians in the United States began to report the effects of cocaine, using themselves as subjects. The use of cocaine as a local anesthetic was pursued. Following Köller's work in Germany, William Stewart Halsted and his colleagues successfully established the ability of injected cocaine to block pain conduction in peripheral nerves, but he paid for this work with an addiction to the drug (Das, 1993; Karch, 1993; Musto, 1992). In 1887 William Hammond was able to chart the dose-effect curve of cocaine administered orally (Hammond, 1974). Hammond also insisted that cocaine was no more addictive than coffee or tea, despite early warnings about its negative effects (Mattison, 1887). This acceptance, combined with the greater availability of the drug in the United States than in Europe, led to its widespread use in this country (Musto, 1992).

Early reports of negative effects attributable to cocaine were found in the literature but were generally dismissed (Johnston, 1853). In the scientific investigation of the drug, however, these negative effects were confirmed. Consequences such as toxic reactions during ophthalmic surgery, cocaine-related stroke, cardiac arrhythmias, and others were reported (Karch, 1993). By 1887 cocaine addiction had been reported in the literature (Mattison, 1887), and by 1888, 90 cases of toxicity, including 6 deaths, had been reported (Karch, 1993). In 1892 a single French scientist reported 261 "accidents with hypodermic injections of cocaine" resulting in 21 fatalities (*New York Medical Journal,* 55 [1892], p. 457).

Nonetheless, between 1884 and 1887 Freud continued to support and even praise cocaine, as well as to prescribe it for his patients, his family, and himself (Spotts and Shontz, 1980). His prescription of the drug to his friend and colleague Ernst von Fleischl-Marxow to "cure" his morphine addiction, however, led to the first reported instance of "chronic intoxication and full-fledged cocaine psychosis" (Spotts and Shontz, 1980, p. 6). By 1887, when Albrecht Erlenmeyer, a fellow psychiatrist, charged Freud with unleashing the "third scourge of humanity" on the world—the first two being alcohol and opiates—Freud had begun to distance himself from his earlier opinion about the drug (Gold, 1992). His last work on cocaine, *Craving for and Fear of Cocaine,* published in 1887, was designed to defend his position on the drug while noting for the first time that individuals had differing physiologic responses to it (Spotts and Shontz, 1980). Although he continued to use it throughout his life, he ceased openly supporting it, and even went so far as to withdraw discussions about this period in his life from his autobiography (Spotts and Shontz, 1980).

The wonder potion of the early 1880s, cocaine had become, for at least some in the European scientific community, the "devil's own device" by the late 1880s (Mattison, 1887, p. 1025). This disenchantment with cocaine was also found in the United States during the 1890s. Books such as *Eight Years in Cocaine Hell* (1902) began to appear, and by 1890 about 400 cases of cocaine addiction, usually in combination with addiction to opiates, had been reported (Das, 1993). In 1894, at the annual meeting of the American Medical Association, this statement was introduced:

> We know the great value of the drug [cocaine] when properly used, the peculiarly delightful effect which it seems to have upon many persons and the baleful effects which have followed its over use. Is it not time, then, that we who have in part been the cause of this state of things should give our attention to the subject?

In view of the present state of the matter, the following propositions are offered:

1. Cocain, one of the most useful of drugs, is capable of being more harmful than even alcohol or opium.
2. The use of cocain is increasing to a serious extent.
3. For this the medical profession is largely responsible.
4. It is the duty of the profession to guard the public by every proper means against the dangers arising from the use of cocain.
5. To this end, it is desirable that this Association place itself on record as distinctively discountenancing the careless use of cocain: a, by the manufacturers of proprietary medicine; b, by the general public; c, by the general profession; d, and, lastly and particularly, by the Department of Rhinology which we represent. (Delavan, 1894, p. 452)

Withdrawal of scientific and popular praise of and support for the drug did little to curb its use. Reports from Europe in the period immediately after World War I indicated widespread use of the drug, perhaps encouraged by the casualness with which physicians had prescribed it prior to the war (Spotts and Shontz, 1980). Cocaine dens were reported in Germany, described as "both disreputable and dirty and also fashionable and up-to-date establishments" (Louis Lewin, 1924, cited in Spotts and Shontz, 1980, p. 11).[7] Cocaine was also said to lead to a change in sexual orientation from heterosexual to homosexual. Some theorized that the dampening effects of the drug on potency, along with a craving for new sensations, was actually responsible for the observed upswing in homosexual behavior.

Concurrent with increased observations of risk and illness, the trend toward professionalization of medicine and pharmacy, calls from progressive activists for reform of food and drugs, and prohibitionist campaigns for abstention led to increasing demands for action against patent medicines and nostrums, including cocaine, in the United States. State action was taken first. In the belief that easy access to cocaine led to addiction,[8] Oregon passed a law in 1887 requiring a physician's written prescription for acquiring cocaine. Between that year and the start of World War I, forty-six states passed laws regulating its use (Young, 1987).

Patent medicines were not covered by these laws, but federal action addressed this shortcoming (Young, 1987). In 1906 the Pure Food and Drug Act required that the contents of all over-the-counter medications be labeled and that food or soda containing cocaine or opium not be shipped across state lines (Spotts and Shontz, 1980). It also restricted the importation of coca leaves. Although the act covered most patent medicines, it appeared not to address those potions made by physicians in their practices. In a report on the composition of Vin Mariani, the American Medical Association itself claimed that the overuse of cocaine, in patent medicines at least, was the fault of the medical profession: "Can we blame the layman for using peruna, wine of cardui, etc., simply because they are advertised, when there are physicians who, for the same reason, prescribe concoctions that are just as quackish and just as useless?" (American Medical Association, 1908, p. 86). The Harrison Narcotic Tax Act of 1914 went substantially further and required that all those handling the drug be registered with the government, pay special taxes, and keep records of each sale. Those who were not registered could obtain cocaine by prescription only. In 1922 the U.S. Congress (wrongly) defined cocaine as an opiate and all but stopped the importation of coca leaves into this country (Spotts and Shontz, 1980).

Cocaine now went underground, much as alcohol did (Ray, 1978; Spotts and Shontz, 1980). Unlike alcohol use, however, cocaine use was not widespread and appeared to be limited to those defined as bohemians, such as musicians and artists, or to affluent members of certain minorities (Sabbag, 1976). Those who used the drug were linked by the media with groups seen as threatening the social fabric, especially African Americans and foreigners (Young, 1987).[9] The drug remained underground for decades.[10] By the 1930s amphetamines were seen as a cheaper and longer-acting substitute.[11] By the 1950s the federal government was claiming success in the war on recreational drugs, at least with regard to cocaine (Das, 1993; Musto, 1992). Even its surgical use was curtailed during the 1920s as a result of the development and introduction of newer, longer-lasting anesthetics (Spotts and Shontz, 1980).

The negative effects of amphetamines, which became the street substitute for cocaine in the 1930s, and the somewhat permissive attitudes toward drug use during the Vietnam War era allowed cocaine to make a resurgence in the late 1960s to early 1970s: "Cocaine, the truly American drug: first used by the Andean Indians, now with its resurgence restating the Yankee energy and vitality of free enterprise . . . even incorporated into our leisure hours ('Coke-time') . . . it is inevitable that cocaine, perhaps the most rapturously euphoric drug known to man, would be rediscovered by the dark experimenters of the Snorting Seventies" (Gay et al., 1973, p. 426; see also Das, 1993; Gold, 1992). Cocaine was again viewed as a "safe" high. The drug was initially used by methadone patients seeking the euphoria not offered by methadone (Spotts and Shontz, 1980), but it soon became the drug of choice for middle- and upper-class individuals (Gold, 1992). In large part, use by these groups resulted from the publicity given cocaine by persons in the public spotlight, which in turn led to a perception that cocaine was not dangerous—the hard-learned lessons from earlier decades concerning the dangers of cocaine having been by this time forgotten (Kleber, 1988; Musto, 1992). Risks from this "Champagne of pharmaceuticals" were seen as minimal (Gold, 1992). Even the 1980 edition of the *Comprehensive Textbook of Psychiatry* stated that cocaine was safe if used only two or three times per week (Grinspoon and Bakalar, 1980). Individual drug use averaged 1 to 4 grams per month, and the high cost of the drug limited its acceptability (Das, 1993).

The current wave of cocaine use began in the late 1960s to early 1970s, initially among middle-class or well-to-do users. Later, during the late 1970s and early 1980s, it became popular among the inner-city poor. During the period 1972–1982 the lifetime prevalence of cocaine abuse in the general population increased from 1.6% to 8.5% for older adults and from 9.1% to 28.3% among younger adults (Abelson and Miller, 1985). After reaching a peak in 1985, a decline occurred in cocaine abuse (Substance Abuse and Mental Health Services Administration [SAMHSA], 1991).[12] During this period increasingly fewer young adults appear to have been initiated into cocaine use (that is, have ever tried cocaine; SAMHSA, 1991). Data from the Drug Abuse Warning Network (DAWN) about cocaine-related emergency room episodes appear to confirm this finding.[13] Between 1989 and 1992, the only increases found in emergency room visits for cocaine use were among those between the ages of 35 and 64 (SAMHSA, 1994a). Preliminary data for 1993 (SAMHSA, 1994c) indicated that between 1990 and 1993, cocaine-related episodes per 100,000 population increased by 49%, from 36 to 54, with most of this increase occurring between 1990 and 1992. Similarly, cocaine-related episodes per 100,000 emergency department visits rose 41% between 1990 to 1993, from 98 to 137. Data from the Drug Use Forecasting system (DUF) also indicated that cocaine remained the most pervasive drug among adult male arrestees, and the rate of use remained largely unchanged (National Institute of Justice, 1994a).[14] In 1993 the rate of testing positive for cocaine ranged from 19% to 66% in various precincts, compared with 16% to 63% in 1992, with the median percentage dropping slightly from 45% to 43%. Similarly, among juvenile arrestees, levels of cocaine use were largely unchanged from 1992 to 1993 (National Institute of Justice, 1994b). Cocaine remains a drug of cities. Data from DAWN indicate a small but consistent increase in the share of cocaine-related emergency room episodes attributable to the 15 largest cities, from 75.6% of all such episodes in 1989 to 77.8% in 1992 (SAMHSA, 1994a).

When "crack" (mass-produced, smokable) cocaine first appeared in the United States in the 1980s, it was alarmingly inexpensive, very potent (albeit with a short duration of action), and highly addictive. Initial use was almost always by inhalation ("snorting"). Crack, or cocaine freebase in a crystalline, ready-to-smoke form, arrived from the Bahamas during the early 1980s, developed largely in response to the absence there of high-quality, inexpensive cocaine (Kleber, 1988). Crack first appeared in major U.S. cities during 1986 and 1987 and rapidly spread to the rest of the country. The drug began to take a firm hold on poor communities and caused high levels of disruption in the social fabric (Dunlap and Johnson, 1992). Transfer of the drug from the middle class to the lower class coincided (perhaps coincidentally) with increased media attention, as well as with increasingly harsh legislation against it (Musto, 1992; Reinarman and Levine, 1989). Despite the laws prohibiting it, the widespread understanding of its negative physical effects and the great difficulty in treating addiction to it, crack remains the drug of abuse for many cocaine users. Cocaine use in the 1880s and 1890s was clearly shown to have damaging and long-lasting physiological effects, particularly those related to addiction. Increased and heightened sexual desire and behavior were also noted (Freud, 1884). Crack use in the 1980s and 1990s has had similar addictive and sexual effects; its overall impact on society, however, has been much greater. Complicating the physiological effects of cocaine itself, crack use has been implicated in new cases of heterosexually transmitted HIV infection (Chaisson et al., 1989; Diaz and Chu, 1993).

Cocaine Use and Users in the United States: An Overview

In 1991 more than 4 million Americans admitted to having used crack and/or cocaine.[15] Almost 1.9 million admitted to current use of cocaine, that is, use within the previous 30 days (U.S. Bureau of the Census, 1994). When synthetic estimation, as opposed to survey techniques, are applied, the latter figure is confirmed, with 2 million Americans estimated to use cocaine weekly (Rhodes, 1993).[16] Cocaine appears to be a drug of the young, with 1.4% of those aged 12 to 25 admitting current use in 1991, as compared with 0.8% of those over age 25 (U.S. Bureau of the Census, 1994). Until 1991 the young (12–25) were also more likely ever to have used cocaine than those over the age of 25 (U.S. Bureau of the Census, 1994). Current (at the time of the survey) cocaine use appears to have peaked in 1985, with 1.5% of those aged 12 to 17 and 7.6% of those 18 to 25 admitting to use (U.S. Bureau of the Census, 1994). In a series of surveys conducted by the Gallup Organization between 1980 and 1985, differences between those enrolled in college and all post–high school students were found for 1980 through 1982, with almost no difference found thereafter (Kozel and Adams, 1986). No additional surveys have been conducted by Gallup that would test differences in use among college and non-college attenders since the appearance of crack.

The National AIDS Demonstration Research (NADR) project (Brown and Beschner, 1993) was, however, able to survey a large number of crack abusers. This multisite project was designed to locate injection drug users in selected cities who were not in treatment, assess their AIDS risk, make assignments into treatment, and evaluate the effectiveness of various intervention strategies. Of the 48,000 injection drug users (IDUs) recruited into the project, more than 22,000 reported lifetime use of crack and heroin (that is, use at some time in their lives). Of these, minority heroin users were most likely to have used crack, with 55.7% being African American, 18.2% Hispanic, and 2.3% Asian or Native American (McBride et al., 1992). More than 51% of crack and/or heroin users were between the ages of 30 and 39, older than would have been expected from national census data (McBride et al., 1992; U.S. Bureau of the Census, 1994).

Cocaine is not usually the first drug to be abused (Jones, Lewis, and Shorty, 1993). A Veterans Administration study (Khalsa, Paredes, and Anglin, 1993) found that marijuana, glue, hallucinogens, amphetamines, and barbiturates were all likely to have been used before an individual tried cocaine. Intranasal use, or snorting, seems to be the primary route for first use of the drug, with 96% of those in at least one study having begun by this route (Kang et al., 1991). Inhalation of crack or freebase is the primary means of use for subjects entering treatment, with between 72% and 88% of admissions reporting this route (Kang et al., 1991; Bunt et al., 1990).

Not every user of cocaine goes on to dependence, a state in which use of the drug is given a much higher priority than other behaviors which once had higher value (Edwards, Arif, and Hodgson, 1981). Dependence among users for nonmedical purposes was found to be 16.7% for stimulants (Anthony, Warner, and Kessler, 1994). Thus, for each cocaine user with a history of cocaine dependence, 5 persons have used cocaine without becoming dependent. This is, however, a relatively high rate when compared with other drugs of abuse, exceeded only by rates for tobacco and heroin. Comparative figures for dependence on other drugs are: tobacco, 31.9%; heroin, 23.1%; alcohol, 15.4%; stimulants other than cocaine, 11.2%; anxiolytics, sedatives, and hypnotic drugs, 9.2%; cannabis, 9.1%; analgesics, 7.5%; psychedelics, 4.9%; inhalants, 3.7%; and all other drugs, 14.7% (Anthony, Warner, and Kessler, 1994).

Cocaine use appeared to peak during the mid to late 1980s. Other measures of its effect on society, however, show a recent increase. Emergency room mentions of cocaine as reported by the Drug Abuse Warning Network continued to rise from a low of under 2,000 in 1976 to a high of approximately 110,000 in 1989. By 1990 this figure had declined to 80,355 mentions. DAWN data for 1992 (SAMHSA, 1994a) indicated a significant increase of 18% in emergency room mentions of cocaine since 1991, from 101,189 to 119,843. This increase was within the context of a 10% overall growth in emergency room drug abuse mentions, from 393,968 in 1991 to 433,439 in 1994 (SAMHSA, 1994a).[17] Preliminary data for 1993, the most recent available at the time of writing, indicated the number of cocaine-related emergency episodes to be approximately 123,000 (SAMHSA, 1994c). The change between 1992 and 1993 was not statistically significant. Medical examiner data follow a similar pattern. Cocaine mentions for the years 1989 through 1992 were 3,520, 2,417, 2,867, and 3,100 (SAMSHA, 1994b). Crack has been the source of much of this increase. Of the emergency room mentions, only 2% were attributable to crack in 1983 as compared with 86% attributable to inhaled or injected cocaine. By 1989, however, 37% of mentions were due to crack, with only 35% due to sniffed or injected cocaine (Homer, 1993). By 1992, only 1.3% of cocaine-related emergency room mentions were attributed to sniffed or injected cocaine, while 75% were attributed to smoked (including freebase) cocaine (SAMHSA, 1994a). The reasons for emergency room visits also differed from those for other drugs. In 1992, 25.7% of cocaine-related emergency room admissions sought detoxification, the highest number for all substances measured. Only 13.6% sought treatment for overdose. This was the second-lowest rate among all 60 drugs named (SAMHSA, 1994a).

Cocaine use has shown a recent statistically significant increase among junior and senior high school students, from 1.6% of junior high school students (grades 6–8) in 1992–93 to 1.9% in 1993–94, and from 3.4% of senior high school students during 1992–93 to 4.0% during 1993–94 (National Parents' Resource Institute for Drug Education, 1993–94, cited in Executive Office of the President, 1995). Cocaine use has also been cited in association with heterosexually transmitted AIDS. A study of drug abusers in the New York–New Jersey metropolitan area found that 84% of non-IDUs (non-injection drug users, mostly crack smokers) were HIV-positive as compared with 54% of IDUs (Pickens et al., 1993). Among women crack use has been found to be the greatest single determinant (14% of variance) of sexual risk behavior (McCoy and Inciardi, 1993). Because the duration of the high from crack is short, a large and continual number of doses is required. For crack addicts needing more drugs, quick acts of prostitution with other crack users may be the most convenient way to obtain the drug (Ratner, 1993). Large numbers of sexual partners are reported, with a consequent increase in the potential for HIV transmission. Increases in crack use have also been related to increases in syphilis rates (Pickens et al., 1993). In data reported by the Suffolk County (New York) Department of Health for 1988, almost 90% of those with syphilis were either crack dealers and/or users, prostitutes who used crack, or those who had sexual contact with dealers or users (Imperato, 1992).

The rate of psychiatric involvement among cocaine users is also high. It has been estimated by the Alcohol, Drug Abuse, and Mental Health Administration that 53% of drug abusers also have a diagnosable mental disorder (Jonas, 1992). The psychiatric diagnoses for those who use cocaine differ from diagnoses for those who use opioids or depressants (Weiss et al., 1988). Among a sample of hospitalized patients, cocaine users, when compared with abusers of other drugs, were found to have significantly higher levels of cyclothymic disorder (11.4% v. 2.7%, p < .001) and attention deficit disorder (4.7% v. 0.7%, p < .02), and lower levels of agoraphobia with panic attacks (0.7% v. 5.8%, p < .01) and antisocial personality disorder (16.1% v. 28.0%, p < .01; Weiss et al., 1988).[18]

Cocaine users frequently use other drugs as well. In the Epidemiological Catchment Study conducted in the 1980s, 84% of cocaine-dependent people were found to be also alcohol-dependent (Gold, 1992). Cocaine use among those using opioids is also common. In a study of people in methadone treatment, illicit opiate use was most common among those on a methadone dose of less than 70 mg and those who were also using cocaine (Hartel et al., 1995). The NADR projects found that among those who used heroin and cocaine more than once a day, 27.6% also reported more than once-daily use of alcohol, as compared with 13.6% of those who did not use crack daily. For those using crack more than once a day, more than 61% also reported snorting cocaine more than once a day. Amphetamine use was also high at 39.9% (McBride et al., 1992). In another study of individuals in treatment for cocaine abuse, about 53% were also found to be dependent on cannabis, using DSM-III-R[19] criteria for such a diagnosis (Klahr et al., 1990). Other studies have confirmed this high rate of co-use. Particularly prevalent were marijuana use (Kleinman et al., 1990) and alcohol use (Khalsa, Paredes, and Anglin, 1993). Rounsaville, Anton, et al. (1991) suggested that the high rate of alcohol use found among cocaine users is not reflective of a step toward harder drugs, as it is with opiate addicts, but may be explained by the anxiety- and insomnia-reducing effects of alcohol.

Cocaine abuse may also indirectly contribute to accidental death. One study found that 59% of reckless drivers not apparently impaired by alcohol tested positive for marijuana and cocaine, and some 83% of those drivers assessed as being moderately or extremely intoxicated tested positive for either marijuana or cocaine, compared with 14% of persons identified as being only mildly intoxicated or not intoxicated (Brookoff et al., 1994).

The Cost of Cocaine Abuse

The retail value of the cocaine "industry" in 1980 ranged from $27 to $32 billion, making it the seventh largest in the United States, using Fortune 500 standards (Van Dyke and Byck, 1982). By 1985 estimates of its worth had reached $50 to $70 billion (Clayton, 1985). For exporting nations, cocaine's value is even more substantial. In 1850 in Bolivia, taxes on the more than 15 million Spanish pounds of coca produced there accounted for one-twelfth of the state's revenue (Johnston, 1853). In 1980 in Bolivia, cocaine revenue exceeded that from tin, the country's leading legal export (Van Dyke and Byck, 1982). In Colombia refined cocaine exports totaled $1 billion, about half the value of that country's coffee crop (Van Dyke and Byck, 1982). In 1991 an estimated 337,100 metric tons of coca leaf were produced worldwide (Bureau of Justice Statistics, 1992).

Until the early 1980s the price of cocaine often served as a powerful disincentive to the abuse of the drug. During the 1980s, however, the costs associated with cocaine dropped dramatically. This drop in cost, coupled with greater availability in an easy-to-use form (crack), resulted in a rapid spread of cocaine abuse. Despite its low price, the costs of cocaine use to the individual can be immense, and the depletion of personal resources can be a contributing factor to the personal and social deterioration seen among cocaine abusers.

As of the time of writing, cocaine is relatively inexpensive. In 1990 pure cocaine sold to investigators by a chemical firm cost about $80 for 5 grams, with 5 grams of freebase cocaine selling for about $43 (Morgan, 1992). Therefore, a unit dose of 100 mg costs $1.60. The cost of a unit dose of illicit cocaine is substantially higher but, surprisingly, has remained remarkably stable since the turn of the century. Between 1907 and 1914, the unit of sale of cocaine in the New York City market was estimated to be 100 mg, sold in powder form for 25 cents. This was the approximate equivalent of the hourly wage of an industrial worker (Musto, 1992). In 1990 the price for 100 mg of cocaine was again approximately one hour's wage, as reflected in the gram price of cocaine ranging from $80 to $100 and an average hourly wage of $10 (Carlson and Siegal, 1991; U.S. Bureau of the Census, 1994). Crack is substantially cheaper per unit dose than powdered cocaine. One study of a midwestern city conducted in the winter of 1990 found that crack sold on the street for $1 to $3 for a "crumb" up to $50 for "working halves" (Carlson and Siegal, 1991). "Cookies," which are larger than "rocks," may cost from $5 to $25 apiece (Chitwood, 1993). It is estimated that a $10 "rock" of crack (about the size of a Tic-Tac) would provide two "hits" each lasting approximately 45 minutes (Carlson and Siegal, 1991).

For the individual user, however, the financial burden can be immense. In a 1991 study by Kang et al., about half the subjects spent more than $400 on cocaine in the month preceding entry into treatment. Of those admitted to a psychiatric inpatient unit who were of lower socioeconomic status, costs averaged $463 per week for the month prior to admission and $338 per week for the year before admission (Bunt et al., 1990). Costs ranged from zero to $2,500 for the week prior to admission and ranged from $120 to $1,500 per week for the month prior to admission. In a study by Boyd and Mieczkowski (1990), the amount spent each week on crack by a group of regular users ranged from $100 to more than $2,100, with a mean of about $940. Some 13% of the sample spent $2,100 or more weekly on cocaine, with no differences found between males and females. Another study found that an average of $9,375 was spent obtaining cocaine by private hospital patients in the six months prior to admission, with men spending more than three times the amount spent by women, although no differences in use were noted (Griffin et al., 1989). Most of the money was raised through criminal activity, with 70% of women and 90% of men reporting the sale of drugs, and 52% of women and 62% of men reporting property and vice crime. Some evidence exists to support the notion that white abusers spend more than African American abusers, with

$1,408 in cocaine buys monthly reported by whites and only $800 by African Americans (Ziedonis et al., 1994). In 1990 at least $18 billion was spent on cocaine by users, though this is considered an extremely low estimate (Bureau of Justice Statistics, 1992).

In addition to the costs to the individual user, costs of cocaine abuse are incurred by the society at large. These can be quantified in five ways: medical costs, costs for treatment and primary prevention, lost productivity costs, crime-related costs, and the costs of control.

Of the approximately 120,000 cocaine-related emergency room visits in 1992, almost 49% resulted in admission to the hospital. In such cases the costs incurred for each hospital stay are likely to be higher than average. In what may be the first study specifically addressing the hospital costs involved in the care of cocaine-exposed infants, Chiu, Vaughn, and Carzoli (1990) estimated that each case incurred $5,110 in hospital care costs, compared to $2,513 for non-exposed infants. Average costs in excess of that for normal full-term infants was $36,481 for those in the neonatal intensive care unit and $801 for those in the regular nursery. Such costs were attributed to a longer-than-average stay in the nursery (6.7 days versus 2–3 days) and neonatal intensive care unit (average stay 21.5 days). Hospital costs for cocaine-exposed infants were greater in all categories (room, laboratory, physician, radiology) but one: pharmacy charges. A figure of $5,200 in additional costs for the hospital care of cocaine-exposed infants was derived by Phibbs, Bateman, and Schwartz (1991). This figure was based on the difference between the costs for the care of cocaine-exposed infants ($7,957) and those for non-exposed infants ($2,757).[20] For adults, additional but largely unmeasurable medical costs are attributable to injuries (including those owing to accidents and criminal activity), outpatient care received in the hospital setting, and other non-hospital medical services (Bureau of Justice Statistics, 1992). A study conducted by Rutgers University estimated that up to 15% of health care costs in the United States are attributable to drug use and drug-related problems (Drug Strategies, 1995).

While the costs specific to cocaine treatment cannot be ascertained, estimates can be made by examining the funds expended for treatment of all drugs of abuse. The total monies earmarked for drug treatment by the federal government increased by 293% between 1981 and 1991, from $446 million to $1.752 billion (Bureau of Justice Statistics, 1992).[21] Since those who abuse cocaine weekly, either solely or in combination with other drugs, are estimated at about 75% of all heroin and cocaine users (Rhodes, 1993), treatment costs for cocaine alone can be estimated at $1.1 billion in 1991. The National Institute on Drug Abuse has estimated that for each dollar spent on treatment, other costs to the public are reduced by $4 to $7, and a savings of $3 in increased productivity is experienced (Drug Strategies, 1995). Expenditures to prevent drug abuse increased by an astounding 1,624% between 1981 and 1991, from $86 million to $1.483 billion (Bureau of Justice Statistics, 1992).

Employment among those who use cocaine is variable. In the NADR study, of all heroin and/or crack users, only 16.6% reported full- or part-time employment, with another 13.9% reporting sporadic employment (McBride et al., 1992). What is more surprising, however, is that 14% of those employed full-time reported use more than once a day, and almost 15% of those employed part-time reported such use. In other studies, employment among cocaine users entering treatment was found to be as high as 67.9% (Means et al., 1989). Using the lower rate of only 32.1% unemployed, with 1.9 million people using cocaine regularly (U.S. Bureau of the Census, 1994), one can estimate a loss of almost $3.2 billion to federal, state, and local treasuries.[22] In addition, an unknown amount in other costs is incurred in public assistance for those receiving the aid because of a drug disability, and/or for the support of their dependents.

Between 1989 and 1991, arrests for the sale or manufacture of cocaine or heroin dropped by 12% but were still more than 800% higher than in 1980 and about 225% higher than in 1985. Arrests for possession in 1991 were the lowest since 1988, but still almost double those recorded in 1985. Arrest rates in the Northeast for manufacture were twice those of the next-highest region, while those for possession were highest in the West (U.S. Bureau of the Census, 1994). In 1983, 20% of crimes committed under the influence of any drug (6% of all crimes) were attributable to cocaine use. By 1989 this figure had risen to 52% of crimes committed under the influence (14% of all crimes). The same source has estimated that daily cocaine users each obtain $7,000 more in illegal income than nonusers (Bureau of Justice Statistics, 1992). If only one-tenth of the 1.9 million current users of cocaine use the drug daily, $426 million per year of illegal income is attributable to their cocaine use alone. Moreover, prison costs of approximately $20,000 per inmate per year for the 150,000 serving time for cocaine-related crime in 1989 add $3 billion to the crime-related costs of cocaine (Bureau of Justice Statistics, 1992; Drug Strategies, 1995; U.S. Bureau of the Census, 1994).

Monies spent for legal control of cocaine abuse is the final category of cost to society. In addition to treatment, prevention, and law enforcement strategies in the United States, the federal government has taken several approaches to controlling drug use. These include interdiction of drugs entering the country and attempts to reduce the production of drugs in other countries. In 1991 more than $10 billion was expended for these purposes (Drug Strategies, 1995).

Entering Treatment

Treatment experience is generally infrequent among cocaine addicts. Some 79% of subjects entering treatment in one study had received no prior treatment for substance abuse (Kang et al., 1991). In another study, 49.4% had never had prior treatment, with 28.4% having had one or two previous treatment experiences and 22.3% having had more than two (Means et al., 1989). Entry into treatment typically occurs in the person's late 20s, although the range of ages at admission may vary substantially. In a study by Dougherty and Lesswing (1989), the average age of admission to an inpatient unit in New York was 27.8 years. Ziedonis et al. (1994) found that ages at entry into treatment were 27 years for whites and 29 years for African Americans. Other studies have reported ages of 29.9 years (range, 20–65 years; Means et al., 1989), 29.7 years (Weiss et al., 1986), and 29.0 years (Helfrich et al., 1983). Women were found to enter their first treatment at a younger age than men (Griffin et al., 1989). For Veterans Administration subjects (all of whom were male), the average age was somewhat higher (mean age, 37 years; Khalsa, Paredes, and Anglin, 1993).

In general, cocaine use is at a high level at the time of treatment entry. Subjects in the Griffin et al. (1989) study reported having used approximately 107 grams of cocaine during the prior six months (just under 5 grams a week). Severe cocaine abusers seeking treatment at the Yale Substance Abuse Treatment Unit were reported to have been using 1.6 grams a week during the three months before the study (range, 0.5–4.0 grams/week; Gawin, Morgan, et al., 1989). Upon entry into treatment, subjects in the Kang et al. (1991) study had used cocaine several times a week or more for at least one month, and 34% had used the drug at least that often for four or more years.

Conclusions

Stimulant abuse problems relating to cocaine, amphetamine, or methamphetamine use are not new to this country.[23] A cyclical pattern of abuse has existed for the last century. The first wave of cocaine abuse began in the mid-1880s and continued through the mid-1930s, when amphetamine was synthesized. Amphetamines replaced cocaine as the stimulant of choice by the 1940s and continued as such until the late 1960s, when cocaine again made a comeback (Musto, 1992; Ray, 1978). In general, these successive waves of wide use have been preceded by the perception that the drug was essentially benign and safe. There has also been a distinct "memory lapse" which prevents users (and the scientific community) from remembering the dangers of the drugs documented during a previous wave of use (Musto, 1992).

In the third and largest stimulant epidemic in this country, the current explosion in cocaine use began in middle and upper socioeconomic groups in the mid-1980s and expanded to the poor within three years. According to Ellinwood (1974), stimulant epidemics run a consistent and predictable course, beginning with a change in perception of the drug from being glamorous to being dangerous. Curbs on availability of the drug resulting from decreased production and prescription (and sometimes from increased enforcement of anti-drug laws as well) begin to have an effect. New use diminishes, and present users run the course of their addiction, causing a simultaneous increase in treatment demand and emergency room contacts. This activity is followed by a quiescent period of 5 to 15 years, after which a misperception of safe use again leads to an epidemic.

As Gawin, Allen, and Humblestone (1989) have observed with respect to the last, and still current wave of cocaine abuse: "The combination of low initial expense, unprecedented availability, and extreme abuse liability has resulted in an epidemic of refractory, recurrent cocaine dependence, making obvious the limits of current cocaine-abuse treatment strategies for crack abuse, and has led to unprecedented levels of public concern" (p. 322).

Overall, cocaine abuse has declined among a number of high-risk populations since having reached its apex during the mid-1980s. For example, Golub and Johnson (1994) found cocaine use to have declined among youthful arrestees in Manhattan since that time. This decline was dramatic, from 69% of arrestees in 1987 to 17% in 1993. There was a similar drop among arrestees up to age 18 from a high of 78% in 1986 to a low of 10% in 1993. Golub and Johnson note, however, that widespread use of cocaine will undoubtedly persist among this group as it ages. This phenomenon has already occurred with heroin addicts first addicted in the 1960s and 1970s, resulting in an aging opiate addict population (Platt, 1995a). In fact, this finding was reported for cocaine addicts by Gfroerer and Brodsky (1993), who compared data from the

National Household Survey on Drug Abuse for 1985 and 1991. They found that since 1985, frequent cocaine users have become older, with fewer in the 12 to 17 (1985: 17.9% versus 1991: 8.1%) and 18 to 25 (44.5% versus 33.1%) age ranges and more in the 26 to 34 (1985: 23.3% versus 1991: 41.6%) and over 35 (14.4% versus 17.2%) categories. Yawn et al. (1994) found a decline in cocaine abuse among pregnant women in Minneapolis–St. Paul from 4.0% to 2.0% from 1989 to 1993.

Yet, this general decline in cocaine use to below the flood level of the 1980s appears to have tapered off, and to have reached a low point during 1990 with a steady increase in rates of cocaine abuse after that (SAMHSA, 1994a, 1994b). Regardless of these general increases and declines in cocaine abuse, there is likely to be an ongoing core of cocaine abuse in this country, as evidenced by figures such as the 16.5% of newborns and 25.1% of other patients (most of whom were males 20 to 39 years of age) admitted to Los Angeles County–University of Southern California Medical Center between July 1 and December 1, 1991, who tested positive for cocaine metabolites (Chan et al., 1993).

2

Administration, Action, and Pharmacology of Cocaine

In its pharmacological action, cocaine—perhaps more than any other of the recognized psychoactive drugs—reinforces and boosts what we recognize as the highest aspirations of American initiative, energy, frenetic achievement, and ebullient optimism even in the face of great odds. On the coin's darker side, of course, are exhaustion, paranoia, and violence.

—Gay et al., 1973, p. 426

Cocaine belongs to a class of drugs called stimulants, the hallmark of which is to produce a temporary increase in functional activity or efficiency. Many drugs belonging to this class are, however, both prescribed and proscribed by society because of their potential for abuse. Among the drugs belonging to this class of stimulants are amphetamine (Benzedrine, no longer made commercially), dextroamphetamine (Dexedrine, Dexampex, Ferndex, Oxydess), methamphetamine (Desoxyn, Methedrine, Methampex), methylphenidate (Ritalin), phendimetrazine (Preludin), and pemoline (Cylert).[1] In the United States the stimulant drugs which are most commonly abused are cocaine in its various forms;[2] the various forms of amphetamine; and the stimulant-like drugs, including methylphenidate (Ritalin) and prescription weight-reduction formulations (Schuckit, 1994).

Other stimulants, rather than being proscribed by society, are widely accepted and used, with very distinct societal differences in preference and use. Caffeine, for example, probably the most widely used stimulant in the world, is consumed in the West as an ingredient in tea, coffee, and soft drinks. Cola nuts (Cola acuminata) or aguarana seeds (Paullinia cupana) are used to make beverages throughout Africa and

South America (Pickering and Stimson, 1994). Some 200 million persons on the Indian subcontinent and in the Pacific use betel (Areca catechu), which contains arecoline (a stimulant-like cholinergic agent), while in the Middle East and Northeast Africa, khat (Catha edulis), a plant which contains cathinone, an alkaloid chemically resembling amphetamine and having similar psychostimulant and euphorigenic effects to both amphetamine and cocaine, is widely used (Kalix et al., 1991; Schechter and Glennon, 1985). Khat is frequently used like coffee, taken at social gatherings at the end of the day, when the stimulant effects of increased alertness, talkativeness, friendliness, and concentration are desirable, like those obtained with coffee taken after meals in our society. As is also the case with cocaine, excessive use can lead to adverse effects, including delusions and psychosis. All of these stimulants are inexpensive and readily available (Kaplan, Husch, and Bieleman, 1994).

Legally available stimulants are widely used for the purpose of maintaining alertness by persons in occupations where such assistance is perceived as necessary. Thus, long-distance drivers, students, and night workers may use stimulants in a controlled fashion to remain awake and alert in order to better perform an occupational task. Stimulants may be prescribed under conditions where a high level of alertness is essential, such as among soldiers in wartime. This use of stimulants by these occupational groups is a means to an end, which may be contrasted with the use of stimulants for their psychological effects, as is the case in recreational or compulsive use of drugs. Stimulants have also been used for therapeutic purposes. Amphetamine, for example, has been used for such varied purposes as the treatment of asthma, narcolepsy, fatigue, depression, and weight reduction (Pickering and Stimson, 1994).

What Is Cocaine?

Cocaine is a alkaloid that occurs naturally in the leaves of the *Erythroxylon coca* shrub, which is indigenous to Peru, Bolivia, Colombia, and Ecuador. As noted in chapter 1, the chewing of coca leaves is still practiced by natives of South America. Coca leaves themselves contain a very low concentration of cocaine, less than 0.5% to 1%, thus providing a natural barrier to ingestion of sufficient cocaine to cause toxicity. For ingestion, the leaves are toasted and then either mixed with an alkaline material, or mixed into an alkali powder (ashes) consisting of the toasted leaves and other burned leaves, and then chewed into a "wad" or "quid," placed between the cheek and gum and chewed continually, sometimes for hours (Verebey and Gold, 1988). The relatively slow absorption rate and the resulting low concentration of cocaine (less than half that obtained by inhalation) results not so much in a high as in a pleasant euphoria (Brown, 1989).[3] Oral use via direct application to the gums is also practiced.

Cocaine has two main pharmacological actions, the blocking of sodium channels in the membranes of excitable neurons and muscle cells, and the blockade of catecholamine reuptake in the brain. The former action produces a local anesthetic effect through interference with the ability of nerve cells to propagate impulses (action potentials), and the latter produces central nervous system effects by increasing the effects of norepinephrine- and dopamine-mediated changes in the nervous system (Commissaris, 1989).

Forms of Cocaine

Cocaine is variously known as "C," "blow," "coke," "flake," "girl" versus "boy" for heroin, "lady," "nose candy," "paradise," "snow," "stardust," "toot," or "white lady." Other street names for cocaine noted by Gay (1981) include "her," "La Dama Blanca," "candy," "jam," and "the pimp's dog." It is most commonly available in a powdered form, cocaine hydrochloride, or in a purer crystalline form (cocaine base), commonly known as "freebase" or "crack." Cocaine hydrochloride is an odorless white crystalline powder having a bitter taste and numbing effect. It is very soluble in water and is also soluble in alcohol (Cox et al., 1983). It is prepared by dissolving pulverized coca leaves in a bath containing alcohol and benzine.[4] This mixture is then shaken, and the alcohol-benzine solution is drained. After hydrochloric acid is added, the mixture is shaken again. Sodium bicarbonate is then added. A precipitate is formed as a result of the rise in pH. This precipitate is then washed with kerosene and chilled, leaving crystals of crude cocaine, or coca paste. The cocaine content of this paste is in the range of 40% to 90% (Inciardi, 1987).

This process produces a water-soluble salt, which can be ground into a fine powder. For sale on the street, this powder may be diluted with a wide variety of adulterants (Inciardi, 1987; Siegel, 1982a; Tanenbaum and Miller, 1992). These are primarily added either to increase the pharmacological effects or to "stretch" the bulk of the cocaine before it is sold. Shannon (1988) identified five general categories of cocaine adulterants: local anesthetics, sugars, stimulants, toxins, and inert ingredients. Adulteration with related but nonpsychoactive local anesthetics (such as procaine, lidocaine, benzocaine, or tetracaine) can contribute to the numbing effect of cocaine on the nasal passages. Sugars such as mannitol, lactose, and glucose (the most common adulterants) add bulk, while stimulants such as caffeine, ephedrine, phenylpropanolamine, and amphetamines provide additional central nervous system effects. Inert adulterants may include insitol, talc, and cornstarch. Finally, other substances which have been found in confiscated cocaine include flour, acetaminophen, ascorbic acid, boric acid, heroin, calcium, methaqualone, pemoline, phencyclidine, potassium, quinine, strychnine, thallium, aspirin, sodium bicarbonate, plaster of paris, magnesium sulfate, brick dust, ether, and leaded gasoline (Inciardi, 1987; Shannon, 1988). Any of these adulterants may be found in any form of cocaine.

Freebase cocaine is extracted from cocaine hydrochloride by first placing it in an alkaline solution and then mixing it with a solvent such as ether or acetone. The mixture then separates into two layers, the upper one containing the dissolved cocaine. Evaporation of the upper layer of the mixture leaves a residue of almost pure cocaine crystals. An alternative method for making freebase involves heating a solution of cocaine hydrochloride in a pan while baking soda is added until a solid "rock" is formed (Laposata and Mayo, 1993; Wallach, 1989).

Crack is prepared by mixing cocaine hydrochloride with baking soda and water, and then heating the mixture to remove the water. The resultant crystals (cocaine base) have a melting temperature of 98°C, and vaporize at temperatures above this point. Thus, the crystals can be smoked. The popping sound produced when the crystals are heated underlies the name "crack" for this form of cocaine (Brown et al., 1992; Laposata and Mayo, 1993). Both freebase and crack are essentially composed of the free radical of cocaine.

Administration and Actions

Cocaine is consumed by diverse routes and over an extremely wide range of doses.
    —Jones, 1987, p. 56

Cocaine may be administered intranasally ("snorted"), taken orally, chewed or used sublingually, smoked as either coca paste or crack, inhaled in vapor form, or injected. Injection may be by either subcutaneous or intravenous routes. Intravaginal use has been reported as well as oral-vaginal insufflation (Collins, Davis, and Lantz, 1994). The drug may also be inserted rectally, to be absorbed by the rectal mucosa (Schrank, 1993). One case has been reported of powdered cocaine being put into the eyes (Ravin and Ravin, 1979). Cocaine is also mixed with heroin in a form called "speedball" and injected.[5] The freebase method became popular in the mid-1970s and peaked in the mid-1980s, with the emergence of crack cocaine following shortly thereafter. It should be noted that the smoking of coca paste has never been very popular in the United States.

In contrast with the late nineteenth century, when oral ingestion in the form of an elixir (Freud, 1884) or injection (*New York Medical Journal*, 55 [1892] p. 457) was preferred, inhalation of cocaine, or snorting, was the most common method of administration after the reintroduction of the drug during the late 1960s (Musto, 1992). Snorting was reported as the method of choice for approximately half of all users during this time (Gay et al., 1973).

One researcher questioned why the nasal route should be so popular, given the similar bioavailability (about 30%) and intensity obtained from both nasal and oral routes. He further found similar intensity and patterns of effects for oral, nasal, and intravenous routes of administration, and suggested that the rate of change in plasma (and therefore, presumably, brain) levels of cocaine may result in an important subjective element in the choice of a route of administration (Jones 1984). Cocaine smoking and intravenous injection of cocaine are equipotent in terms of peak plasma effects (Fischman, 1988). Furthermore, cocaine smoking (including crack smoking) does not carry the stigma and risks of injection (Johanson and Fischman, 1989). Nevertheless, crack cocaine smoking may be the most dangerous change in substance abuse to have appeared in the 1980s owing to its increased availability and acceptance, and to the illusion of safety of use (Gawin, Khalsa, and Ellinwood, 1994).

Injection

As noted earlier, injected cocaine is the form of the drug used much more commonly by addicts than by occasional users. When administered by injection, one-tenth to one-quarter gram of cocaine (although experienced users may inject up to a gram on each occasion) is typically placed in a spoon. Water is added, and the resulting mixture is strained, drawn up into a syringe, and injected. Euphoria follows almost immediately. Injection of cocaine may occur in episodes of highly intensive use, called "runs." A run of cocaine injection may require the expenditure of large sums of money for the drugs needed to sustain the high (Weiss and Mirin, 1987; Weiss, Mirin, and Bartel, 1994), and is also likely to result in neglecting one's job, family obligations, nutrition, and sexual function, all of which are secondary to users while they are maintaining the drug-induced high (Pearsall and Rosen, 1992).

The use of injected cocaine among individuals identified as injection drug users (IDUs) exceeds injection use of heroin. Data from the National AIDS Demonstration Project indicate that more IDUs have tried cocaine than any other injectable drug, and that a larger number had injected cocaine alone than any other single drug, including heroin. Alcohol was the only substance used more frequently than injected cocaine. Even in Hispanics over age 40, the only group in which use of injected heroin alone exceeded use of injected cocaine alone, the margin of heroin use over cocaine use was very narrow. Only when frequency of use is examined does injection use of heroin exceed injection use of cocaine. Although variations are noted in the combined use of heroin and cocaine as a function of race and age, injection use of heroin and cocaine combined ("speedballing") is consistent: over 96% of those who had used the combination had injected it (Feucht, Stephens, and Sullivan, 1993).

Injection use of cocaine carries with it the risks associated with the injection of any illegal substance, including infection caused by contaminated needles or the presence of adulterants. Such complications may include local abscesses, bacterial endocarditis, hepatitis, malaria, and HIV. (See Chapter 6 of this volume; also Platt, 1986, chap. 6, and Platt, 1995b, chap. 6 for further discussion of the risks associated with injection use of illicit drugs.) Whereas injection use of heroin may result in scarring caused by the presence of contaminants and adulterants, this is not typically the case with cocaine use, except as the result of subcutaneous bleeding. Recent cocaine injection sites typically appear as needle puncture marks surrounded by a halo of normal skin, then a very prominent bruise. This characteristic sign likely results from the vasoconstrictive effects of cocaine in the area of the injection site. The backup of blood within capillaries surrounding this area results in their rupture, producing the ecchymosis. This process does not result in a scar, except in the case of repeated use of the same site(s) for injection. The presence of numerous round or oval scars in intravenous cocaine users may arise from the same processes that result in perforation of the nasal septum (see Chapter 6), or may result from a lack of adequate healing of unrelated local infections caused by a disruption of circulation as a result of cocaine's vasoconstrictive effects. Necrotizing fasciitis, in which large areas of skin slough from injection sites (found in the case of other injection drugs), may also be present in injection cocaine use.

Although rare, if this condition is left untreated, partial and complete autoamputations may result (Wetli, 1993). Cellulitis and pronounced lymphedema may accompany this condition, which may result in erosion down to the muscles and tendons.

Intravenous use of cocaine produces a peak "high" within 10 to 15 minutes after injection, lasting for about 30 to 45 minutes. Intense effects can be achieved with injection of much smaller doses than those that are administered orally (Rowbotham and Lowenstein, 1990). Sudden death in the case of injection use may occur rapidly as a result of respiratory collapse. By comparison, death resulting from oral or nasal use of the drug may not occur for up to an hour after administration, following the appearance of generalized seizures (Wetli and Wright, 1979).

Inhalation

Intranasal use ("snorting" or "sniffing") remains a very popular route for administering cocaine. It was the primary route of first use of cocaine for 96% of those in the study by Kang et al. (1991). Cocaine, when obtained by the user in its crystalline cocaine hydrochloride form, is prepared for inhalation by placing it on a shiny surface, such as a mirror or glass-topped table, where it is then finely chopped with a razor blade and arranged in "lines" about one-eighth inch in width and one to two inches long. A line of cocaine consists of approximately 20 to 30 mg (Commissaris, 1989; Cox et al., 1983). Thus, one gram of cocaine (typically costing from $50 to $100) can be used to make 30 to 50 lines. The cocaine is then inhaled through a rolled-up bill (often of a large denomination, reflecting the "status" assumed to be associated with cocaine use) or a hollow, straw-like tube called a "tooter." Sometimes, a "coke spoon" is used to hold sufficient cocaine to inhale in one nostril. Great ceremony may accompany the inhalation procedure, and the objects used in it (that is, the razor blade, spoon, mirror, and straw) may be made of valuable metals such as gold or platinum (Weiss and Mirin, 1987; Weiss, Mirin, and Bartel, 1994). Administration may be repeated two or three times an hour over several hours. Very heavy inhalation users have been reported to use up to 10 pure grams (10,000 mg) daily (Cox et al., 1983).

Following inhalation, there is rapid absorption of cocaine into the bloodstream through the capillary-rich nasal mucosa, and blood levels rise quickly (within 30 seconds to 2 minutes), with peaks at 15 minutes to an hour after inhalation (Higgins et al., 1990; Resnick, Kestenbaum, and Schwartz, 1977; Van Dyck et al., 1976; Weiss and Mirin, 1987; Weiss, Mirin, and Bartel, 1994). Effects on mood are evident within 15 to 30 minutes after intranasal administration, and cardiovascular effects, including increased heart rate and blood pressure, appear within 15 to 20 minutes. These effects have generally been found to wear off within 45 to 60 minutes, although cocaine metabolites may still be present in the bloodstream for 4 to 6 hours after administration (Javaid et al., 1978; Resnick et al., 1977; Weiss and Mirin, 1987; Weiss, Mirin, and Bartel, 1994), although Higgins et al. (1990) found that cardiac measures, including heart rate and blood pressure, remained significantly elevated for up to 3 hours. This finding was attributed to intrasubject variability, the prolonged effects of frequent performance testing reflecting an interaction effect resulting either from the additive effect of cocaine dosages or from sensitivity to cocaine's effects by subjects who used cocaine only infrequently.

Intranasal use of cocaine is rarely as effective as other routes of administration in producing dependence, although approximately half of those persons presenting themselves at treatment programs used this route exclusively (Kleber and Gawin, 1984). Inhalation can, however, result in sudden death during recreational use, even when the same amount of drug is used as on previous occasions (Wetli, 1993). In such cases death is likely the result of pharmacological "kindling," a phenomenon in which repetitive subthreshold stimulation (either of an electrophysiological or pharmacological nature) of the same brain sites results in increasing central nervous system electrical activation and behavioral arousal (Goddard, McIntire, and Leech, 1969). This process eventually results in the onset of major motor convulsions in response to stimulation which previously did not produce an effect (Post and Kopanda, 1976).[6] Wetli (1993) has suggested that delayed absorption may be the mechanism underlying sudden death. In cases of death resulting from inhalation, a delay of approximately 25 to 30 minutes between the last dose of the drug and the final seizure suggests delayed absorption from the nasal passages. Initially, vasoconstriction would have limited absorption; sudden vasodilation could then have resulted in a surge of cocaine into the blood, resulting in the onset of convulsions when the drug reached the central nervous system.

Freebasing

Cocaine in its hydrochloride powder form decomposes at a relatively low temperature. Thus, it is inefficient to smoke it. A chemically altered form, alkaloidal cocaine, or cocaine base ("freebase"), is typically prepared for smoking, although the popularity of this form of cocaine, which involves risks in preparation, has diminished with the ready availability of crack cocaine.[7] Cocaine freebase is 37% to 96% pure (Weiss and Mirin, 1987; Weiss, Mirin, and Bartel, 1994), depending on how carefully its preparation is carried out. The freebase form of cocaine, while soluble in alcohol, acetone, oils, and ether, is nearly insoluble in water. Heating it at low temperatures results in liquefaction and the release of fumes, which can then be inhaled. This is typically accomplished with the aid of a small glass pipe heated with a butane lighter or stick dipped in alcohol or rum which is then lit, with a resultant dosage per inhalation of about 1/15 gm or 70 to 80 mg, with a range of about 50 to 120 mg (Gay, 1982; Khalsa, Tashkin, and Perrochet, 1992; Siegel, 1980). Heating cocaine hydrochloride in aluminum foil until it first liquefies and then volatilizes is also practiced, although the liquid cocaine base is colorless, and its low cohesion causes it to behave like mercury on smooth, metallic surfaces such as foil. For this reason, a little heroin is sometimes added to give the liquid some color (Grund and Blanken, 1993). The addition of heroin also results in a mixture that is more cohesive and easier to manage as well as one that is less volatile. (For descriptions of the mechanics of cocaine preparation, see Grund and Blanken [1993], as well as any one of a number of popular "underground" publications, including Lee's *Cocaine Handbook* [1983]). Freebasing can be a highly dangerous pursuit because of the risk of explosion resulting from combustion of the ether used in the processing, traces of which still remain, and the presence of open flames. This is particularly the case when flames from butane or acetylene torches are employed by intoxicated users to heat the mixture (Weiss and Mirin, 1987; Weiss, Mirin, and Bartel, 1994).[8]

Freebase smoke consists primarily of cocaine particles, which account for 93.5% of the smoke; the remaining 6.5% is cocaine vapor (Snyder et al., 1988). Inhalation of freebase smoke results in absorption through the large surface area provided by the alveoli in the lungs, from where it is carried directly to the heart and then, via the aorta, to the brain. This relatively direct passage to the brain accounts for a more rapid onset of pharmacological action than when cocaine is injected, in that injected cocaine must first travel through the venous system before entering the heart (Miller, Gold, and Millman, 1989).

Inhalation of crack or freebase was the primary route of use for subjects entering treatment in a number of studies. In the Kang et al. (1991) study, 72% reported using this route on admission, while in the Bunt et al. (1990) study, the figure was 88%. Freebasing was first introduced in the Los Angeles area during 1976–1983, and its popularity increased rapidly. Freebasing then became popular in the New York area during the early 1980s. Until the emergence of crack smoking, freebasing was the most common form of cocaine smoking in the United States (Khalsa, Tashkin, and Perrochet, 1992).

Smoking

COCA PASTE

Cocaine may be smoked either as coca paste or in the more frequently used crack form (cocaine freebase sold in a crystalline, ready-to-smoke form). Coca paste, also known as "base," "basuco," "susuko," "pasta," "pasta basica de cocaina," "pistillo," and "bubble gum" (derived from the similarity of the brand name "Bazooka" to "basuco"), is a partially purified extract of coca leaf. Coca paste is thus an intermediate product of the processing of the coca leaf into cocaine (Inciardi, 1987). It consists of a highly variable mixture of cocaine sulfate, kerosene, sulfuric acid, and sodium carbonate which is filtered and dried. In effect, it is an impure form of freebase which may contain kerosene and other solvents used in the processing. The cocaine content of coca paste varies from 20% to 91% (Brown, 1989; Weiss and Mirin, 1987; Weiss, Mirin, and Bartel, 1994). The paste, which may be gray-white or brown in color, is allowed to dry, and is placed at the end of a tobacco or marijuana cigarette, lit, and inhaled.[9]

The cocaine content of the inhaled smoke is rapidly absorbed, and the concentration of cocaine in the blood rises quickly. Since inhalation results in delivery of a dose of cocaine to the brain within only a few seconds, an intense, although relatively brief, state of intoxication may occur after only one or two inhalations. Plasma cocaine concentrations may reach levels as high as 462 nanograms per milliliter (ng/ml) after only three minutes of smoking cigarettes laced with coca paste. After having reached such an initially high plasma level, experienced coca paste smokers can maintain a smoking pace for over an hour or more at levels very close (within 5%) to the value reached after the first four or five cigarettes by smoking approximately one every fifteen minutes (Paly et al., 1982).

As is the case with the use of other forms of cocaine, subjective feelings of euphoria, gregariousness, and well-being generally result from initial use of coca paste. Prolonged use, however, may result in diminished feelings of euphoria, accompanied by anxiety, hostility, and extreme depression. This may lead to increased alcohol intake in order to decrease the anxiety and rapid mood change induced by smoking coca paste (Weiss and Mirin, 1987; Weiss, Mirin, and Bartel, 1994). Continued use of coca paste may lead to a number of symptoms, including numbness in the mouth, burning sensation in the eyes, pounding heartbeat, tremulousness of limbs, headache, insomnia, dizziness, abdominal pain, and profuse sweating. Prolonged use may result in visual and auditory distortions, overwhelming anxiety, aggressiveness, severe depression, hallucinations, and paranoia. Long-term use may result in a condition which has been labeled "coca paste psychosis," which is characterized by extreme hypervigilance, paranoid delusions, and hallucinations, during which overdose, suicide, and homicide can result (Weiss and Mirin, 1987; Weiss, Mirin, and Bartel, 1994).

CRACK

Crack (or "rock") is cocaine freebase which is prepared before sale to the consumer by processing cocaine hydrochloride with ammonia or baking soda and water and then heating it to a boil to remove the hydrochloride. Usually available in the form of small chips, the "rocks" are 75% pure when sold. Crack may be purchased on the street in the form of "rocks" or larger "cookies." The cost of cookies may range from $5 to $25 each, depending on their size (Chitwood, 1993). The high degree of purity, accompanied by a low price, makes use of this very addictive form of cocaine a significant risk, particularly to the young.[10] Typically sold in vials, a dose or "hit" has a cocaine content usually between 50 and 150 milligrams. Khalsa, Tashkin, and Perrochet (1992) found that most of their sample of cocaine smokers purchased crack rather than making the drug by freebasing it themselves. Only 14% freebased it, and 2% smoked the powdered form.

Crack has the property of melting at 98°C and volatilizing at higher temperatures (Gold, 1984). Typically, inhalation of the ignited crack (so called because of the crackling sound sometimes heard when it is lit) in a glass pipe or water pipe results in very low yields, with somewhere in the neighborhood of 1% to 5% of the cocaine content actually being inhaled. Like coca paste, crack can be smoked in a tobacco or marijuana cigarette (Weiss and Mirin, 1987; Weiss, Mirin, and Bartel, 1994). Crack cocaine is characterized, perhaps to a greater extent than any other drug, by the ability to induce persistent and intensive drug-seeking behaviors (DuPont, 1991).

Smoking of crack (or freebase, which is very similar to crack in its physiological effects) typically results in physiological changes and subjective effects very much like those produced by smoking coca paste.[11] These include a rapid rise in the cocaine content of the blood, which reaches a peak some five to ten minutes after inhalation. A rise in blood pressure, body temperature, heart rate, and respiratory rate then occurs (Weiss and Mirin, 1987; Weiss, Mirin, and Bartel, 1994). These physiological events are accompanied by an intense euphoria, followed by a "crash" consisting of severe depression, agitation, and cocaine craving about ten minutes later. The user may attempt to stave off the crash by smoking constantly. This sequence is called a "spree" (this term is also applicable to the use of cocaine by other routes of administration). The term "run" has also been increasingly applied to such sequences of events, although it originated in association with amphetamine use.

Among injection drug users of cocaine and/or heroin, the use of crack is also very popular. Crack abuse rapidly increased during 1986 and 1987 in major cities such as New York, Miami, Detroit, and Washington, D.C., where it came to dominate the illicit drug market (Johnson et al., 1990). A description of the cocaine-smoking epidemic of the 1980s from the perspective of a cultural anthropologist can be found in Hamid (1992). Data reported in the National AIDS Demonstration Research (NADR) study (Brown and Beschner, 1993) indicate that over half the IDUs in this study had used crack in the previous six months.[12] Such use was particularly heavy among African American IDUs, of whom 61.2% had used crack recently. This figure approached that for recent injection use of heroin (69.3%). Daily crack use was also much more common among African American IDUs (20.9%) than among Hispanics (5.8%), whites (9.3%), or other ethnic groups (12.4%). Hispanic IDUs were the group least likely to have used crack, with only 27.1% having done so in the previous six months (Chitwood, 1993).

In the NADR study, frequent (particularly daily) use of crack was positively associated with the current frequency of injection use of cocaine alone, and negatively associated with the frequency of heroin use alone. This relationship also held for crack use within the previous six months, in that persons who had injected cocaine during this time were also more likely to have used crack, and persons who had injected heroin during the previous six months were less likely to have used crack. Crack users were also more likely than other IDUs to have used alcohol and marijuana and to have snorted cocaine frequently. The smoking of crack was also related to higher levels of cocaine inhalation or snorting (Chitwood, 1993).

Crack has been called "the fast-food variety of cocaine" by Inciardi (1992), who explained its popularity this way: "It is cheap, easy to conceal and vaporizes with practically no odor; the gratification is swift and is commonly described by users as an intense, penetrating, almost sexual euphoria" (p. 305). Crack users will spend as much as $500 on a three- or four-day binge, sometimes called a "mission," marked by an almost constant smoking of crack, from 3 to 50 "rocks" per day. The user rarely sleeps or eats during a "mission" and ignores basic hygiene, thus compromising his or her health. Physical appearance deteriorates; scabs may appear on the face, arms, and legs as a result of burns or of picking at the skin to remove imaginary crawling insects. Burned facial hair, lips, and tongue may result from contact with hot pipe stems, and a constant cough may be present (Inciardi, 1992).

Although medical problems associated with cocaine smoking are discussed in detail in Chapter 6, it should be noted here that smoking crack results in a high frequency of acute respiratory symptoms attributable to both deep, prolonged inhalation of the smoke and employment of a Valsalva maneuver (a forced expiration of air with closed mouth and nose) to increase air pressure in the lungs. This results in the potential for rupture of alveolar blebs (blisters) and dissection of free air into the mediastinum (the space between the pleural sacs) and/or pleural cavity (Khalsa, Tashkin, and Perrochet, 1992).

Finally, it should be noted that another form of crack, "space-base," consists of crack with the addition of liquid PCP, LSD, heroin, or other drugs which are believed by users to extend the cocaine high. This combination began to appear in the United States in 1986 (Inciardi, 1987).

Topical Application

Topical application of cocaine hydrochloride, the only licit route of administration, is used in nasal, nasopharyngeal, mouth, throat, and ear surgery anesthesia (Brown, 1989; Ritchie and Greene, 1990). Because of insufficient cutaneous absorption, no psychotropic effect results from this route of administration (Brown, 1989).

Purity of Illicit Cocaine

There is great variability in the purity of cocaine actually obtained in street purchases. This variable purity is most likely the result of the drug's having been diluted, or "cut," at one or more levels of distribution in order to increase the quantity available for sales to the end user. The level of purity of course determines the amount of the drug in a dose.

Thus, a "line" of cocaine made from a 10% pure purchase will result in a dose of approximately 3 mg of the active drug, while a 50% pure purchase will result in a line containing 15 mg of cocaine (Weiss and Mirin, 1987; Weiss, Mirin, and Bartel 1994). The bioavailability of cocaine varies as a function of the form used and the site of entry into the body. For example, orally or intranasally administered cocaine is only 30% to 40% as available as cocaine intravenously administered in the same individual (Jones, 1984). Local vasoconstriction produced by the drug itself may actually inhibit a high degree of absorption when cocaine is taken intranasally (Wilkinson et al., 1980). Low levels of purity in intranasally administered cocaine may result in doses which cannot be distinguished from a placebo, thus suggesting the presence of other factors (for example, expectations, learning, and so on) in the "cocaine experience" in addition to the actual pharmacological effects of the drug (Weiss and Mirin, 1987; Weiss, Mirin, and Bartel, 1994).

Latency and Duration of Action

The route by which cocaine is administered directly affects the speed with which peak euphoric effects of the drug are experienced. Inhalation of freebase cocaine results in the most rapid onset of action, with the euphoric effects (the "high") being experienced within as little as 5 to 10 seconds, and certainly within 1 minute of intake. Next in rapidity of action is intravenous use, with the euphoric effects associated with this method of use being experienced within 30 to 120 seconds. The onset and peak highs associated with injection use occur in about 5 to 10 minutes and last for approximately 30 to 45 minutes. This euphoria precedes peak plasma levels and wears off while cocaine is still detectable in plasma (Miller, Gold, and Millman, 1989; Resnick, Kestenbaum, and Schwartz, 1977). Peak levels of cocaine in plasma following inhalation are reached at 15 to 60 minutes, and cocaine persists in the plasma for 4 to 6 hours. This persistence in the plasma may be explained by the presence of residual cocaine on the nasal mucosa for approximately 3 hours, resulting in continuous absorption secondary to cocaine's vasoconstrictive action (Van Dyke et al., 1976).

With oral use of cocaine, measurable absorption takes slightly longer: it does not reliably occur until 30 minutes after administration, a time lag that likely reflects a delay in absorption into the bloodstream until the cocaine reaches the alkaline environment of the small intestine. The peak subjective high thus occurs sooner after intranasal administration

(15–60 minutes) than after oral administration (45–90 minutes). Orally administered cocaine may also be experienced more intensely. The peak plasma concentration, however, is similar to that obtained with intranasal administration, possibly because of the similar half-lives of cocaine in plasma after oral administration (about 0.9 hours) and intranasal administration (1.3 hours; Van Dyke et al. 1978). These findings contradicted the then existing "conventional wisdom" of both cocaine users and others that cocaine is rendered ineffective when administered orally (see, for example, Ashley, 1975; Brecher, 1972) as a result of its being hydrolyzed (decomposing) in the gastrointestinal tract (Ritchie and Cohen, 1975; Osol and Pratt, 1973). The traditional Indian experience of chewing coca leaves would also be inconsistent with this belief. Absorption could occur through the mouth itself, however.

Regardless of route of administration, the duration of cocaine's euphoric action is relatively short, reflecting the brief half-life of cocaine. Half-lives under 1 hour have been reported by a number of investigators (Barnett, Hawks, and Resnick, 1981; Chow et al., 1985; Isenschmidt et al., 1992; Javaid et al., 1983). Van Dyke and associates (1982) reported a half-life of 0.8 to 1.3 hours and Jones (1984) 61 to 80 minutes, although Kogan et al. (1977) estimated a half-life of up to 2.8 hours. This duration of action is significantly shorter than that for other major drugs of abuse, including other stimulants. As noted earlier, amphetamine, for example, has a half-life of more than 4 hours, with a duration of action as long as 10 to 30 hours (Goff and Ciraulo, 1991). The mood-elevating effects of amphetamines may last 8 to 10 hours (Änggård et al., 1973). In general, the peak euphoric effects of cocaine occur prior to peak plasma levels being reached and while plasma levels are rising (Van Dyke et al., 1982), as is the case for many other psychoactive drugs (Jaffe, 1990).

Finally, it should be noted that choice of route of administration may in part be a function of the personal characteristics of the user. Hall, Havassy, and Wasserman (1991) found both ethnic and/or cultural and gender differences in the routes by which cocaine was administered. African Americans tended to smoke crack (82%, versus 17% for whites), while whites were more likely than African Americans to have used cocaine intranasally (63% versus 2%). Females, regardless of ethnicity, were also more likely to use cocaine intranasally than were males, a finding confirmed by Griffin et al. (1989). Nurco et al. (1988) found that in New York, cocaine was the leading nonnarcotic drug of abuse for both African Americans and Hispanics. For whites, cocaine was the second most frequently abused drug, after marijuana. In Baltimore, cocaine was the second most frequently abused nonnarcotic illicit drug among African Americans (following marijuana) and the third most frequently abused nonnarcotic illicit drug among whites (following marijuana and diazepam).

The Neurobiology of Cocaine

Effects on Neurotransmitters and Synaptic Transmission

Peripherally, cocaine produces local anesthetic effects which are due to its capacity to produce a blockade of electrical impulses within nerve cells. This action is caused by cocaine's ability to react with the neuron membrane, producing a rapid depolarization and an influx of sodium ions. This blocks ion channels and prevents further ion exchange, the mechanism for conduction of electrical impulses along the neuron membrane. Because conduction is prevented, the sensory signal is not transmitted to the central nervous system (Brown, 1989).

In addition to its local anesthetic effects, cocaine has two other primary peripheral effects: the production of localized ischemia or vasoconstriction through the blockade of norepinephrine reuptake at sympathetic nerve terminals in the periphery; and marked changes in cardiovascular functioning, primarily increased blood pressure and alteration of cardiac rhythm. These effects are the result of the blockade of norepinephrine reuptake and sodium channels in the vasculature, together with the cardioaccelatory effects resulting from increasing catecholamines at sympathetic terminals in the heart (Commissaris, 1989).

At the systemic level, cocaine alters the endogenous neurotransmitter system. Centrally, cocaine acts upon catecholaminergic neurotransmission, including both noradrenergic and dopaminergic pathways. Noradrenergic pathways appear to be important in mediating the nonspecific activating effects of stimulants, including cardiovascular complications and the appearance of symptoms which follow discontinuation of stimulant use (Gawin and Ellinwood, 1988; Kosten, 1990). Dopaminergic brain circuits appear to be important in stimulant-induced euphoria and the reinforcing effects which maintain stimulant abuse (Shepherd, 1988; Wise, 1984). Serotonergic pathways may also play a role in cocaine abuse, although this has not been firmly established (Kosten, 1990; Shepherd, 1988).

The central mechanism in the action of cocaine and other stimulants with high abuse potential appears to be their stimulation of dopaminergic reward pathways in the brain (Gawin and Ellinwood, 1988; Goeders and Smith, 1983; Yokel and Wise, 1975). According to Kosten (1990), the following actions take place at the synapse during stimulant action: the release of catecholamines from presynaptic terminals; the blocking of dopamine, norepinephrine, and serotonin uptake, the major mechanisms for inactivating neurotransmitters; and changes in receptor sensitivities with chronic use. Chronic use may result in effects other than just those resulting from increased availability of catecholamines and serotonin. These include sensitization ("reverse tolerance") and tolerance. The former has been demonstrated in the laboratory with respect to locomotor and stereotypic effects of cocaine (Segal and Mandell, 1974; Stripling and Ellinwood, 1977). This phenomenon, which can persist for weeks or months, can occur after only a few days of cocaine administration (Post and Rose, 1976; Post et al., 1981). The mechanism underlying sensitization is not well understood, but it likely involves the dopaminergic system. Behavioral sensitization may be localized in the nucleus accumbens, although other neural systems may mediate the acute motor effects of cocaine (Kalivas and Duffy, 1990). Sensitization can be blocked by haloperidol (Weiss, Post, Pert, et al., 1989).[13] While administration of apomorphine, a dopamine receptor agonist, has been shown to prevent the development of a sensitization response to amphetamine in mice (Riffee, Wanek, and Wilcox, 1987), apomorphine did not prevent sensitization induced by subchronic cocaine administration (Riffee, Wanek, and Wilcox, 1988), suggesting that sensitization to these two stimulants may involve different processes.

Tolerance to the effects of cocaine can develop through decreased inhibition of reuptake with chronic use; decreased release of the neurotransmitters catecholamine and serotonin, perhaps owing to depletion at the presynaptic terminal (although this mechanism has not been confirmed); or changes in receptor sensitivity at either presynaptic or postsynaptic sites leading to neuronal autoinhibition (Kosten, 1990; for a fuller discussion of the pharmacology and neurobiology of cocaine and other stimulants, see Johanson and Fischman, 1989; Kosten, 1993).

Specifically, cocaine blocks the reuptake of norepinephrine and dopamine at presynaptic locations, thus increasing the concentration of these transmitters at postsynaptic receptor sites. This concentration of dopamine is particularly increased in the reward pathways (Bozarth and Wise, 1981). Activation of the sympathetic nervous system also occurs, accounting for cocaine's activating effects. These include tachycardia, increased systolic blood pressure, mydriasis, and other sympathetic effects (Ritchie and Greene, 1990).

As noted earlier, the "dopamine hypothesis" seeks to explain the reinforcing properties of cocaine. It proposes that cocaine binds at the dopamine transporter and inhibits neurotransmitter reuptake. As a result, dopaminergic neurotransmission is potentiated in mesolimbocortical pathways, leading to reinforcement of events associated with cocaine binding and inhibition of intake at the molecular level (Kuhar, 1992). As other drugs, such as nicotine and alcohol, also activate the mesolimbic pathway, this may serve as the final common pathway for a number of psychoactive substances even if their initial site of action is at another place in the nervous system (Kuhar, Ritz, and Boja, 1991).

Although substantial evidence for the dopamine hypothesis is available for animals, less evidence is available for humans. At the animal level, for example, Ritz et al. (1987) reported evidence that dopamine transport inhibition is likely the primary mechanism responsible for the reinforcing effects of cocaine, and thus the "receptor site," or the site of action where the events resulting in the reinforcing effects are initiated, although other sites could not be ruled out. Among the lines of evidence available for this explanation at the human level, Kuhar, Ritz, and Boja (1991) list the following: positron emission tomography (PET) studies showing similarity in time course between cocaine receptor (dopamine receptor) occupancy and cocaine effects; the presence of paranoia and psychosis in both prolonged or high-dose cocaine abuse and in schizophrenia, a disorder believed to involve the dopaminergic limbic pathway; the action of indirect dopamine receptor stimulators such as methylphenidate or bromocriptine in successfully reducing initial cocaine craving, suggesting that dopaminergic agents can influence the same processes as cocaine (Dackis et al., 1987; Khantzian et al., 1984); the preference shown for dopamine uptake blockers in choice studies (Chait, Uhlenhuth and Johanson, 1987); and the suggestion that flupenthixol decanoate, a dopamine receptor blocker, can decrease craving (Giannini et al., 1986; Gawin, Kleber, et al., 1989).

The administration of other dopamine blockers such as chlorpromazine or haloperidol did not reduce cocaine-induced euphoria or self-administration, but did reduce psychotic symptoms (Gawin, 1986a). Haloperidol also failed to attenuate the cocaine "rush," only modestly influenced the subjective effects of cocaine, and attenuated cocaine-induced systolic and diastolic blood pressure (Sherer, Kumor, and Jaffe, 1989). Both of these findings suggest that the blockade of D_2 receptors (a subset of dopamine receptors of which haloperidol is a primary antagonist) did not strongly affect cocaine euphoria, although pretreatment with dopaminergic receptor blockers prevented amphetamine-induced euphoria. These results suggest the possibility that dopaminergic mechanisms are involved in initiation of cocaine use but not in later phenomena such as dependence and craving. Using single photon emission computed tomography, Pearlson and associates (1993) found that intravenously administered cocaine produced subjective effects (self-ratings of "rush" and "high") corresponding with regional decreases in cerebral blood flow to sites rich in dopaminergic terminals, suggesting dopaminergic system involvement in producing these subjective states.

While the effects of cocaine on the dopaminergic neuronal systems in the brain are thought to be mediated by short-term blockage of dopamine reuptake, long-term use results in depletion of dopamine at these same sites (Volkow et al., 1990). This depletion may result in disruption of dopaminergic transmission, causing dysphoria and drug craving. The Volkow et al. (1990) study, however, demonstrated a recovery of postsynaptic dopamine receptor availability to normal levels in detoxified cocaine abusers after a drug-free period of one month. A more recent study also examined the possibility that cocaine exposure alters the dopamine transporter and concluded that regulation of the dopamine transporter is highly sensitive to cocaine dosing regimens and withdrawal intervals (Little et al., 1993).

Several aspects of the mechanisms described herein form the basis of pharmacological interventions for cocaine abuse. For example, when dopamine pathways are antagonized by neuroleptics which act as dopamine blockers (Phillips, Broekkamp, and Fibiger, 1983), or when these same pathways are destroyed chemically or are surgically ablated (Bozarth and Wise, 1986; Roberts, Corcoran, and Fibiger, 1977), the behavioral effects of cocaine are eliminated. Cocaine's reinforcing and euphoric qualities may also occur as a result of the drug's effects on serotonin, although the mechanisms involved are not yet known. Cocaine administration increases the neurotransmitter serotonin at synaptic sites by inhibiting reuptake, in much the same way as dopamine and norepinephrine are affected (Hall, Talbert, and Ereshefsky, 1990), likely resulting in reduced serotonin turnover. Serotonin levels are also reduced by cocaine. Thus, agents that modulate serotonin may influence the action of cocaine (Johnson and Vocci, 1993). It is also known that μ agonists such as morphine and methadone stimulate dopamine transmission in the mesolimbic system, while κ agonists reduce it to the same extent. Since buprenorphine (a μ-partial agonist) suppresses cocaine self-administration in rhesus monkeys to the same extent that it suppresses opioid self-administration, the possibility exists of a link between the opioid system and the system(s) responsible for producing the reinforcing effects of cocaine in non-human primates (Johnson and Vocci, 1993).

The central nervous system actions of cocaine may be divided into euphoric and noneuphoric effects. Noneuphoric effects, particularly the marked hyperactivity and anorexia (decreased appetite) seen in cocaine use, also appear to be related to the blockade of dopamine reuptake. Other effects, including derangements of the anterior pituitary function, may occur as a result of both acute and chronic administration of cocaine. These effects are also not entirely clear, however. For example, a decrease in plasma prolactin (hypoprolactinemia) was reported in male cocaine abusers by Gawin and Kleber (1985a). Yet hyperprolactinemia following initiation of abstinence has also been reported in male chronic cocaine abusers (Cocores, Dackis, and Gold, 1986; Dackis and Gold, 1985b). The latter probably results from an increase in synaptic dopamine in the brain (Commissaris, 1989), a finding suggesting to Dackis and Gold (1985b) that cocaine acutely activates dopamine neuronal activity, whereas with chronic use dopamine is inhibited. Since cocaine blocks dopamine reuptake (Ross and Renyi, 1966; Taylor and Ho, 1978; Taylor, Ho, and Fagan, 1979), and dopaminergic systems modulate prolactin secretion (Tuomisto and Mannisto, 1985), prolactin would be expected to be suppressed by cocaine and to rebound under cocaine withdrawal (Mendelson et al., 1988). Nonetheless, Mendelson et al. (1988) found continued prolactin elevation in 5 of 8 subjects during protracted cocaine abstinence, leading them to suggest a protracted cocaine abstinence syndrome, with plasma prolactin as a useful marker for relapse potential. Although a later study (Mendelson et al. 1992) also found a decrease in prolactin levels following cocaine administration, this effect may have been the result of inhibition of luteinizing hormone-releasing hormone (which stimulates both prolactin and luteinizing hormone) by cocaine. Cocaine also stimulates the release of ACTH (Borowsky and Kuhn, 1991; Mendelson et al., 1992), an action which may also reflect cocaine's effects on dopaminergic mechanisms (Johanson and Fischman, 1989; Ritz et al., 1987).

Similarities and Differences between Cocaine and Amphetamines

Although the two are structurally dissimilar, the amphetamines share many pharmacological properties with cocaine. These shared properties make the subjective effects virtually indistinguishable in some respects (Brown, Corriveau, and Ebert, 1978; Fischman et al., 1976). The pharmacological properties resulting in this similarity include (to varying degrees) the common influence of both cocaine and amphetamines on monoaminergic neurotransmission (Kosten, 1990; Wise, 1984). Both types of drugs result in enhanced dopamine, norepinephrine, and serotonin release (Kosten, 1990; Moore, Ciueh, and Zeldes, 1977; Wise, 1984).

The two drugs differ, however, with respect to duration of action. Cocaine has a plasma half-life of 90 minutes. The half-life for euphoric effects is significantly shorter, under 45 minutes, largely owing to a rapid decline in effects (Gawin and Ellinwood, 1988). By contrast, amphetamines have a half-life and a euphoric effect lasting four to eight times longer (Änggård et al., 1973). This difference results in variable patterns of abuse, particularly during binges, when cocaine may be taken as frequently as every 10 minutes (Gawin and Kleber, 1985b), whereas one or more hours may elapse between administration of successive doses of amphetamines (Kramer, Fischman, and Littlefield, 1967). Cocaine binges may last up to 7 days, although 12 hours is more typical (Gawin and Kleber, 1985b), while amphetamine binges typically last for 24 hours or more, and a length of up to 5 days is not unusual (Kramer, Fischman, and Littlefield, 1967). Overall, with the exception of duration of action, and resultant patterns of use, the amphetamines and cocaine produce similar, though not identical, neurochemical and clinical effects.

Cocaine Metabolism

Cocaine is metabolized through three pathways: plasma cholinesterase, and to a lesser extent hepatic cholinesterase, by hydrolysis, which converts cocaine to an inactive metabolite (ecgonine methyl ester) that accounts for 32% to 49% of cocaine's metabolites excreted in urine (Inaba, Stewart, and Kalow, 1978); nonenzymatic hydrolysis of cocaine in the blood, resulting in the formation of benzoylecgonine, the major active metabolite of cocaine, which accounts for 29% to 45% of cocaine excreted in urine (Fish and Wilson, 1969); and norcocaine, an active metabolite of cocaine, which is formed by a process of N-demethylation, although norcocaine accounts for less than 5% of the total cocaine metabolites (Inaba, Stewart, and Kalow, 1978; Stewart et al., 1977; Stewart et al., 1979).

Cholinesterase activity is essential for cocaine metabolism to take place, since approximately 50% of cocaine is metabolized through this pathway (Inaba, Stewart, and Kalow, 1978). There is an inverse relationship between the symptoms of cocaine intoxication and plasma cholinesterase activity, and the life-threatening effects of cocaine toxicity are increased in the presence of low plasma cholinesterase activity (Hoffman et al., 1992). Schrank (1993) has noted the need for further study of the role of individual variability in plasma cholinesterase activity with respect to the risk of adverse reactions to cocaine.

Cocaine has an elimination half-life of about 75 minutes when administered intranasally and 48 minutes when administered orally (Wilkinson et al., 1980). The drug may be detected on the nasal mucosa for up to 3 hours following administration (Van Dyke et al., 1982), while unmetabolized cocaine in the serum, with a half-life of about 1 hour (range, 16–87 minutes; Chow et al., 1985), appears to be detectable in the blood for up to 2 to 3 hours, and possibly as much as 24 hours (Kogan et al., 1977). Benzoylecgonine and ecgonine methyl ester, the primary metabolites of cocaine, have half-lives in blood of 7.5 hours and 3.6 hours, respectively, and are almost fully eliminated by approximately 45 and 21.6 hours after use (Verebey, 1987). Benzoylecgonine has, however, been detected in urine for up to 10 to 22 days after cessation of use in very high dose cocaine abusers (Weiss and Gawin, 1988). Detection of cocaine in humans using these markers is limited to a time frame of up to 5 to 6 days following exposure when sophisticated technology (gas chromatography/mass spectrometry [GC/MS] and radioimunoassay [RIA] have the greatest sensitivity) is used (Verebey, 1987). In the case of heavy users, and depending on the method used, 2 to 3 days is a conservative limit for detection of cocaine metabolites in blood, particularly when the less sensitive enzyme-multiplied immunoassay (EMIT) technology is used. At times, however, this window of detection may be less than one day, since the level of benzoylecgonine drops rapidly. In the case of 24-hour levels of benzoylecgonine in urine below 125 ng/ml, the GC/MS or RIA techniques are likely to be required. Thus, Verebey (1987) recommends thin-layer chromatography confirmed by EMIT for routine detection of cocaine, EMIT for intermediate-level screening, RIA or GC/MS for detection of low-level use, and GC/MS for forensic-level analysis.

Laboratory Determination of Cocaine Use

Laboratory determination of cocaine use is accomplished by measuring cocaine metabolites in the urine, primarily through detection of benzoylecgonine and ecgonine methyl ester. Cocaine itself is not usually present in sufficient quantities to test for, since plasma concentrations decrease rapidly, and only about 10% is excreted unchanged in the urine

(Verebey, 1987). Methods used for detection of cocaine and its metabolites include *chromatography,* including thin layer chromatography, gas liquid chromatography, high-pressure liquid chromatography, and gas chromatography with mass spectrometry; and *immunology methodology,* including enzyme multiplied immunoassay (EMIT) and radioimmunoassay (RIA). EMIT, because it is relatively inexpensive with moderate to good sensitivity, is commonly used as the primary screening procedure. Confirmation, if needed, is then obtained by gas chromatography with mass spectrometry (Pollack, Brotman, and Rosenbaum, 1989). Problems associated with obtaining accurate laboratory detection of cocaine and its metabolites have been discussed by Hansen, Caudill, and Boone (1985) and Lehrer and Gold (1987), although wider use of chromatographic and immunoassay analytical techniques ultimately will eliminate these problems.

Hair analysis has been proposed as an ideal research tool for retrospective determination of illicit drug use, since measurement of drug use history typically relies on what Marques, Tippetts, and Branch (1993) have called the "flimsiest and most distrusted variable in all of science— self reported use" (p. 160). Hoffman and associates (1993) found that hair analysis detected more cocaine abusers than did self-report or urinalysis. This finding was attributed to the larger window of detection for this method. In addition, the level of self-reported cocaine use over the preceding 30 days was strongly correlated to the amount of cocaine metabolite found in hair. Magura et al. (1992) compared radioimmunoassay of hair (RIAH) with two other measures (confidential EMIT urinalysis and self-report of cocaine use) for 134 patients in methadone maintenance treatment and found "confirmation" of findings by RIAH by urinalysis or self-report for cocaine and heroin in 87% and 84% of cases, respectively. By contrast, Hindin and associates (1994), using two samples of substance abusers (one entering residential treatment, the other a posttreatment group), found that self-reported illicit drug use closely paralleled RIAH results at treatment entry but not at follow-up. Among treatment entrants, 89% of RIAH cocaine positives and 96% of RIAH heroin positives were confirmed by self-report, whereas at follow-up, only 51% of cocaine positives and 69% of heroin positives were confirmed by self-report. The results of this study would have been even more useful had the same sample been utilized at both points.

Using undamaged maternal hair, Marques et al. (1993) found a strong and significant relationship between cocaine levels in mothers' and in infants' first hair, accounting for 40% of variance in mother-child hair pairs; this relationship, however, was not present for maternal hair damaged by hair care products. Maternal urine benzoylecgonine and hair cocaine levels were significantly related ($r = .41$), while self-report measures did not relate to hair and urine levels, although this failure may be accounted for by the use of continuous data versus the dichotomous data used in other studies. Marques et al. (1993) concluded that third trimester maternal cocaine use was reflected in cocaine levels in infants' hair, and that where hair is undamaged, hair analysis can provide a quantitative measure of infants' exposure to cocaine. Hair color may also influence the accuracy of hair analysis, since benzoylecgonine seems to be more efficiently incorporated into darker hair, in the relative order black > brown > blond, paralleling the presence of melanin content (Reid, O'Connor, and Crayton, 1994). Thus, lightly pigmented hair may be less appropriate as a sample for benzoylecgonine analysis.

Despite the positive evidence for the validity of hair analysis, such methods still need to be perfected. Contamination by other drugs of abuse in the air may produce many false positive findings, and hair products may damage hair, resulting in decreased accuracy. A report by the U.S. General Accounting Office acknowledges these threats to validity of the procedure while recommending the use of hair analysis as a diagnostic procedure (General Accounting Office, 1993). As with other laboratory procedures for determining the presence of drugs of abuse, there may be substantial interlaboratory variability in accuracy of findings (Welch, Sniegoski, and Allgood, 1993).

Use of Cocaine with Other Drugs

Cocaine use frequently takes place in the presence of other substance abuse. Consequently, effects resulting from the interaction of cocaine with other substances are common. Effects from the interaction of cocaine with alcohol, heroin, sedatives, and marijuana are reviewed in this section.

Cocaine and Alcohol

Alcohol abuse and cocaine abuse are frequently found in combination, with between 2.4% and 6.1% of the general population concurrently abusing the two drugs. Grant and Harford (1990), for instance, estimated that in the general population about 4 million persons had abused cocaine and alcohol at the same time or on the same occasion during the preceding month, with 9 million persons abusing the two drugs during the previous year. With respect to concurrent use of both substances during these time periods, 5 million had used both during the past month, while 12 million had used both during the past year. In one study, two samples of cocaine-dependent inpatients were also found to be 68% and 89% alcohol-dependent, respectively (Miller, Gold, and Klahr, 1990). Alcohol use, however, may not be any more prevalent among cocaine abusers than among abusers of opioids and depressants (Weiss et al., 1988).

Use of alcohol in combination with cocaine is the most frequent substance abuse pattern among persons presenting at emergency rooms in metropolitan areas with two drugs present in their systems, according to the Annual Emergency Room Data for 1992 collected by the Drug Abuse Warning Network (SAMHSA, 1994c). In 1992 this combination accounted for 52,476 (37%) of 141,773 cases of alcohol in combination with another drug. Cocaine alone accounted for 119,843 cases. Of a total of 433,493 drug abuse episodes in hospital emergency rooms, alcohol in combination with other drugs accounted for 32.7% of all cases, and alcohol in combination with cocaine for 12.1% of all cases, while cocaine by itself accounted for 27.7% of all cases.

In the Kang et al. (1991) study, 26% of those seeking admission to outpatient cocaine treatment had drunk alcohol to intoxication at least three times per week for one month or more at some time in their lives. In the Khalsa, Paredes, and Anglin (1992) study of male cocaine users, 76% reported drinking the equivalent of at least 2 ounces of ethanol a day during approximately half of the time between first use of cocaine and treatment entry. This reflected both a heavy use of alcohol before first use of cocaine and a high rate (more than half) of meeting DSM-III-R alcohol dependence diagnoses. The Weiss et al. (1988) study found that a lifetime diagnosis of alcoholism was equally common in both cocaine abusers and abusers of opiates and central nervous system depressants. Thus, alcoholism is not necessarily more frequently associated with abuse of cocaine than with abuse of depressant drugs.

Some studies, however, do indicate a relationship between alcoholism and cocaine use. The current and lifetime rates of alcoholism in the sample of cocaine abusers studied by Rounsaville, Anton, et al. (1991) were found to be 28.9% and 61.7%, respectively, or twice the rates seen in opiate addicts. Furthermore, the diagnosis of alcoholism was found generally to occur after cocaine abuse, whereas most opioid addicts had an onset of alcoholism before opiate abuse. The same study suggested that this finding likely reflected different roles of alcohol for the two groups. For the opiate addicts, alcohol was part of the route toward use of harder drugs such as opiates. In the case of cocaine addicts, alcohol and sedatives may be used to reduce the anxiety and insomnia produced by cocaine. Detoxification from alcohol may thus be necessary in the early stages of cocaine treatment. A greater need for alcohol treatment was found among whites in comparison to African Americans, as reflected in higher scores on the ASI (3.2 on this scale for whites versus 2.3 for African Americans; Ziedonis et al., 1994). This discrepancy may be explained in part by white and African American cocaine abusers' attempting to cope differently with withdrawal. Rounsaville, Anton, et al. (1991) have suggested that whites use alcohol to relieve cocaine intoxication or withdrawal, while African Americans use other drugs for this purpose.

Cocaine reverses some of the effects of alcohol on psychomotor performance as well as increasing some of the pleasurable subjective effects associated with either drug alone (Farré et al., 1990; McCance-Katz et al., 1993). Under laboratory conditions, subjects reported greater increases in "good effects" and "feeling good" after use of cocaine and alcohol in combination than when either alcohol or cocaine was used alone (Farré et al., 1990, 1993; McCance-Katz et al., 1993). The use of cocaine and alcohol in combination may result not only in an enhanced and prolonged euphoria but also in greater toxicity. This greater toxicity, in turn, can result in a higher prevalence of cocaine-related emergencies requiring acute medical care (Hearn, Rose, et al., 1991), and may account for the many cocaine-related fatalities in which relatively low blood cocaine levels are found at postmortem (Wetli and Wright, 1979). The risks associated with combined cocaine and alcohol use are increased by the possibility that the positively perceived subjective and performance effects of combined cocaine and alcohol intoxication could lead to underestimating their true toxicity (Farré et al., 1990).

A number of responses result from the interaction of orally ingested alcohol and intranasally ingested cocaine. These include greater cardiovascular effects (that is, elevated heart rate and blood pressure) than those attributable to either substance alone (Farré et al., 1993; Foltin and Fischman, 1988; Higgins et al., 1992). Alcohol in combination with cocaine attenuates the subjective perception of sedation and the disruption of psychomotor performance resulting from alcohol alone (Foltin et al., 1993; Higgins et al., 1993a). This subjective effect could lead to increased use of such combinations and result in underestimates of alcohol impairment. Given the cost of cocaine, however, and the fact that alcohol does not always increase the subjective effects produced by cocaine, Foltin et al. (1993) considered it unlikely that these drugs are used in close temporal proximity for any reason other than their availability.

The use of alcohol in conjunction with cocaine may significantly increase the risk of adverse reactions by the production of cocaethylene in the liver, through the process of transesterification (conversion of one ester into another). Cocaethylene is an active metabolite of cocaine which is formed in the liver in the presence of alcohol (Jatlow, 1993; Rafla and Epstein, 1979). Formation of cocaethylene occurs through the transesterification of benzoylecgonine (Jatlow et al., 1990). Studies suggest an even higher lethality of cocaethylene than cocaine in animals (Katz, Terry, and Witkin, 1992), and a relationship between cocaethylene and violent agitation in humans (Schrank, 1993). In fact, many of the enhanced effects seen when alcohol is used in combination with cocaine might be the result of the formation of cocaethylene. Cocaethylene may be stored in body tissues (Hearn, Flynn, et al., 1991), and increased quantities of cocaethylene may accumulate relative to cocaine during binge use. The effects noted by Farré et al. (1990) and McCance-Katz et al. (1993) may be the result of the production of cocaethylene. Cocaethylene likely has greater euphorigenic effects than cocaine alone (Farré et al., 1990), and in animal studies has been found to be equipotent with cocaine in producing convulsions (Hearn, Rose, et al., 1991; Katz, Terry, and Witkin, 1992). The increased toxic effects of cocaethylene may be due to this compound's blockade of dopamine reuptake at the synaptic cleft, thus further inhibiting the reuptake of dopamine produced by cocaine (Hearn, Flynn, et al., 1991). This targeted action may thus be the basis of the high abuse liability of the cocaine-alcohol combination through the additive effects of cocaethylene.

The order of ingestion of cocaine and alcohol may influence the effects resulting from their interaction. When alcohol is ingested prior to cocaine inhalation, there are significant increases in plasma cocaine concentration and in cocaine's subjective and heart rate effects. By contrast, when cocaine is ingested prior to alcohol, Perez-Reyes (1994) found it not to alter blood alcohol levels or subjective ratings of cocaine intoxication, and to result in slower formation and smaller quantities of cocaethylene. Furthermore, the appearance of cocaethylene in plasma did not alter the decline of subjective and heart rate effects resulting from cocaine, nor did it raise plasma concentrations of cocaethylene.

The lethality of the cocaine-alcohol combination is underscored by the fact that 124 of the 237 cases of cocaine-related deaths in Dade County, Florida, between January 1989 and February 1990 involved use of these two substances in combination. Cocaethylene was detected in 62% ($N = 77$) of those cases in which both cocaine and alcohol were present (Hearn, Flynn, et al., 1991). This combination may also contribute indirectly to mortality among cocaine abusers, since cocaethylene appears to stimulate HIV replication in human blood (Peterson et al., 1991; Shapshak et al., 1993).

The prevalence of a lifetime diagnosis of alcohol dependence among persons with a diagnosis of cocaine dependence has been found to range between 30% and 94% (Miller, Gold, and Belkin, 1990; Miller, Millman, and Keskinen, 1989; Miller, Summers, and Gold, 1993). Data from the Epidemiologic Catchment Area study of 20,000 persons from the general population found cocaine and alcohol dependence to be more highly correlated than associations between alcohol and any other drug (the alcohol dependence rate among users of stimulants was 62%, compared to 84% among cocaine abusers). Miller, Gold et al. (1989), for example, found the prevalence of current alcohol dependence to be 68% and 89%, respectively, in retrospective and prospective studies of cocaine-dependent inpatients. Employing Research Diagnostic Criteria, alcoholism was found by Carroll, Rounsaville, and Bryant (1993) to be the most frequently diagnosed current and lifetime psychiatric disorder in both treatment-seeking and community samples of cocaine abusers, with current rates of 29% for both. Lifetime rates of psychiatric disorders were also highly similar for the two samples, with 62% for the treatment-seeking and 68% for the community sample. These rates of alcoholism were almost twice the rate seen in opiate addicts. Schnoll et al. (1985) found that, among people admitted to inpatient or partial treatment programs who had used cocaine, some 89% had used alcohol in conjunction with cocaine; only 5% had never used alcohol. About half (51%) of a clinical sample of cocaine-dependent men in a Veterans Administration facility studied by Khalsa, Paredes, and Anglin (1992) also met the criteria for alcohol dependence.

Individuals with alcoholism rather than drug abuse as their primary addiction tend to be older, better educated, and of higher socioeconomic status, to have higher rates of affective disorders, and to have begun the use of other substances following the onset of alcohol abuse (Carroll, Rounsaville, and Bryant, 1993; Lesswing and Dougherty, 1993). Hesselbrock, Meyer, and Keener (1985) did not, however, find this true of women in their study of hospitalized alcoholics, who reported abusing other substances before the onset of alcohol abuse and/or dependence. There is also conflicting evidence whether cocaine abusers are more severely impaired than alcoholics who later develop cocaine dependence (Carroll, Rounsaville, and Bryant, 1993; Hesselbrock, Meyer, and Keener, 1985). Two comparisons of cocaine- and alcohol-addicted individuals obtained similar patterns of psychopathology on psychological tests (Johnson, Tobin, and Cellucci, 1992; Lesswing and Dougherty, 1993), although the cocaine abusers in the study by Lesswing and Dougherty tended to be somewhat more distressed, showing higher levels of agitation, turmoil, confusion, and paranoid trends. Brown, Seraganian, and Tremblay (1993) found cocaine-dependent alcoholics, when compared with "pure alcoholics," to be younger, more likely to be unmarried, and likely to have had more extensive substance abuse histories and more frequent prior treatments. Cocaine-dependent alcoholics may also have more difficulty in achieving abstinence during treatment.

One study found a greater likelihood of cocaine abusers' being cross-addicted to alcohol and other drugs (85%) than of alcoholics' using other drugs (only 18% abused other substances; Lesswing and Dougherty, 1993). Individuals who are both cocaine- and alcohol-dependent may be different from those who use cocaine alone. In the Khalsa, Anglin, and Paredes (1992) study, patients with combined cocaine and alcohol addictions, compared with patients abusing only cocaine, reported a larger number of fathers, siblings, and other relatives with alcohol problems. The cocaine-alcohol abuser group also contained a higher proportion of whites and Hispanics, while the cocaine-only group contained a higher proportion of African Americans. The cocaine-plus-alcohol group had used a wider range of drugs, and preferred intravenous injection, suggesting greater deviance. This group also had delayed treatment entry longer and had a lower level of education than the cocaine-only group. Otherwise, there were few differences between the two groups with respect to demographic characteristics, level of functioning, and progression of cocaine use. Both groups showed significant reductions in alcohol use and antisocial behavior one year after treatment. Carroll, Rounsaville, and Bryant (1993) found greater use of other drugs in addition to cocaine and alcohol, more severe drug dependence, and worse psychological functioning in alcoholic cocaine abusers in contrast with non-alcoholic cocaine abusers. Although this finding differs from those of other investigators, who have found higher rates of psychiatric disorders in combined alcohol-drug abuse (Hesselbrock, Meyer, and Keener, 1985; Weiss et al., 1988), the use of a sample whose principal diagnosis was cocaine dependence in the Carroll, Rounsaville, and Bryant study may account for this divergence.

While cocaine addiction and alcoholism have much in common, they differ from each other clinically in significant ways. Washton and Stone-Washton (1993) suggested that it was inappropriate both "to view the cocaine addict as just an alcoholic who happened to get involved with a different drug" (p. 18) and to believe that "all addicts are alike" and to treat them on that basis. They provided a number of important differences between addiction to cocaine and to alcohol. These include the contrasting psychoactive effects produced by cocaine (a central nervous system stimulant) and alcohol (a central nervous system depressant), resulting in different relapse triggers, with cocaine amplifying sensory experience and alcohol modifying it; the strong sexual component associated with cocaine (that is, sexual fantasies, sexual acting-out, and occasional sexual compulsion), any one of which may trigger relapse if not addressed early in treatment; the relative lack of psychomotor impairment (that is, impaired speech, gait, and posture) during cocaine use, making such use more difficult to detect than alcohol use; the smaller number of medical problems and deaths associated with cocaine use, resulting in fewer referrals to treatment for medical problems alone; the legal status of cocaine as opposed to alcohol, causing cocaine users to be labeled as deviants or criminals rather than sick people requiring treatment, with such attitudes often influencing treatment personnel; the more rapid onset (a few weeks to a few months) of addiction to cocaine than to alcohol, particularly in the case of crack cocaine, thus resulting in rapid onset trauma as opposed to progressive, insidious debilitation; the immediate sense of feeling better following cessation of cocaine use, resulting in an equally rapid dissipation of motivation to remain in treatment; and the "awesome" power of cocaine in conditioning of cues (whether people, places, or events) as triggers for onset of powerful cravings.

Cocaine and Heroin

SPEEDBALLING

As noted earlier, "speedballing" is the practice of mixing cocaine and heroin and then injecting the combined mixture. This practice results in a dampening or "mellowing out" of the stimulant effects of cocaine with the more sedating qualities of heroin. In addition to being reported as a very pleasing combination for users (Kosten, Rounsaville, and Kleber, 1987, 1988), cocaine mixed with heroin is also believed by users to protect against the dysphoria or depression which often follows use of cocaine alone. (Conversely, cocaine is also used with heroin to counteract "the nods," or sleepiness, which follows opiate use.) The combination of heroin and cocaine may be a highly risky one, since the depressant effects of heroin on the respiratory system may be intensified by cocaine (Weiss and Mirin, 1987; Weiss, Mirin, and Bartel, 1994).

Speedballing is very common among injection drug users. Data from the National AIDS Demonstration Project, or NADR (Feucht, Stephens, and Sullivan, 1993), indicate that at least 96% of IDUs who had used the combination of cocaine and heroin had injected it. Among injection drug users seen in Newark and Jersey City, New Jersey, as part of the NADR study, 37.5% were found to inject speedballs on a daily basis, and another 6.1% used the combination daily by non-injection routes, primarily smoking (Bux et al., 1993). Among a sample of injection drug users in methadone maintenance treatment in New York City, 46% had "speedballed" within the previous month (Magura et al., 1989). The practice of speedballing appears to follow initiation of injection use of both drugs, although the evidence on this point is not certain. It is more common among women than men, and more common among African Americans and Hispanics than among other racial groups. As is the case for both cocaine use alone and heroin use alone, injecting heroin and cocaine in combination four or more times daily is most common among women and Hispanic IDUs (Feucht, Stephens, and Sullivan, 1993). Cocaine plus heroin or morphine was the second most frequently mentioned drug combination (following alcohol in combination) among emergency room admissions during 1992, with 15,517 such mentions, accounting for 3.6% of all mentions.

The practice of speedballing is highly associated with the seroprevalence of the human immunodeficiency virus (Siegal, Carlson, and Falck, 1993). More than three-quarters (76%) of injection drug users in high seroprevalence areas engaged in this practice, compared with 48% of respondents in low seroprevalence areas. For African American injection drug users, the frequency of daily speedballing was 42% in high prevalence areas and 18% in low prevalence areas; for Hispanic injection drug users these percentages were 57% and 20%. By contrast, white injection drug users in both high and low seroprevalence areas reported the lowest percentages of daily speedball injection (17% and 13%, respectively). In general, speedball users have been characterized in the literature as having more severe psychopathology, as well as being more maladjusted, compared to opiate and cocaine abusers (Dolan et al., 1991; Malow et al., 1992).

SMOKING COCAINE AND HEROIN ("CHASING THE DRAGON")

While smoking cocaine and heroin in combination is not a new practice, its frequency has increased in recent years. A change from the practice of snorting heroin after snorting cocaine to smoking a mix of the two may explain this increased frequency. Kramer et al. (1990) reported that 40% of patients on two drug detoxification wards in Brooklyn, New York, had engaged in this practice. According to one patient, "To chase the dragon, you put a rock of crack in the pipe, sprinkle some heroin, then another rock, then some heroin" (p. 65). This practice combines the "brief exhilarating high" of cocaine and the lasting effects and dissipation of the crash provided by heroin.

HEROIN AND COCAINE USE AND DEPENDENCE COMPARED

Abuse of cocaine appears to occur more frequently during periods of narcotic addiction than during periods of non-addiction (Nurco et al., 1988). Mean days of cocaine use during periods of narcotic addiction were 152.7 for African Americans, 134.8 for Hispanics, and 58.1 for whites. Conversely, mean days per year of cocaine use during periods of non-addiction to narcotics were 23.1 for African Americans, 34.9 for Hispanics, and 25.2 for whites.

Although drawing direct analogies from the results of animal studies to humans must be done with caution, the results of an animal study comparing the effects of long-term intravenous self-administration of heroin and cocaine in rats are interesting. In this study animals allowed continuous free access to cocaine showed excessive cocaine self-administration alternating with brief periods of abstinence (Bozarth and Wise, 1985). Animals who were allowed continuous free access to heroin showed stable drug administration, with a gradual increase in daily heroin intake over two weeks. There was a marked difference in the general health of animals in the two conditions. The animals in the heroin condition maintained grooming behavior, pre-test body weight, and a good state of physical health. By contrast, those in the cocaine condition tended to cease grooming behavior, to lose up to 47% of pre-test body weight, and to show a pronounced deterioration in general health. After thirty days of continuous testing, 90% of rats self-administering cocaine had died, versus 36% of rats self-administering heroin. The investigators concluded that "these results suggest that cocaine is a much more toxic compound than heroin when animals are given unlimited access to intravenous drugs" (p. 81). The implications for human users were clear: long-term use resulting in higher concentrations of the drug is likely to result in higher rates of fatalities.

Addressing the question whether cocaine and heroin dependence differed, Hasin et al. (1988) compared the levels of use in groups of each among polydrug abusers on an alcohol treatment unit. No difference between the two groups was found in this study, which employed the Diagnostic Interview Schedule (DIS), on indicators such as subjective judgments of dependence, loss of control, tolerance, or withdrawal, or in number of unsuccessful attempts to cut back.[14] The results of this study thus suggested that cocaine had a dependence potential similar to that of heroin. Anthony and Petronis (1989), however, who also compared heroin and cocaine users in a multisite epidemiological study, found that cocaine users were less likely to report similar dependence-related problems. These differences in findings were attributed either to the lesser willingness of polydrug users in alcohol treatment to give a complete self-report about drug-related problems, or to the general unreliability of substance abuse treatment samples in providing information as to the frequency of risk associated with drug use in the community. The authors did not, however, conclude that their findings contradicted the dependence liability associated with cocaine use.

Craig (1988) compared cocaine and heroin users among drug abusers on a Veterans Administration inpatient unit and found that cocaine addicts did not differ significantly from opiate addicts with respect to personality traits. Based on results from the MMPI and the Adjective Check List,[15] both opiate and cocaine addicts were characterized by acting-out traits, rebelliousness, depression, anxiety, alienation, and hyperactivity, although the cocaine users had modulated levels of severity. The study concluded that "drug treatment programs need not consider the cocaine patient as a unique entity who needs special programming based on psychological characteristics" (p. 605). A similar study, employing the Millon Clinical Multiaxial Inventory,[16] also found very few differences between cocaine and heroin addicts, although the cocaine addicts appeared to demonstrate more features consistent with antisocial personality, while the opiate addicts demonstrated more problems with alcohol abuse and anxiety and had more somatic complaints (Craig and Olson, 1990). This finding is inconsistent with both the finding of greater antisocial personality disorders in cocaine addicts (Malow et al., 1989) and the findings of increased alcohol problems among cocaine abusers.

Cocaine and Benzodiazepines

At times benzodiazepines may be used to blunt the dysphoric effects of declining cocaine levels. Not only may this practice prolong altered mental states, but also it decreases the risk of seizures resulting from cocaine toxicity. This practice, however, also increases the risk of respiratory depression (Schrank, 1993).

Cocaine and Marijuana

Marijuana, as a "gateway" drug, is frequently found in close association with cocaine abuse. In one study of psychiatric inpatients and outpatients, some 53% of cocaine-dependent individuals were found to have a concurrent diagnosis of cannabis dependence (Miller et al., 1990). In another study, 53% and 46% of retrospective and prospective samples of inpatients with a diagnosis of cocaine dependence were also found to have diagnoses of marijuana dependence (Miller et al., 1989). Of a sample of cocaine smokers studied by Khalsa, Tashkin, and Perrochet (1992), 20% also currently smoked marijuana, and an additional 48% had smoked marijuana in the past, while 32% had never smoked marijuana. These are not surprising findings, given that 98% of cocaine addicts report having used cannabis before becoming addicted to cocaine (O'Malley, Johnston, and Bachman, 1985). Schnoll et al. (1985) reported that among patients who had been treated for cocaine dependence, 76% had also used marijuana, and 42.9% reported having used marijuana daily. In the Kang et al. (1991) study, 71% of respondents had smoked marijuana at least three times per week for at least five months or more at some time in their lives. Miller, Gold, and Belkin (1990) found, in two samples, that 46% to 53% of patients with a diagnosis of cocaine dependence also had a diagnosis of cannabis dependence. Marijuana is the substance most often smoked mixed with cocaine. In the study by Khalsa, Tashkin, and Perrochet (1992), this combination accounted for 67% of cases in which cocaine was smoked in combination with another substance, while another 12% of respondents smoked both marijuana and tobacco mixed with cocaine.

Cocaine in combination with marijuana, regardless of the route by which cocaine was administered (intravenous or intranasal), elevates heart rate to a greater extent and for a longer period of time than either drug alone (Foltin et al., 1987; Foltin and Fischman, 1990). Yet, increases in blood pressure were found to be similar to those obtained with cocaine alone (Foltin and Fischman, 1988). As is the case for marijuana in combination with smoked d-amphetamine (Evans et al., 1976), the subjective effects of marijuana (self-ratings of "stimulated" or "high") in combination with intravenous cocaine are also prolonged, although for the marijuana-cocaine combination, in contrast with the amphetamine combination, the magnitude of such effects is small. The temporal proximity of cocaine and marijuana may also play a role in prolonging subjective effects, a factor that may play a significant role in the decision to use the drugs in combination (Foltin et al., 1993).

In considering the physiological, performance, and subjective effects of heroin, marijuana, and alcohol in combination with cocaine, it is well to keep in mind the admonition of Foltin and associates (1993) that the small doses used in laboratory studies of drug interactions probably underestimate the actual decrements seen outside the laboratory, where larger single doses, or multiple doses taken during binges, are more likely to be the case.

Conclusions

Cocaine, which belongs to the stimulant class of drugs, is extracted from the leaves of the Erythroxylon coca *shrub, which is indigenous to a number of South American countries. It is available in powdered hydrochloride, partially purified paste, and crystalline freebase ("crack") forms. Cocaine may be administered by injection, by absorption through the mucous membranes, as well as by respiratory, gastrointestinal, and genitourinary routes.* Regardless of route of administration, cocaine is readily absorbed by body tissues (Goldfrank and Hoffman, 1993). Peak onset of action resulting from absorption from intravenous and inhalation routes is typically 30 seconds to 2 minutes. Subjective peak effect resulting from intranasal administration usually occurs within 15 to 30 minutes, while from the gastrointestinal tract absorption may take 90 minutes. The route by which cocaine is administered affects the length of time which elapses before the subjective effects of the drug are experienced (Javaid et al., 1978).

The duration of cocaine's effects is relatively brief and is a direct function of the plasma half-life of cocaine's active metabolites. The resultant half-life of plasma concentrations is typically 15 to 30 minutes when the drug is administered intravenously or inhaled, 1 hour when administered intranasally, and up to 3 hours after absorption from the gastrointestinal tract (Goldfrank and Hoffman, 1993; Resnick, Kestenbaum, and Schwartz, 1977).

Cocaine is usually used as part of a pattern of polysubstance abuse. Alcohol is the most commonly abused substance in connection with cocaine, and alcoholism represents a common event in the lives of many cocaine abusers, with approximately one-third of cocaine abusers meeting the criteria for a current diagnosis of alcohol abuse, and two-thirds the criteria for a lifetime diagnosis (Rounsaville, Anton, et al., 1991). These rates of alcoholism are approximately twice those for opiate abusers.

Substances of abuse taken in combination with cocaine are often used for their interactive effects with other drugs. For example, opiates (typically heroin) are used in combination with cocaine in order to dampen the effects of cocaine, while marijuana is used to augment the high obtained with use of cocaine and in the belief that it will protect against the dysphoria which often follows cocaine use. Such combinations of drugs increase the risks associated with cocaine use. Marijuana augments some of the physiological effects of cocaine (Foltin et al., 1987, 1990), while benzodiazepines dampen cocaine's dysphoric effects, although the latter carry (as does heroin) the risk of respiratory depression. The use of cocaine and alcohol in combination, for example, results in the formation of cocaethylene, a compound which increases cocaine's lethality.

In addition to its central effects, cocaine's peripheral effects include localized ischemia and vasoconstriction as well as marked changes in cardiovascular functioning, primarily increased blood pressure and altered cardiac rhythm. Cocaine exerts its central actions through alteration of the endogenous neurotransmitter system, acting primarily by enhancing dopaminergic activity in reward pathways and blocking dopamine reuptake (dopamine reuptake inhibition) in the brain (Johanson and Fischman, 1989). It has been suggested that cocaine shares with other drugs of abuse the stimulation of the mesolimbic system, which may serve as the final common pathway for a number of substances (Kuhar, Ritz, and Boja, 1991).

II

Behavioral Aspects

3

The Subjective Experience, Course, and Parameters of Cocaine Abuse

Subjective and Related Effects

Acute Subjective Effects

Acute subjective effects of cocaine use, regardless of route of administration, include feelings of profound well-being, euphoria, enhanced alertness, intensified awareness of the environment, intense energy, magnification of normal pleasures, decreased anxiety, increased self-confidence, increased perception of mastery, a reduction in social inhibition, increased interpersonal communication, heightened sexual drive, and diminished fatigue and reduced need for sleep (Gold, 1984). In fact, it has been suggested that the acute effects of cocaine provide an excellent model of mania (Post and Weiss, 1989). Gawin (1991) described the fundamental subjective effect of cocaine as "the magnification of the intensity of almost all normal pleasures" (p. 1581), while perceptions of the environment, although intensified, remain undistorted. In a study by Seecof and Tennant (1986), the subjective effects of the cocaine "rush" were characterized for both male and female users by increased excitement, pleasure, thirst, strength, and anxiety. There were, however, some gender differences. Males ranked subjective feelings of power obtained from cocaine use very high, while females ranked high feelings of satisfaction, warmth, and relaxation obtained from using cocaine. (It should be noted that these subjective differences in experience also reflect societal gender role norms.) Both males and females ranked low subjective feelings of sexual orgasm in association with cocaine rushes. This study, however, was done with heroin addicts, so the results may not be completely generalizable to exclusive users of cocaine.

There is a need to differentiate between the euphoric "rush" and the "high" produced by cocaine. The high is characterized by a state of alertness, activation, and subjective feelings of well-being (Resnick, Kestenbaum, and Schwartz, 1977). In contrast, the rush is characterized by subjective feelings of power, excitement, extreme pleasure, strength, and anxiety (Seecof and Tennant, 1986). The feelings associated with the rush have also been likened to those accompanying orgasm (Siegel, 1982b). The presence and strength of both of these subjective phenomena is dependent on route of administration. While both are present during intravenous use of cocaine and inhalation of freebase, the rush is largely absent during intranasal administration ("snorting") of powdered cocaine. Additionally, the effects are experienced less intensely and have a slower onset during intranasal administration (Fischman, 1984). This difference likely accounts for the preference among experienced cocaine abusers for intravenous over intranasal administration of cocaine (Kumor et al., 1989; Spotts and Shontz, 1976).

The high obtained from cocaine may well result from the rate of change in cocaine brain levels. If this were not the case, noted Brown (1989), the cocaine "blues" would not begin at the moment when cocaine concentration in the brain reaches a high point. Furthermore, increases in the brain plasma levels of cocaine in an individual with stimulant concentrations present will not be as intense as in a stimulant-free individual.

Cocaine, even if not used to the point of intoxication, but particularly in the case of repeated use, as may occur during a run or spree, can cause compulsively repeated actions, extreme psychomotor agitation, and poor judgment, as well as enhancement of emotions and sexual feelings. Such effects may lead to accidents, illegal acts, or atypical sexual behavior (Gawin and Ellinwood, 1988, 1989; Washton, 1989a). As the amount of cocaine used and the duration of a binge increase, pleasurable effects are replaced by disagreeable side effects. These may include agitation, anxiety, and panic attacks, as well as some of the effects observed during intoxication, such as pacing, stereotyped movement, grinding of the teeth and jaws, insomnia, loss of sexual drive, and inattention to personal hygiene. Paranoid delusions and visual and auditory hallucinations may also appear. Medical complications, including seizure, cardiac arrhythmia, and respiratory arrest, become more likely.

Gawin and Ellinwood (1988, 1989) have suggested that the euphoria seen in early use of stimulants is largely the result of the increasingly positive external feedback to the user rather than the result of direct pharmacological effects of the drug. This results in a perception on the part of the user that the source of euphoria is in the environment rather than in the drug. At lower doses cocaine may enhance interactions with the environment, allowing increased performance and confidence, or at the least reversing fatigue-induced performance decrements (Fischman and Schuster, 1980), and more likely giving the subjective impression of increased efficiency. Evidence suggests, however, that increased performance does not extend beyond initial levels (Resnick, Kestenbaum, and Schwartz, 1980), and performance has been shown to deteriorate with continued use of cocaine (Fischman, 1978).

DYSPHORIA

The restless irritability seen following the high has been labeled "anguish" as a result of its aversiveness. This feeling, together with a desire to maintain the high, results in repeated administration of cocaine, as well as in the use of speedballs to take the edge off the "down" (Brown, 1989).

Higher levels of anxiety, suspiciousness, and dysphoria are likely to occur with increasing use of cocaine. Following discontinuation of cocaine use, the "crash," a state resembling an acute onset of agitated depression, occurs (Gawin and Kleber, 1986a; Gold, 1984; Roehrich and Gold, 1991). This crash, also referred to as "the post-coke blues," is characterized by rapid decreases in mood and energy levels, anxiety, agitation, depression, and a desire for more cocaine. Fatigue and exhaustion, as well as a craving for sleep and hypersomnolence, are also very characteristic (Gawin and Kleber, 1986a; Resnick, Kestenbaum, and Schwartz, 1980). These acute effects are followed by decreased activation, lack of motivation, intense boredom, and anhedonia or the absence of pleasure in acts that would normally provide it (Gawin and Ellinwood, 1988, 1989). These effects have been characterized as a "cocaine withdrawal syndrome," described in detail later in this chapter. The presence of such adverse responses may explain in part the simultaneous use of opiates to modulate such effects (Post, 1975). Cocaine dysphoria may also be characterized by attentional dysfunction, including the inability to concentrate, difficulty in maintaining thoughts during verbal behavior, ignoring relevant stimulation, and a general preoccupation with personal problems (Post, 1975; Siegel, 1978).

Frequency of Occurrence of Cocaine-Related Symptoms

The relative frequency of occurrence of both psychological and physical symptoms of cocaine abuse are evidenced in the results of a survey of 500 callers to the 800-COCAINE hot line (Washton, Gold, and Pottash, 1984). In order of decreasing frequency, psychological effects reported by callers included depression (83%), anxiety (83%), irritability (82%), apathy and laziness (66%), paranoia (65%), difficulty concentrating (65%), memory problems (57%), lack of sexual interest (53%), and panic attacks (50%). Reported physical effects, in order of decreasing frequency, were sleep problems (82%), chronic fatigue (76%), severe headaches (60%), nasal sores and bleeding (58%), chronic cough and sore throat (46%), nausea and vomiting (39%), and seizure and loss of consciousness (14%).

Cocaine Intoxication

Cocaine intoxication can be of sudden onset and have fatal consequences. The first signs of onset of cocaine intoxication may be agitation accompanied by dysphoria or other alterations of mood and autonomic nervous system functioning. Other symptoms may include euphoria, increased alertness, decreased appetite, sleep disorder, enhanced energy, rapid heartbeat, and hyperkinesis, anxiety, and sweating. Accompanying or following these symptoms may be assaultive behavior, paranoid ideation, delirium, syncope, nausea, vomiting, chest pain, tremors, seizures, hypertension, hyperthermia, respiratory paralysis, cardiac arrhythmias, and, ultimately, death. When fatal consequences do not occur, cocaine intoxication may be self-limiting, with recovery taking place within twenty-four hours (Cregler and Mark, 1986a).

Hallucinations

Hallucinations can result from continued use of cocaine. In a condition called *formication,* hallucinatory "cocaine bugs" may be perceived. This condition is a form of paresthesia or tactile hallucination typically reported by long-term cocaine abusers in which the user believes that there are insects crawling under the skin.[1] The intensity of the sensation may be so great that the user will attempt to cut out the imagined insects with a knife. In the laboratory, monkeys given cocaine may develop skin ulcerations from attempts to bite, pick, and scratch their skin

(Brown, 1989). The basis of formication may lie in stimulation of nerve endings in the skin, the action of cocaine on the noradrenergic innervation of the somatosensory cortex in humans, or drug-induced degradation of pyramidal cells in the sensory motor cortex (Brown, 1989).

Siegel (1978) interviewed 85 recreational cocaine abusers, aged 21 to 38, all of whom had used a minimum of one gram of intranasal cocaine every month for one year. Thirty-seven (43.5%) had experienced perceptual phenomena relating to cocaine use, mostly consisting of increased sensitivity to light, halos around bright lights, and difficulty in focusing the eyes. Hallucinatory experiences relating to vision, touch, smell, hearing, and taste were present in 15 subjects. These had typically appeared after six months of cocaine use, especially during periods of intensive use. Visual phenomena, primarily flashes of light (which Siegel labeled "snow lights," since they were described as resembling the "twinkling of sunlight reflected from frozen snow crystals" [p. 310]), were present in 13 subjects and had appeared first, followed by geometric patterns seen when the eyes were open. Other visual hallucinations typically consisted of the sensation of objects moving at the corners of the visual field (that is, subjects reported, "Something just flew by," "Something or someone just moved over there"). Siegel described cocaine-induced visual hallucinations as sharing many characteristics with migraine hallucinations. These visual hallucinations were followed immediately by tactile hallucinations, at first itching of the skin, primarily of the hands (but also of the legs and back), followed by the sensation of foreign particles moving under the skin, small insects crawling over the body, particularly on the hands and face, and people brushing against the body. Siegel characterized these as "pseudohallucinations," since none of his subjects believed that insects or objects were actually present. Tactile hallucinations were in turn followed by olfactory (smells of smoke, gasoline, natural gas, feces, urine, and garbage), auditory (voices calling, whispering), and, finally, gustatory hallucinations.[2] Siegel's description of cocaine-related hallucinatory events is quite interesting and deserves reading.

Paranoia

Paranoid symptomatology resulting from stimulant use has been the object of descriptive studies and even laboratory induction (Angrist and Gershon, 1970; Angrist et al., 1975; Bell, 1973; Ellinwood, 1967; Jaffe, 1985; Kramer, Fischman, and Littlefield, 1967). Although most of this literature relates to suspiciousness and other symptomatology associated with amphetamine use, at least one experimental induction of such symptomatology following cocaine infusion in the laboratory suggests that symptoms seen following cocaine use are not very different from those following amphetamine use. Such symptoms may appear within ninety minutes of cocaine use, while euphoria is still present, and may not be dose-related (Sherer et al., 1988). Cocaine-induced paranoia may be of two types. One is a transient or binge-limited form confined to the cocaine use episode and not present after emergence from the post-binge hypersomnia or "crash." Typical symptoms may include suspiciousness or beliefs that dealers or the police are in pursuit, and misinterpretation of stimuli as supporting such a delusion. Actual perceptual hallucinations and bizarre delusions are rare (Satel, Southwick, and Gawin, 1991). Paranoia has been noted to be common, but not universal, in samples of cocaine users. In one study of adolescent middle-class users, 74% of heavy crack smokers, 65% of intermediate smokers, and 46% of experimenters were characterized by pervasive suspiciousness and mistrust (Schwartz, Luxenberg, and Hoffmann, 1991). In a study of 50 cocaine-dependent men without other Axis I disorders, Satel and Edell (1991) found that 68% had experienced paranoid episodes following cocaine use. Thus, a substantial percentage of, but certainly not all, cocaine abusers are likely to develop cocaine-related paranoia.

In the study by Satel, Southwick, and Gawin (1991), most paranoid episodes associated with cocaine were found to be limited to the period of use. Thus, one way in which cocaine-induced paranoid episodes may differ from the paranoid episodes characteristic of amphetamine use is that the latter may be of a persisting nature, sustained for days, weeks, or longer following the crash. In this study of 50 cocaine-dependent males admitted to a treatment program, 68% had experienced transient paranoid states while using cocaine. The authors concluded that such states were a common feature of cocaine dependence, and not simply a result of exceeding a threshold of use. Typically, these states became more intense and were manifested earlier in the course of the binge as cocaine use continued. Furthermore, increased severity and rapidity of onset with continued use of cocaine were consistent with a sensitization model of cocaine-induced paranoia, and did not reflect the quantity (either duration or amount) of cocaine use, route of administration, or concurrent use of other drugs, although use of hallucinogens prior to becoming cocaine-dependent may have been a predisposing factor. Heavy cocaine users (more than 5 grams per week) who display transient paranoid symptoms (binge-limited cocaine-induced paranoia) while intoxicated appear, in general, to be at higher risk of developing psychosis. It was not clear from this study, however, whether this finding reflects drug-induced neurobiologic changes or expresses an intrinsic vulnerability to paranoia in individuals who are otherwise asymptomatic (Satel and Edell, 1991).

Obsessive-Compulsive Behaviors

Chronic use of stimulants, including cocaine, can result in stereotyped obsessive-compulsive behaviors. Such behavior can include repetitious examining, searching, and sorting behaviors, which have been labeled by cocaine abusers as "punding," "hung-up activity," and "knick-knacking" (Ellinwood, Sudilovsky, and Nelson, 1973). Rosse et al. (1993) described compulsive foraging behavior associated with intense cocaine craving, often following exhaustion of a supply of crack cocaine. Also referred to as "chasing ghosts" or "geeking" by patients, a search, often intensive, is conducted for pieces of crack cocaine which the individual believes may have fallen to the floor while crack was being smoked. This behavior may include repeated examination of the floor, carpet, furniture, or path, as well as repeated checking of pockets, clothes, and even shoes and socks. A careful examination is made of anything which may resemble rock cocaine, including pebbles, candle wax, food crumbs, plaster, paint chips, and so on. Although this behavior may be described by cocaine abusers as bizarre, amusing, and even annoying when observed in others, it may be difficult for them to resist the impulse to search themselves. Rosse et al. (1993) examined this behavior in 41 cocaine-dependent patients and found it to be more than simply a consequence of intense cocaine craving. Rather, it is more like a compulsion, though too complex to be a stereotype, and may possibly be a "pure" form of compulsive behavior. It appears in the context of heavy cocaine use and lasts at most a few hours but does not involve other compulsive acts such as hand washing. Evidence from the Epidemiological Catchment Area Survey suggests that cocaine-abusing patients are at increased risk for the later development of obsessive-compulsive behavior, although the evidence in support of such a link still remains tenuous (see, for example, Rosse et al., 1994).[3]

Cocaine Craving

Craving, or intense urges for additional doses of the drug, represents a major factor in relapse to cocaine abuse following abstinence. Although craving also plays a similar role in opioid addiction, it may be an even stronger motivation to resume use in the case of cocaine (O'Brien, Childress, et al., 1992).[4] Craving is readily elicited by stimuli associated with prior use of the drug. These stimuli or cues may include people (for example, a friend with whom one has used cocaine), places (for example, a location where the drugs have been used), objects (for example, a powdery substance such as sugar or talc), odors, or internal mood states and emotions such as euphoria or dysphoria (Childress, McLellan, and O'Brien, 1986a, b; Rohsenow et al., 1990–91). Frequently, cravings are accompanied by arousal and palpitations, and an anticipatory high may be present even before the drug is ingested. The presence of such strong associations should not be surprising, given the many links to cues which are likely to have developed over months or years of drug use. Nonetheless, about one-third of patients being treated for cocaine dependence show no reactivity to cocaine-related cues (O'Brien et al., 1993).

Craving is frequently triggered by shifting internal mood states. For example, a study by Satel and Gawin (1989) describes two patients whose cocaine craving paralleled and was likely triggered by seasonal dysphoria. By contrast, Voris, Elder, and Sebastian (1991) found no association between craving and mood or depression scores. In rats with established behavioral repertoires in response to cocaine, the administration of cocaine has been shown to lead to rapid and sustained increases in target behaviors (de Wit and Stewart, 1981). In a laboratory study of craving following the administration of cocaine, Jaffe et al. (1989) found that the actions and stimulus properties of cocaine itself were a major factor in increasing the motivation to further use of drugs. Significant increases in the urge to use drugs occurred as early as fifteen minutes after intravenous cocaine administration, while mood elevations resulting from drug use were still present.

Craving following termination of cocaine use seems to be significantly diminished when treatment is provided in inpatient settings. In a study of a group of inpatient cocaine addicts, Voris, Elder, and Sebastian (1991) found relatively low levels of craving for cocaine. Similarly, Flowers et al. (1993) found little craving and depression among the groups of cocaine-addicted Veterans Administration inpatients evaluated after an unspecified period of detoxification. Other investigators have reported similar, relatively rapid decrements in craving in inpatient settings (Margolin, Kosten, and Avants, 1992; Weddington et al., 1990). It is likely that there are simply fewer previously salient cocaine cues in the hospital environment to elicit craving. It is surprising that internal cues that could elicit craving, such as mood state, could have changed so rapidly, although one study found a rapid decline in depression on the Beck Depression Inventory after admission to treatment, even though it was outpatient treatment (Iguchi et al., 1994).[5] In any event, such declines in craving are, unfortunately, likely to be short-lived, since return to environments associated with cocaine abuse very often results in a rapid return of craving and drug use (Childress, McLellan, et al., 1988; Margolin, Kosten, and Avants, 1992).

Cocaine craving may result from disruption of dopamine neurotransmission. It has been suggested that cocaine craving may be the psychological and behavioral manifestation in humans of the neuronal sensitivity or "kindling" seen in animal studies. Such kindling has been shown to occur in the animal limbic system, specifically in the amygdala and hippocampus, but has yet to be demonstrated in humans. Halikas and Kuhn (1990) have labeled this proposal the "kindling hypothesis of cocaine craving."

Craving is frequently elicited by cues associated with past drug use, both internal and external. Responses to exposure to cocaine-related cues may, through the process of classical conditioning, actually elicit physiological responses. These may include decreased skin temperature, increased heart rate, and increases in skin conductance. Classification of reactions to cocaine-related cues is not as readily apparent as is the case for opioid-related cues (O'Brien et al., 1993). While some patients show effects indicative of a drug-induced high, others may show feelings associated with a cocaine "crash."

Cues with drug-related content have been shown to elicit both physiological and subjective responses when compared with cues without drug content. Several studies have demonstrated that, in the case of heroin users, heroin cues (heroin paraphernalia, sites where heroin "copping" takes place, and so on) elicit decreases in skin temperature and skin resistance and increases in self-reports of craving and withdrawal (Childress, McLellan, and O'Brien, 1986a, b; O'Brien, Ehrman, and Ternes, 1986). Since such associations are believed to result from past classical conditioning, treatments have been directed toward attempts to reduce the strength of such conditioned associations (O'Brien et al., 1990a). Similar Pavlovian conditioned responses have been demonstrated in cocaine-abusing patients. Ehrman et al. (1992), in a sample of cocaine abusers who freebased and smoked the drug but who did not have a history of opiate injection, found cocaine-related but not opiate-related or neutral stimuli to elicit conditioned responses associated with cocaine use. These included decreases in skin temperature and resistance, as well as increases in heart rate, self-reported cocaine craving, and self-reported cocaine withdrawal. The study concluded that the presence of such physiological and subjective responses were likely the product of Pavlovian conditioning.

Is Cocaine Addicting?

How addicting is cocaine, if it is addicting at all? Although there are few, if any, workers in the field who would deny that cocaine possesses a high addiction liability, there is some evidence that addiction is not a uniform outcome of cocaine use. In an eleven-year exploratory follow-up study of a small network of cocaine users ($N = 27$ at baseline and 24 at follow-up), Murphy, Reinarman, and Waldorf (1989) found that, despite the potential for serious abuse, long-term controlled use was possible. Four types of career cocaine use patterns were identified:

1. *Continuous controlled use* was demonstrated by one-third of the sample, who made regular use of modest amounts (not exceeding 0.25 to 1 gram weekly), often on weekends, but sometimes not for weeks at a time.

2. *Controlled use to heavy use to controlled use,* also reflecting one-third of the sample, consisted of peak periods of daily use for months or years of 2 to 3 grams weekly, followed by periods of low use (about 0.25 gram per week), with shifts in pattern of consumption triggered by physiological side effects and influenced by other life events (such as the need for money and so on).

3. *Controlled use to heavy use to abstinence,* reflected in the patterns of one-quarter of the sample, consisted of moderate use for an average of 5 to 6 years, followed by escalation to levels perceived as uncontrolled and detrimental. This pattern was marked by high levels of cocaine-related problems (including involvement in cocaine-related activities), use of alcohol and other drugs, and physical side effects (convulsions, hallucinations), and characterized by guilt and strained relationships, until family pressure, guilt, or external events (for example, pregnancy) led to cessation of drug use.

4. *Uncontrolled use to abstinence* was the least common of the four patterns. Cessation of cocaine use occurred after very long periods of use (up to ten years) of modest amounts of cocaine (0.25

gram weekly, with rare 1-gram weekly binges) without any cocaine-related problems, but in which the nervousness and edginess produced by cocaine, as well as the cost, eventually became aversive.

As the authors of this study note, these types of cocaine abuse patterns may be more typical of the white middle-class user than of the increasingly more common users from poor and minority backgrounds.

Noting that *dependence* on cocaine has not been fully established, in part because of a lack of distinct physical symptoms upon cessation of regular use, Erickson and Alexander (1989) focused on the behavioral attributes of *addiction* to cocaine, preferring the term *addiction liability* to represent the likelihood that the use of cocaine will be followed by addiction, in the sense of a behavioral disorder according to one of several definitions. These include Wesson and Smith's "compulsion to use the drug, loss of control over the amount used, and continued use in spite of adverse consequences" (1985, p. 200); Gawin and Kleber's (1985b; 1986a) idea of "a recurrent pattern of cyclic binges, rather than continuous daily use and withdrawal symptoms modeled on alcohol and heroin abuse" (Erickson and Alexander, 1989, p. 251); and the World Health Organization's "syndrome manifested by a behavioral pattern in which the use of a given psychoactive drug, or class of drugs, is given a much higher priority than other behaviors that once had higher values" (Edwards, Arif, and Hodgson, 1982, p. 10; cited by Erickson and Alexander, 1989, p. 251).

The lines of evidence for the position developed by Erickson and Alexander (1989) include the following:

1. *Animal studies* of cocaine self-administration, in which animals either demonstrate preference for cocaine when given periodic access or continuously self-administer cocaine to the point of death or debilitation (see Johanson, 1984), are not truly representative of humans, who have infinitely more behavioral choices.

2. *Studies of the effects of cocaine on the reward centers of the brain* (for example, Frawley, 1987; Wise, 1984) have been contested (for example, *Science,* 1988) and lack evidence that cocaine is more reinforcing, under normal circumstances, than other reinforcers.

3. *Clinical studies* have not demonstrated that cocaine is, by itself and apart from multiple drug use, capable of creating addiction

problems for the majority of persons who use it. Thus, problem cocaine users may be a small, relatively self-selected sample.

4. *Data from survey research studies* such as the NIDA National Household Survey (Abelson and Miller, 1985) and the NIDA National High School Senior Survey (O'Malley, Johnston, and Bachman, 1985) indicate that most persons who have tried cocaine use it infrequently, and have not progressed to more regular use.

5. *Community studies* of persons neither in treatment nor in prison who appear to have experienced significant fluctuation between periods of compulsive and controlled use (see, for example, Erickson et al., 1987; Murphy, Reinarman, and Waldorf, 1989) suggest that social norms regarding cocaine abuse and personal concerns about health constrained actual use.

On the basis of these reported wide variations in patterns of cocaine use, Erickson and Alexander (1989) suggest that cocaine is like other substances which people use to excess, that it is not a uniquely addictive drug, and that fewer than 5% to 10% of users will progress to more intensive use. Thus, they conclude, "The likelihood that cocaine users will become addicted has been greatly overstated" (p. 263).

While many of the points they make are well taken, one wonders if the greater danger of cocaine lies in *underestimating* its effects. The fact that cocaine is *severely* addicting (for there are degrees of addiction, as measured, for example, by involvement in the "drug life") in the case of a small percentage of users—say 10%, if we accept the upper end of their estimate—does not make it any less risky to that 10%, very few of whom are likely to recognize their addiction liability before they begin to use the drug, and for whom addiction may be disastrous. Furthermore, it is a dangerous drug—no less for the experienced user than for the novice, for both of whom it may in fact be deadly. Such danger may be a direct result of the often unpredictable and potentially fatal physiological effects of cocaine, or it may be a result, also potentially fatal, of involvement in drug dealing, in which a high proportion of cocaine users engage. Thus, while Erickson and Alexander (1989) are correct in noting the range of addiction liability which exists with respect to cocaine, and the overstatement of cocaine's dangers for some persons in some cases, the portrayal of the risks for even a relatively small proportion of users as severe is still warranted.

The Course of Addiction

Initiation into Cocaine Use

There are many reasons for the first use of cocaine. Reasons for initial use reported by male addicts (Khalsa, Paredes, and Anglin, 1993) included to satisfy curiosity (36%); to facilitate socialization at parties (34%); to "have fun or celebrate" (34%); to relieve dysphoric states such as depression and anxiety (15%); to get "high" (7%); easy availability (6%); and to enhance sexual pleasure or to procure sex partners (3%). In the study by Griffin et al. (1989), the reasons given by both men and women for initiation of cocaine use included taking it to help cope with depression; to increase sociability; to help cope with anxiety; to cope with health problems; and, for women alone, to decrease guilt feelings. Women were more likely to cite specific reasons for using cocaine than men, while men were more likely not to cite any reason for initiating cocaine use. Subjects in the Griffin et al. (1989) study were asked if the drug was effective in meeting these needs. Apparently it was, at least symptomatically. A surprising number of both men and women (58%) who took cocaine to help cope with depression found that it helped elevate their mood. Women experienced more relief from guilt than did men (47% versus 23%), who experienced *more* guilt while intoxicated. A majority of both men and women experienced an increase in sociability (57%), while relief from anxiety occurred in 40%. These findings underline the highly reinforcing qualities of cocaine use.

The theme of self-medication for aversive internal states by using cocaine and other drugs has been suggested by a number of writers as a factor in cocaine use. For example, Nunes et al. (1990) suggested that some cocaine-using patients with social phobias may use the drug to increase their self-confidence, while others may use it to ameliorate depressive symptoms.

Introduction to cocaine use by friends and/or acquaintances is common. In one study, 76% of cocaine users were first introduced to the drug by friends or acquaintances, 8% by a parent or relative other than a sibling, 4% by a girlfriend or wife, 4% by a sibling, and 8% by a dealer or prostitute. Some 40% of those persons introducing the subject to cocaine were cocaine-dependent themselves (Khalsa, Anglin, et al., 1993). In another study by the same team of researchers, it was found that for almost all respondents (85%), their first supply of cocaine was free (Khalsa, Paredes, and Anglin, 1993). Crack cocaine use in adolescence has been described as "contagious" by Schwartz, Luxenberg, and

Hoffmann (1991), who found that 39% of teenage cocaine "snorters," 57% of crack experimenters (use of crack fewer than 9 times), and 80% of intermediate (use of crack 10 to 50 times) and heavy (use of crack more than 50 times) users had persuaded at least one friend to try cocaine for the first time. This pattern of initiation also held true in the case of sex partners of more frequent crack smokers.

With respect to initial route of administration, intranasal use was the most common (76%), followed by smoking (11%), intravenous use (4%), and freebasing (3%). Another 5% smoked cocaine as "primo" (marijuana cigarettes spiked with cocaine) or as "rails" (tobacco cigarettes laced with cocaine; Khalsa, Paredes, and Anglin, 1993).

With continued use and the development of dependence, the route of administration changes. While most cocaine users start out with intranasal use or smoking crack in a social setting, this pattern may vary over time. Intranasal use, the most common route of administration at initiation of cocaine use, decreased to 10% at time of entry into treatment. At the same time, the proportion of the sample using crack increased from 11% at initiation to 70% upon entering treatment. Crack use increased rapidly over the 6 to 7 years preceding entry into the study, while percentage of time using cocaine at a "severe" level also increased rapidly, regardless of route of administration, coinciding with increased use of crack. Time from first use of cocaine to treatment entry averaged 11.5 years (Khalsa, Paredes, and Anglin, 1993).

Some users stay at their initial level and route, maintaining low rates of use, while others lose control over their use of cocaine (Murphy, Reinarman, and Waldorf, 1989). These individuals may go on to experiment with smoking freebase or crack in order to enhance the high gained from the use of the drug. Some go on to injection use, either of cocaine alone, or of cocaine in combination with other drugs such as heroin. Pearsall and Rosen (1992) have pointed out that what often starts as a "social drug" to be used at parties and with friends can become in many cases "an all powerful obsession leading to social isolation, loss of relationships with non–drug-using friends, and strained or broken relationships with spouses or significant others" (p. 315).

As is the case with heroin abusers, the seeking and use of cocaine can be a pervasive, consuming activity in a drug abuser's life. Abusers in the study by Khalsa, Paredes and Anglin (1993) used cocaine 75% or more of the time they were not incarcerated between their first use of cocaine and entry into treatment. With such a pattern of use, job performance and attendance may become erratic and unpredictable, and the user is likely to become moody, irritable, and even paranoid. Health, including personal care and hygiene, nutrition, and attention to medical needs, is neglected as well. The strength of the drive toward compulsive use is well illustrated by animal models in which an animal will press a lever thousands of times for a single dose of cocaine (Johanson, 1984).

Following the usually highly positive subjective and social experiences associated with initial use of cocaine, continued use typically develops into a pattern of bingeing on high doses, frequently carried out in isolation (Gawin and Ellinwood, 1988; Siegel, 1982a). At this point there is little recognition on the part of the user of the negative external contingencies associated with use of cocaine, and there is little to distinguish the compulsive user from other users. Increased use, as a result of either increased availability of the drug (perhaps through selling it) or increased availability of funds for purchasing it, may lead to compulsive, uncontrolled use (Gawin and Ellinwood, 1989). The route of intake may now change from inhalation to smoking or injection in order to produce a more intense experience. Use of these routes is likely to bring extreme euphoria. During the periods of dysphoria associated with non-use, such episodes of euphoria leave memories which can trigger craving and further use (Gawin and Ellinwood, 1988).

A useful cross-section of cocaine abuse patterns among out-of-treatment injection drug users is provided by the National AIDS Demonstration Research study. Cocaine abuse among the NADR population was very high, with reported injection use of cocaine among those who had ever used cocaine at 95.6% for males and 93.8% for females. The figures for injection use within the previous six months for those who had used cocaine within that period were 92.1% for males and 91.2% for females, and of these individuals, 35.4% of males and 41.4% of females had injected at least once a day. Injection use of cocaine four times a day or more in this group was reported by 12.5% of males and 18.7% of females. The percentages who had ever combined heroin and cocaine in the entire group was 72.2% for males and 72.9% for females. Injection use of combined heroin and cocaine among those who had ever used this combination was very high, with 97.8% of males and 97.4% of females reporting this route. Injection use for those who had used combined heroin and cocaine in the previous six months was reported by 83.9% of males and 85.4% of females, and of these individuals, 40.2% of males and 50.1% of females had injected at least once a day. Injection use four times a day or more of combined heroin and cocaine in this group was reported by 14.2% of males and 24.0% of females (Feucht, Stephens, and Sullivan, 1993).

Even with such patterns of heavy use, a period of abstinence during a crack use career is not an unusual event. Khalsa, Paredes, and Anglin (1993) found that 86% of abusers reported a period of abstinence of at least one month's duration during their dependence careers. As is the case for addiction to heroin, the proportion of time spent in abstinence decreases as addiction progresses.

Yet, many Americans appear to have used cocaine without encountering serious problems. One explanation may reside in the social context of cocaine use. Employing a "snowball" sampling methodology, Kaplan, Bieleman, and TenHouten (1992) identified a group of "casual users" in the Netherlands. Such users were identified as those who had cocaine contacts within a wide scope of settings, and whose social network involvement with other cocaine users could not be characterized solely by shared cocaine use most of the time. In contrast, compulsive cocaine users had a high degree of involvement with other cocaine contacts with whom they used cocaine most or all of the time. These researchers suggested that the "controlled" user also had a low degree of involvement in his or her cocaine network, perhaps reflecting an attempt to check drug use by avoiding the "social euphoria" brought on by sharing cocaine frequently within a social setting.

Ultimately, many cocaine abusers enter treatment, which they seek for a variety of reasons. These include the presence of depression and other drug-related problems, as well as the severity of cocaine use (Chitwood and Morningstar, 1985; Helfrich et al, 1983). These may not, however, be the salient variables which lead to seeking treatment, since their presence alone was found in one study not to differentiate between treatment-seeking and non–treatment-seeking cocaine addicts (Carroll and Rounsaville, 1992). For cocaine addicts, the perception of negative consequences of cocaine use (loss of relationships, loss of employment), together with either the presence of support or the pressure to enter treatment, may be among the most important reasons for doing so (Carroll and Rounsaville, 1992). Also, the feeling that one has lost control over one's cocaine use, rather than the specific amount or frequency of that use, seems to be a very salient factor in the decision to seek treatment (Gawin and Kleber, 1985b).

Prior treatment experience is generally infrequent among cocaine addicts entering treatment. Some 79% of subjects in the Kang et al. (1991) study had received no previous treatment for drug abuse. In the study by Means et al. (1989), 49.4% had never had treatment, while 28.4%

had one or more previous treatment experiences, and 22.3% had more than two.

Time before treatment entry may vary substantially. Schnoll et al. (1985) reported that, for patients entering cocaine treatment in Chicago between 1979 and 1983, 87% had been using cocaine for less than 4 years, and 37% for less than 6 months. These data suggest the wide range of progression to cocaine abuse at levels leading to the decision to seek treatment. Some 65% had tried to stop using cocaine, 17% three or more times without success, and 58.4% had not been able to remain drug-free for more than a week. Gawin (1991) also reported, on the basis of a sample of admissions to treatment (Gawin and Kleber, 1985b), that about 2 to 4 years passed between initial exposure to cocaine and the development of addiction. This study found that treatment entry appeared to be a function not of daily cocaine use, or of any specific level of use, but rather of the experience of extended cocaine binges, which resulted in the recognition that one's use of cocaine was out of control.

These times to treatment entry can be contrasted with the 11.5 years reported by Khalsa Anglin, and Paredes (1992) and Khalsa, Paredes, and Anglin (1993) for crack cocaine users seeking treatment in the Veterans Administration system. Gawin, Khalsa, and Ellinwood (1994) noted a lapse of 18 to 48 months between first intranasal use of cocaine and presentation for treatment. Almost all subjects in this study had used cocaine at a "severe" level, although a large number had also been abstinent at some point in their drug use careers. Aggregate lengths of time in each of these states was 4.5 years for severe use and abstinence for almost 5 years. The average time from first severe use of cocaine to treatment entry was 83 months, with the longest continuous period of severe use being 37 months in length. Not only may the progression of addiction to crack be longer than that for abuse of other forms of cocaine, but also in the case of crack use in the African American community there may be less psychopathology on the part of abusers (Platt et al., 1989), thus resulting in a slower progression of the addiction. While this has been shown to be the case for opiate addiction, the factor has yet to be demonstrated with cocaine abusers.

Finally, both time to treatment entry and number of prior treatment experiences appear to be lower for primary cocaine abusers than for primary opiate abusers. Calsyn and Saxon (1990) reported that primary cocaine abusers entered Veterans Administration substance abuse treatment after an average of 5.2 years of cocaine use and 1.6 treatment episodes, while primary opiate abusers entered treatment after 11.4 years of opiate use and 5.7 prior treatment episodes.

Patterns of Abuse

A number of typologies of cocaine abuse patterns have been developed. One describes the progression of use to treatment entry, while another describes cocaine abuse patterns among controlled abusers. A third typology describes major subtypes among cocaine abusers based on psychopathology.

In their study of the natural history of cocaine abuse, Khalsa, Anglin, et al. (1993) identified four patterns of progression from initiation of cocaine use to entry into treatment: initial occasional use, not out of control, progressing to severe use (Mild–Moderate–Severe, accounting for 16% of the sample); mild initial use, progressing to severe use with no intervening period of moderate use (Mild–Severe, 44%); initial moderate-to-severe use (Moderate–Severe, 10%); and immediate severe use (Instantly Severe, 29%). Severe use was defined as daily use, for at least a month, of any quantity, with weekly binges of at least three days a week for at least a month, or very heavy biweekly binges during which at least 10 grams of cocaine were used. Not surprisingly, initial mild use resulted in a much longer period (both Mild–Moderate–Severe and Mild–Severe, 141 months) of cocaine use prior to treatment than initial use at a moderate (Moderate–Severe, 109 months), or severe level of use (Instantly Severe, 111 months). Thus, the Instantly Severe group experienced the shortest time lapse between initiation into drug use and treatment entry. In demographic terms, the Mild–Moderate–Severe group contained the largest proportion of young subjects, African Americans, and subjects over age 50; the Moderate–Severe group the highest proportion of whites; and the Instantly Severe group the highest proportion of subjects with more than a twelfth-grade education.

Schwartz, Luxenberg, and Hoffmann (1991) found three patterns of crack use among middle-class adolescent polydrug abusers. "Experimenters," who had used crack 1 to 9 times, accounted for 67% of their sample; an intermediate group, who had smoked crack 10 to 50 times, accounted for 15% of their sample; and heavy users, who had used crack more than 50 times, accounted for 18%. Preoccupation with obtaining and using the drug, inability to modulate such use, and rapid development of pharmacological tolerance were characteristic of about half the experimenters and nearly all the heavy users. Suspicion, mistrust, and depression increased as level of crack use increased. Heavier crack use was also associated with injection use of cocaine, with nearly one-fourth (23%) of the intermediate and heavy users engaging in this practice, versus 7% of the experimenters.

As for use of other drugs prior to treatment entry in the four types of cocaine users identified by Khalsa, Anglin, et al. (1993), the Mild–Moderate–Severe group showed the lowest level of marijuana use as well as the lowest level of excessive alcohol and narcotic use. The Mild–Severe group was characterized by the highest level of daily marijuana and amphetamine use; the Moderate–Severe group by infrequent marijuana use but by high levels of narcotic and amphetamine use; and the Instantly Severe group by the lowest levels of marijuana and amphetamine use. In general, as time of cocaine use increased and treatment entry approached, time spent in severe use increased, along with a shift to crack use from use of cocaine by other routes, and excessive use of alcohol and other drugs decreased.

As has previously been noted, Murphy, Reinarman, and Waldorf (1989) have described four types of sustained, controlled long-term use: continuous controlled use, controlled to heavy to controlled use, controlled to heavy use to abstinence, and controlled use to abstinence. It is likely that more ethnographic studies will define other patterns of cocaine abuse as the disorder is studied in the various strata and subcultures of our society.

Weiss et al. (1986) identified three major subtypes among heavy cocaine abusers: patients with an established history of major depression or attention deficit disorder who may use cocaine to self-medicate; patients with cyclothymic or bipolar disorder who use cocaine when endogenously euphoric in order to intensify and prolong pleasurable symptoms; and patients with primarily characterological psychopathology. Each of these subgroups likely requires different treatment strategies, thus necessitating a careful diagnostic workup.

Temporal Parameters of Abuse

Time between first use of stimulants and abuse can be up to 4 to 5 years (Gawin and Kleber, 1985b), although this period of time may be significantly shorter in the case of crack abuse (Schwartz, Luxenberg, and Hoffmann, 1991). Gawin and Kleber (1985b) suggested that the time period between initial stimulant use and development of dependence was typically 2 to 5 years. The consensus among a number of clinical observers is that only after the shift from controlled to uncontrolled use of cocaine occurs are clinical consequences noticed (O'Malley and

Gawin, 1990). This shift is characterized primarily by extended binges of cocaine use, during which cessation of use occurs only when available supplies of the drug are exhausted. In the case of crack use, Schwartz, Luxenberg, and Hoffmann (1991) found that more than 60% of heavy crack users in their largely white, middle-class sample of suburban teenagers went from initiation to weekly or more frequent use within 3 months.

There appears to be a temporal relationship between the onset of cocaine abuse and other psychiatric disorders, although there is considerable variability in the course of development of cocaine abuse. One study found that for cocaine abusers with major or minor depression, mania or hypomania, and alcoholism, onset of these disorders took place primarily after the start of drug abuse or in the same year as the start of abuse for some two-thirds of the sample. For cocaine abusers with generalized anxiety disorder, the onset of symptoms occurred in almost even proportions before and after onset of drug abuse. Phobias, anxiety disorder, and attention deficit disorder were predominantly diagnosed before the onset of drug abuse. This was true for 68% of patients with anxiety disorders and 87% of those with phobias. Alcoholism preceded drug abuse in only 21% of patients (Rounsaville, Anton, et al., 1991).

Binges, Sprees, and Runs

For many users of cocaine, such use frequently involves periods of repetitive self-administration during which a significant amount of cocaine is consumed. Such episodes are referred to as "binges." Binges are characterized by as many as ten administrations of the drug over a period of one hour (Gawin, Khalsa, and Ellinwood, 1994; Gold, 1984). Dependence on cocaine usually involves intractable cyclic binges of 12 to 36 hours in length. Binges may occur when the rapid decline in cocaine's effects, coupled with the immediate memory of the euphoric effects, results in a tremendous desire to re-create the experience (Gawin and Ellinwood, 1988). Typically, binges are followed by periods of limited cocaine use or no use lasting from 2 to 5 days in length. Eventually, however, gradually increasing withdrawal symptoms and craving for the elation associated with prior binges, particularly when these occur in the context of the dysphoria of daily life without cocaine, lead to another binge cycle.

The term "spree" has also been used, typically when large amounts, in excess of several grams, have been taken over a period of hours. Sprees generally cover a considerably shorter period of time than do "runs" of amphetamine use, but are otherwise similar (Cox et al., 1983). Although cocaine binges may last for days, they are more likely to have a duration of approximately 12 hours (Gawin and Kleber, 1985b), with a range of 8 to 24 hours. They may occur daily for several days, followed by a period of abstinence several days in length, or, less frequently, may occur over the course of a Friday night or a weekend (Wallace, 1990a). During cocaine binges, there is likely to be an exclusive focus on obtaining and using crack, to the exclusion of any attention to hygiene, nourishment, sleep, family and loved ones, work, and other responsibilities. Only physical exhaustion, or the exhaustion of funds, and thus loss of access to supply of stimulants, will result in cessation of the binge (Wallace, 1990a).

While cocaine binges are similar to amphetamine runs, the latter typically involve longer periods between administrations (perhaps several hours), less variability of mood (more continuity of the "high"), more intense and sustained abuse, and a longer total duration (from 3 to 6 up to 12 days; Kramer, Fischman, and Littlefield, 1967). Cocaine binges may occur 1 to 3 times a week in abusers, and may last from 8 to 24 hours each, with cocaine being administered every 15 minutes in order to maintain the rush of cocaine euphoria. Gawin, Khalsa, and Ellinwood (1994) observed that amphetamine use involves less frequent administration and lower total overall use than cocaine. When their lower cost, greater availability, and greater potency (some ten times greater than that of cocaine) are taken into account, amphetamines make prolonged high-intensity use more likely, although this outcome is mitigated by the somewhat reduced availability of amphetamines. Gawin, Khalsa and Ellinwood (1994) also note that similar intensity and duration of cocaine use, as can occur with cocaine smoking, as well as the availability of large supplies, can result in clinical profiles which are indistinguishable from those of amphetamine users.

Cocaine binges are characterized by a loss of interest in sex, nourishment, sleep, safety, survival, money, morality, loved ones, or responsibilities. Binges may be followed by from half a day to 5 days of abstinence from cocaine (O'Malley and Gawin, 1990). Not surprisingly, the frequent administration of cocaine during binges, up to 4 times an hour, and the repeated insults to the brain's homeostatic mechanisms, specific brain centers, and hemodynamic functioning, may result in acute (as well as chronic) effects on mood, neuropsychological functioning, and the central nervous system and circulatory system (O'Malley and Gawin, 1990).

Four adverse outcomes may result from cocaine sprees or runs. The first is *stimulant-induced psychosis,* similar to that occurring after spree use of amphetamines, and characterized by marked hyperactivity and stereotypical behavior (for example, repetitive motor activities such as pacing and/or head bobbing), delusions of parasitosis (that is, insects under the skin), visual hallucinations (commonly "snow lights" or "snow blindness," shimmering bright slivers of light in the peripheral visual field),[6] a fascination with mechanical devices and a desire to tinker (perhaps by dismantling household appliances), and aggressive or assaultive behaviors (frequently associated with paranoid delusions and excitement, often involving dangerous or belligerent actions toward oneself and others). The other potential outcomes are *convulsions and death,* resulting from accidental overdose, usually from respiratory depression;[7] the permanent loss of midbrain dopamine (and dopamine neurons), resulting in *neuroendocrine dysfunction,* perhaps underlying the phenomenon of craving; and the *cocaine "crash,"* characterized by irritability, a ravenous appetite, excessive sleep, depression, and even suicidal ideation (Commissaris, 1989).

Thus, a critical objective for treatment interventions is the induction of initial abstinence and the disruption of binge cycles (Gawin, Kleber, et al., 1989). Cocaine binges are likely indicative of severe dependence (Gawin and Kleber, 1985b).

Tolerance

Tolerance, which refers to the diminished effects of the drug after repeated administrations or decreased responsiveness to its effects over time, occurs with cocaine use on both an acute and a chronic basis. That is, the size of cocaine doses or "hits" must be increased to achieve the same effects, both during a given series of administrations and with repeated use over longer periods of time. Fischman (1984), for example, found that without an increase in dose every six to ten minutes, subjective effects of the drug decreased with repeated administrations. Repeated chronic administration also results in an increase in the baseline dose needed to produce the desired euphoric effect. Dackis and Gold (1985b) have suggested that tolerance develops as a function of the inability of dopamine-dependent reward pathways in the brain to replenish dopamine. Thus, there is a need for increased activity to continue blocking the reuptake to sustain sufficient extracellular dopamine to produce euphoria.

The development of "virtually complete" tolerance to the euphorigenic and other subjective effects of cocaine has been demonstrated pharmacologically in the case of acute administration by Ambre et al. (1989). They reported pharmacological confirmation and quantification of the subjective reports of cocaine users on a spree that repeated use eventually failed to produce the desired "high." Such highs came to be replaced by a global sensation of "feeling bad." One study suggested the existence of quantitative electroencephalographic evidence for neuroadaptation in response to chronic cocaine use (Alper et al., 1990).

With chronic administration, tolerance to the physiological effects of cocaine also develops. After the first few doses, repeated administration does not uniformly result in further increases for all of cocaine's physiological effects. For example, with repeated administrations of cocaine, heart rate may initially increase then either slow in rate of increase or reach a plateau, while blood pressure may continue to increase until administration of the drug is terminated (Foltin et al., 1988; Fischman and Schuster, 1982). Sensitization, or reverse tolerance, can also develop to the stimulant effects of cocaine. Such sensitization is characterized by long-lasting behavioral responses, including motor hyperactivity and stereotypy, and can affect both rapidity of onset and magnitude of response (Post et al., 1987).

Acute tolerance, that is, tolerance developing within the course of a single administration of a drug, has been found to occur with cocaine. This mechanism is reflected in the more rapid decline in some effects (in particular, the subjective [euphoric] and cardiovascular effects) than in the decline in blood levels of cocaine (Chow et al., 1985; Fischman and Schuster, 1982). Ambre et al. (1988) found the euphoric effects of cocaine (the "high") to intensify to a peak at about one hour after injection and then to decline toward baseline at four hours, despite the presence of relatively constant plasma levels (which, of course, may not correspond entirely with brain levels). It is likely that there is substantial inter- and intra-individual variability in responses to cocaine, including the development of acute tolerance (Hatsukami et al., 1994; Isenschmidt et al., 1992). Other studies have also demonstrated the development of acute tolerance to the pleasurable effects of cocaine, in particular the "rush," in response both to administration of a single dose (Chow et al., 1985; Javaid et al., 1978) and steady-state cocaine infusion following administration of a bolus, a procedure designed to maintain a peak plasma concentration (Kumor et al., 1989). Acute tolerance to the physiological and subjective effects of cocaine appears to dissipate within twenty-four hours (Fischman et al., 1985).

Symptoms of Abstinence

While some writers (Grinspoon and Bakalar, 1980; Estroff and Gold, 1986) are uncertain whether an actual abstinence syndrome appears in response to discontinuation of cocaine after a period of abuse, others (Jones, 1984; Gawin and Kleber, 1986a; Gold and Verebey, 1984) are of the opinion that such a phenomenon does exist. The cocaine abstinence syndrome was first described by Gawin and Kleber (1986a) as triphasic in nature, beginning with the *crash,* which lasts anywhere from 9 hours to 4 days, which is followed by the stages of *withdrawal,* lasting from 1 to 10 weeks, and *extinction,* which may last for years (Gawin, 1991; Gawin and Kleber, 1986a; Satel et al, 1991).

Phase 1: The "Crash"

Phase one, labeled the "crash" by Gawin and Kleber (1986a), consists of a rapid decrease in mood and energy levels immediately following cessation of a binge. This phase is characterized by a rapid intensification of cocaine craving, accompanied by feelings of depression, agitation, and anxiety. Suspicion and paranoia are likely to be present (Sherer et al., 1988). Exhaustion and a craving for sleep build over a period of up to eight hours, during which the further use of cocaine is rejected.[8] Attempts are made to bring on sleep through the use of other substances, such as marijuana, sedatives, opiates, or alcohol. When sleep does occur, hypersomnolence, accompanied by hyperphagia (increased appetite) during brief periods of wakefulness, may be present for several days. Mood then begins to normalize. The exhaustion, depression, and hypersomnolence of the crash probably reflect acute depletion of neurotransmitters, with recovery being dependent on the time needed for neurotransmitter synthesis and repletion. The duration of the crash is directly proportional to the duration and intensity of the binge which preceded it (Gawin and Ellinwood, 1988, 1989). Gawin and Ellinwood (1988) have compared the crash to an alcohol hangover rather than withdrawal from chronic use of opiates or alcohol.

Phase 2: Withdrawal

The crash occurring immediately after cessation of cocaine use is followed in turn by a protracted dysphoric syndrome, characterized by decreased activation, amotivation, intense boredom, and anhedonia (Gawin and Ellinwood, 1988, 1989). These symptoms, which are more subtle and less dramatic than those which follow the crash, and are thus less often recognized, appear within half a day to four days after the crash. The symptoms seen during this phase are similar to those present in withdrawal from other drugs of abuse, with the exception that in the case of cocaine, gross physiological symptoms are not present. With abstinence, anhedonic symptoms will disappear within two to twelve weeks (Gawin and Ellinwood, 1988, 1989; Gawin and Kleber, 1986a). Here, as in phase 1, the severity and duration of symptoms are dependent on the intensity of cocaine abuse.

Thus, abrupt cessation of cocaine use does not appear to precipitate as clearly identifiable a physiological "withdrawal syndrome" as does withdrawal from alcohol or heroin and other opiates. As a result, it is not clear whether the body develops a physiological dependence or "need" for cocaine in order to maintain physiological homeostasis, as is the case with these other drugs. Additionally, the bingeing, or alternation of cycles of high-intensity use of the drug with periods of abstinence or less intensive use, characteristic of heavy cocaine abuse is a very different pattern from that seen in alcohol and opiate dependence. This is not to say that cessation of cocaine use is symptom-free. Unpleasant "rebound symptoms," such as dysphoria, lethargy, and other neurovisceral symptoms, are likely to occur after such cessation, but it is not clear if these are truly withdrawal symptoms reflective of physiological dependence (Satel et al., 1991). Such symptoms are likely the result of depletion of the brain's store of dopamine and other neurotransmitters necessary for maintenance of a normal mood state. Such symptoms usually decrease in intensity over the period of a few days to a week.

The absence of a clearly defined and universally recognized withdrawal syndrome has contributed to the popular perception that cocaine is less dangerous than other drugs in that it is only psychologically and not physically addicting. Such a perception undoubtedly contributed to the rapid and widespread use of cocaine during the 1980s. This, of course, is not the case, since in reality continued use of cocaine and other stimulants leads to sustained neurophysiological changes in the brain systems that underlie and regulate psychological processes, particularly mood states and the experience of pleasure (Gawin and Ellinwood, 1988). O'Malley and Gawin (1990) observed that cocaine dependence does not result in *gross* physiological withdrawal symptoms when use of the drug is discontinued. Rather, brain systems that regulate psychological processes, such as the mesolimbic and mesocortical dopaminergic pathways, adapt to cocaine use. These systems are part of the general reward system. Subsensitivity and multiple receptor alterations have been noted in such systems in animal models following chronic cocaine use. Thus, these changes may parallel the reward subsensitivity (anhedonia) observed in chronic cocaine users. Such findings have led to the suggestion that while chronic, high-dose cocaine use produces an addiction which is expressed *psychologically*, there is a true underlying *physiological* addiction.

Dackis and Gold (1985 a, b, c) have proposed that dopamine depletion, with resultant postsynaptic receptor supersensitivity, may be the basis for the withdrawal symptoms seen after discontinuation of cocaine. The "dopamine depletion hypothesis" postulates a (chronic) depletion of dopamine, although cocaine causes an acute increase in dopaminergic transmission. This depletion inhibits the functioning of central dopamine circuits, resulting in craving. The basis for this hypothesis resides in the fact that cocaine blocks dopamine reuptake and decreases presynaptic vesicular binding (Taylor and Ho, 1978). This, in turn, results in an acute increase in synaptic dopamine concentration, which is then metabolized to 3-methoxytyramine and excreted (Verebey and Gold, 1985). Therefore, dopamine depletion likely occurs more rapidly than the transmitter can be synthesized by the brain (Memo, Pradhan, and Hanbauer, 1981), and a dopamine deficiency develops (Gold and Dackis, 1984).

The dopamine depletion hypothesis has led to the employment of pharmacological agents that act at dopamine receptor sites or affect dopamine availability. Bromocriptine, for example, is a dopamine agonist which facilitates binding of dopamine to postsynaptic receptors. Early promise shown by this agent (Dackis and Gold, 1985a; Giannini and Billet, 1987) was not borne out by later studies, primarily because of side effects leading to treatment dropout (Sherer, Kumor, and Jaffe, 1989; Tennant and Sagherian, 1987). Amantadine, a dopamimetic agent which increases dopaminergic transmission, has been shown to decrease craving (Morgan et al., 1988). It is not yet clear, however, whether this action occurs through an increase in dopamine release or a decrease in dopamine uptake. Another dopamimetic agent, methylphenidate, has also been employed in treating cocaine abuse. Although this agent at first promised to be particularly useful in the case of cocaine abusers with attention deficit disorder (Khantzian, 1983; Khantzian et al., 1984), it has been shown to have no effect in cases where attention deficit disorder was not present (Gawin, Riordan, and Kleber, 1985). Additionally, a number of antidepressants and similar agents have been evaluated for their ability to increase central nervous system monoamine function, decrease postsynaptic receptor sensitivity, and relieve abstinence symptoms. This group includes phenelzine (Golwyn, 1988), bupropion (Margolin et al., 1990), and trazodone (Small and Purcell, 1985), among others.

Gawin and Kleber have focused on the mechanism underlying withdrawal symptoms (for example, post-euphoria cocaine craving and dysphoria) as the primary neurophysiologic mechanism for relapse to cocaine abuse (Gawin and Ellinwood, 1988; Gawin and Kleber, 1984). Since tricyclic antidepressants block uptake of serotonin and norepinephrine, they produce effects opposite to those produced by long-term stimulant self-administration. These effects include the induction of catecholamine receptor subsensitivity and dopamine autoreceptor subsensitivity, thus reversing chronic stimulant-induced anhedonia (Gawin and Kleber, 1984). Hence, tricyclic agents such as desipramine, imipramine, trazodone, and maprotiline have been extensively employed in pharmacological studies. Anti-Parkinsonian agents (benztropine mesylate, amantadine, bromocriptine, tyrosine), which increase dopaminergic transmission, have also been employed.

Hospitalization is generally not essential for withdrawal from cocaine use, though it may contribute to a better outcome. In addition, the potential medical sequelae of cocaine abuse are substantial (see Chapter 6), particularly in the case of injection use, where the user is subject to the same risks as the injection user of heroin (see Platt, 1986, chap. 6 and 1995b, chap. 6 for a discussion of these risks).

Phase 3: Extinction

The extinction phase has no specific duration and generally has no characteristic symptomatology. During this phase, which may last for several years, conditioned craving may continue to occur, on an intermittent basis, perhaps for several years. Such craving is likely to occur in the presence of objects, persons, or events which were temporally paired with cocaine use (Gawin and Ellinwood, 1988, 1989). In the absence of continued cocaine use, extinction of such craving is likely to occur over time.

Cocaine Abstinence Syndrome: Evidence and Views

As noted earlier, it is generally, although not entirely, accepted that the symptoms of the cocaine abstinence syndrome represent genuine physiological withdrawal, and thus indicate the existence of a "true" physiological dependence to cocaine. Brower and Paredes (1987), for example, suggested that the distinction between the "crash" and withdrawal was arbitrary in that the former was simply an early stage of withdrawal. Concerns raised by these authors focused on methodological issues in the collection of the data on which the conceptualization was developed, particularly the use of naturalistic observation, which may have limited the validity and reliability of their findings. They also faulted a lack of description of physical signs and symptoms and inconsistencies with DSM-III[9] criteria regarding definition of phases, in that the term "withdrawal" was applied to protracted psychological abstinence phenomena (for example, anhedonia), rather than to those immediate post-binge symptoms which are accompanied by physical distress. Kleber and Gawin (1987), in reply to the concerns raised by Brower and Paredes (1987), agreed to many of these concerns, noting that their study was indeed a naturalistic one, intended to provide a framework within which further work could be conducted, and that, in disregarding DSM-III criteria, they were anticipating the shift in emphasis in DSM-IV[10] from tolerance and withdrawal to craving and dyscontrol, a shift which is more useful in understanding cocaine abuse. With respect to their inclusion of the crash in the withdrawal phase, Kleber and Gawin suggested that the crash can be present in extended first-time stimulant use, given sufficient duration and dosage, and that failure to include it would not reflect the broader view of tolerance, withdrawal, and dependence needed to understand drugs of abuse such as cocaine. Additionally, "withdrawal" has a clinical meaning, aside from its pharmacological meaning, which is reflective of postwithdrawal symptoms that require attention.

Several studies have documented the course of abstinence symptoms in patients recovering from cocaine addiction. Weddington et al. (1990) conducted a longitudinal study of 12 male cocaine addicts on a closed inpatient research unit, most of whom had been using cocaine intravenously. This study found craving to be most intense on the day prior to entering treatment, with the highest level of mood disturbance on day 1. A gradual linear improvement in mood state, craving, nighttime awakening, and clearheadedness took place over the course of the study, which lasted twenty-eight days. Rather than reflecting a "crash" or cyclical or phasic symptomatology, the symptoms during this period were seen as a continuation of those observed during active cocaine use. These symptoms extended into initial abstinence and steadily decreased over the period of the study. This pattern was very different from that following abstinence from alcohol, opiates, benzodiazepines, and nicotine, where increases in distress, sometimes dramatic, occur during the initial period of withdrawal. Nor was there the "euthymic period" reported by other investigators (for example, Gawin and Kleber, 1986a; Brower and Paredes, 1987). Findings consistent with those of Weddington et al. (1990) were obtained by Satel et al. (1991), who also found generally mild somatic, behavioral, and psychological symptoms in a sample of cocaine-dependent inpatients following abrupt cessation of cocaine use. This subjective symptomatology relating to craving, drug withdrawal, physical discomfort, anxiety, and depression gradually decreased over the three-week period of the study.

Given the similarity of the two treatment regimens (that is, inpatient treatment) with resultant absence of both exposure to environmental cues and interceptive exposure to cocaine-related cues, it may well be that in the absence of such cues, a pattern of generally mild and linearly decreasing withdrawal symptoms can be expected. Both the Weddington et al. (1990) and Satel et al. (1991) studies failed to confirm the presence of a phasic model, as described by Gawin and Kleber (1986a). Reasons suggested by Weddington et al. and Satel et al. include the absence of exposure to cocaine-related cues in inpatient as opposed to outpatient settings, the occurrence of the crash before entry into treatment, and the possible differential application of the triphasic model to inpatient and outpatient settings. Miller, Summers, and Gold (1993), while confirming the existence of a cocaine abstinence syndrome, found it to be "medically and psychiatrically benign," and concluded that it required no pharmacological intervention in an inpatient setting. In common with other studies, symptoms found in this study were transient craving, hyperactivity, slight tremor, insomnia, and apprehension.

Evidence relating to patterns of sleep and mood during cocaine termination has been collected for both acute and chronic administration of cocaine. Watson et al. (1989) studied the effects of one to two grams of cocaine on the sleep of three recreational cocaine abusers. The first night after cocaine use was characterized by reduced total sleep time, time spent in REM sleep, and percentage of sleep time spent in REM. REM latency and sleep latency were both increased. The second and third nights were characterized by an increased percentage of REM sleep and shorted REM latency. By the fourth night, changes attributed to cocaine had all been resolved.

Kowatch et al. (1992) followed nine cocaine patients admitted to an inpatient unit for cocaine withdrawal and treatment. During the first week of withdrawal, a significantly shortened REM latency, an increased percentage of time spent in REM sleep, and a long total sleep period were observed. By the third week, REM latencies were very short, and total percentage of time spent in REM sleep was increased. Week 3 was characterized by a long sleep latency, an abnormally increased total waking time after onset of sleep, and poor sleep efficiency. This pattern is similar to that found in chronic insomnia. Patient ratings of cocaine craving and depression fell dramatically after the first week of withdrawal, and were within normal levels by week 3. The authors of this study noted the similarity of their findings to those obtained in sleep studies of patients with major depression. The Kowatch et al. (1992) study partially confirmed Gawin and Kleber's (1986a) findings regarding a period of hypersomnolence following initiation of withdrawal. Gawin and Kleber (1986a), however, reported that this period lasted up to four days, with sleep normalizing after the first week, whereas Kowatch et al. (1992) observed hypersomnolence through day 9 of withdrawal, disappearing by day 15, while insomnia persisted through the third week of withdrawal. Kowatch et al. suggested that the use of EEG measures in their study may have resulted in greater sensitivity than the semistructured interviews employed by Gawin and Kleber.

Of cocaine abusers seeking treatment in one study (Brower and Parades, 1987), 62 of 75 reported the presence of at least one physical symptom associated with withdrawal, including muscle pains (56%), chills (50%), twitching (48%), and tremors (47%). The severity of the abstinence syndrome also appears to vary as a function of gender. Griffin et al. (1989) observed that the severity of withdrawal symptomatology was greater for women than for men, particularly during early abstinence. Newly abstinent female cocaine abusers in their study did not recover from their depressive symptoms as quickly as did males, a finding noted by Griffin et al. as consistent with data collected on opiate addicts (Moise, Reed, and Ryan, 1982). It was possible, however, that the female cocaine abusers, who had started their addictions at an earlier age than the males, who had a lower overall level of adjustment, and who had entered treatment at an earlier age following a shorter period of addiction, were more severely addicted or were less well adjusted before the onset of addiction.

Finally, it should be noted that Kleber and Gawin (1987) have urged more precise terminology in place of the term "withdrawal," given its dual (pharmacological and clinical) meanings, as this term was not necessarily appropriate for the syndrome seen in cocaine abusers. Weddington et al. (1990) have expressed a preference for the designation "short-term abstinence" to describe this set of phenomena, based on their failure to find a classic withdrawal pattern in the case of cocaine. Observing that the evidence for a clear-cut, predictable cocaine withdrawal syndrome was not fully convincing, Estroff and Gold (1986) compared it to the sequence of events following cessation of amphetamine abuse. These include a crash, characterized by depression, followed by a day or two of increasing irritability, psychomotor retardation, continued depression, and hypersomnia. Irritability peaks at five days, at which point the addict is most likely to leave treatment owing to intense cocaine craving. After five days, irritability begins to decrease and reasonableness begins to be restored. Thus, features of the cocaine abstinence syndrome(s) include depressive symptomatology accompanied by intense cocaine craving (Gawin and Kleber, 1986a, b; Tennant and Sagherian, 1987). Roehrich and Gold (1991) have suggested that the abstinence syndrome can assume clinical importance and a central role in cocaine abuse and addiction because the dysfunction associated with it, combined with cocaine craving, may be instrumental in leading to relapse.

The fact that gross physiological withdrawal does not result from the cessation of cocaine, and that "classic" drug abuse constructs (for example, physiological withdrawal, tolerance, and physical dependence) may not be directly applicable to cocaine abuse throws into question what many have heretofore considered the physiological elements necessary for addiction to take place (Gawin, 1991). Even in heroin addiction, however, relatively few addicts enter treatment with full-fledged physiologically based addiction to opiates. Today's substance abuser is more likely to be involved in the use of a number of mind-altering substances without being truly *physiologically* addicted to any, and, in the absence of a desire for a specific drug or effect, will use whatever is available. Undoubtedly, as Gawin (1991) has suggested, there are physiological adaptations to drug abuse, particularly in the case of cocaine abuse, which lie at the basis of cocaine-related phenomena such as cocaine craving. Thus, although cocaine abuse is not governed by the "classic" constructs of drug abuse, there is undoubtedly a strong neurophysiological basis for continuation of the addiction.

Theoretical Explanations of Cocaine Abuse

A large number of theoretical explanations exist for abuse of drugs in general, and cocaine in particular. In 1980, Lettieri, Sayes, and Pearson provided a compendium of forty-three theories of drug abuse, and Platt (1986) categorized those pertaining to the maintenance and development of heroin addiction into four *conditioning theories* (two-factor theory, simple learning theory, drive theory, and peer-group learning theory); *metabolic deficiency theory,* as proposed by Dole and Nyswander (1965); *sociologic theories,* including deviance theory, anomie, and social deviance; *family theory; psychoanalytic theories;* and *psychosocial theories.* More recently, there has been much less emphasis on such theorizing with respect to cocaine abuse. In general, there has been a very noticeable decline in invoking theoretical explanations for drug use in favor of empirical work, particularly in the case of cocaine use. In the few more recent papers addressing such theory, the two explanations which have been invoked with respect to cocaine abuse have been the self-medication hypothesis and the psychoanalytic viewpoint.

The Self-Medication Hypothesis

The self-medication hypothesis invoked to explain why individuals abuse drugs essentially states that "the specific psychotropic effects of [heroin and cocaine] interact with psychiatric disturbances and painful affect states to make them compelling in susceptible individuals" (Khantzian, 1985, p. 1259). Studies cited by Khantzian in support of the self-medication hypothesis include those which suggest that addicts use cocaine as well as opiates to self-medicate for anxiety or depression (for example, Dorus and Senay, 1980; Rounsaville, Weissman, et al., 1982a; Rounsaville, Weissman, et al., 1982b; Weissman et al., 1976; Woody, O'Brien, and Rickels, 1975), to overcome the fatigue and depletion states associated with depression (for example, Khantzian, 1975), to increase feelings of assertiveness, self-esteem, and frustration tolerance (for example, Wieder and Kaplan, 1969), or to "*augment* a hyperactive, restless lifestyle and an exaggerated need for self-sufficiency" (Khantzian, 1979, p. 100). Khantzian (1985) concluded that a number of factors might predispose an individual to initiate and maintain cocaine dependence, including preexisting chronic depression, depression resulting from cocaine abstinence, hyperactivity or attention deficit disorder, and cyclothymic or bipolar disorder. Thus, addicts, in using heroin and cocaine, "are attempting to medicate themselves for a range of psychiatric problems and painful emotional states" (p. 1263).

The self-medication hypothesis has been evaluated in a group of 494 hospitalized cocaine, opioid, and sedative- and hypnotic-dependent patients (Weiss, Griffin, and Mirin, 1992). Most (63%) reported that they had used their drug of choice for self-medication of depressive symptomatology. This finding was relatively consistent across drugs as follows:

cocaine (59%), opioids (66%), and sedative-hypnotics (64%). More such use of drugs for self-treatment of depression was noted among women, however, than among men (76% versus 58%). Patients diagnosed with major depression used drugs in response to feeling depressed more often than did those not suffering depression (89% versus 60%), although this pattern was statistically significant only for opioid abusers (92% versus 63%).

A similar pattern of drug use in response to depression existed for cocaine abusers (86% versus 57%), although the small sample size precluded a meaningful statistical comparison. When males and females (regardless of which drug was abused) were examined separately, the likelihood that those with a diagnosis of major depression would initiate drug use because of depression held true for males (100% of men with this diagnosis versus 55% of men without this diagnosis), but not for females (81% versus 75%). In the absence of a diagnosis of major depression, however, women were significantly more likely than men to use drugs for depression (75% versus 55%). More than two-thirds (68%) of patients reported that drug use improved their mood, while 26% reported a worsening of their depression after they had used drugs of abuse. Weiss, Griffin, and Mirin (1992) concluded that their findings suggested that patients used drugs to combat depressed mood without necessarily having major depression; that these results argued against the pharmacological specificity sometimes associated with the self-medication hypothesis; and that women tended to self-medicate for depression, even in the absence of major depression, while men were more likely to do so in its presence. Though neither confirming nor rejecting the self-medication hypothesis, these results provide more specificity concerning self-medication behaviors and suggest the need for further research on this issue. In addition, Weiss and Mirin (1986) found patients with bipolar or cyclothymic mood disorders to use cocaine more frequently when "endogenously high" than when depressed or euthymic. Mood states involving elation or a "high" were apparently enjoyable, and the patients sought to prolong this euphoria by using cocaine to augment them.

Psychoanalytic Explanations

Several authors (Khantzian and Khantzian, 1984; Schiffer, 1988; Spotts and Shontz, 1984) have suggested that cocaine abusers suffer from continuing emotional pain relating to hidden childhood psychological trauma. Schiffer argued that the cocaine abusers he successfully treated had been victims of some form of unrecognized psychological trauma or abuse in childhood. The interpretation he offered for drug use on the part of these patients was that "cocaine abuse, in addition to functioning as a form of self-medication, was functioning as a component of a repetition compulsion in which old psychological traumas were symbolically recreated in the post-drug dysphoria" (p. 131). The self-induced re-creation of these problems then allowed the patient to obtain a sense, although false, of having mastered them.

Resnick and Resnick (1984) observed that chronic cocaine abusers often had a fragile and fragmented sense of self and inadequate relationships with others. They traced this to the first three years of life, "when the cohesion of internalized self and object representations normally occurs" (p. 725). As a result of traumas, "deficient self-soothing mechanisms and limited inner resources with which to cope with adversity and stress" (p. 725) are developed. Cocaine use then serves to relieve chronic tension, and to help the individual avoid inner despair and feelings of emptiness. Often, borderline or narcissistic disorders are present.

Conclusions

Cocaine is a highly addicting substance. Initially, its use produces subjective effects (including a "high") which are highly pleasurable, as well as enhancing self-confidence, reducing inhibition, and generally increasing interaction with the user's immediate environment. These effects are highly reinforcing. Continued use carries with it increased tolerance to these positive effects and the emergence of negative subjective states, including anxiety, dysphoria, exhaustion, and agitation. Also accompanying continued use is the development of a craving for more cocaine to eliminate these negative states and to restore the pleasurable state which accompanied initial cocaine use.

Initiation into cocaine use, as is the case with other drugs of abuse, may occur for many reasons, including out of curiosity, as a response to social (interpersonal) pressure, or as a means of self-medicating aversive internal emotional states (Khantzian, 1985). Introduction to cocaine by friends, acquaintances, or relatives is typical (Khalsa, Anglin, et al., 1993). Initial route of use is usually by inhalation, later changing to crack smoking.

Cocaine abuse may remain level, or it may escalate rapidly to a point where it is compulsively engaged in and goes out of control. It is not completely clear why such differences in outcome occur. They may reflect individual differences in addiction liability, or the degree to which an individual is enmeshed in a cocaine-abusing network (Kaplan, Bieleman, and TenHouten, 1992).

The subjective effects associated with cocaine use (that is, the experience of intense anxiety, including panic attacks, paranoia, and apathy), or the fear of losing control because of the drug's effects, may lead some experimenters not to proceed with further use of the drug. Later on, perceived risks in relation to health, social disapproval, establishment of relationships, and even loss of interest in drugs may also be salient factors in stopping, or decreasing, cocaine use (Erickson et al., 1987). Erickson and Murray (1989) found that cocaine users who perceived "great harm" from regular use of the drug were more likely to quit than to continue use (65.2% versus 36%). "Fear of addiction," defined as ever having experienced an uncontrollable urge to use cocaine, was also more likely to be associated with quitting (19.2% versus 16.3%).

Toxic reactions are often associated with continued use, or use of high-dose levels of cocaine. These include intoxication (fatal in some cases), which may be accompanied by a wide range of psychiatric symptoms, including hallucinatory experiences, paranoia, and obsessive-compulsive behaviors.

There are agreed-upon patterns of abuse. Levels of abuse later in a cocaine abuse career typically correspond to levels of use upon initiation. Thus, mild levels of use at entry may remain at this level, although some proportion of abusers will progress to heavy use. Engaging in high levels of cocaine abuse and being relatively older at entry both typically result in a more severe pattern of abuse (Khalsa, Paredes, et al., 1993). Cocaine abuse frequently involves periods of intense, repetitive cocaine use. Such "binges" are similar to amphetamine "sprees," with the exception of being shorter in duration, likely a function of the shorter duration of action of cocaine.

Many, but far from all, cocaine abusers ultimately seek treatment. This may result from recognition of the loss of significant relationships and changing roles in the abuser's life (for example, family acceptance, other relationships, employment), or from the recognition that one has lost control over cocaine use. Length of time before seeking treatment varies substantially, from under four years (Schnoll, Daghestani, and Hansen, 1984) to over eleven (Khalsa, Anglin, and Paredes, 1992). Many cocaine abusers attempt, often unsuccessfully, to quit cocaine use on their own.

Cocaine craving remains an elusive concept, particularly as it is employed in experimental studies. Craving as measured in the laboratory over brief periods of time during clinical trials may be very different from the acute craving which occurs following use of cocaine (see, for example, Gawin, Kleber, et al., 1989). It is clear that more work is needed on this issue.

Relapse to cocaine abuse is the rule rather than the exception. Cocaine craving plays an important role in relapse. Intense craving for cocaine, even in abstinent persons, may be triggered by cues associated with prior cocaine use. Such cues may include shifts in internal mood states, as well as the presence of persons, locations, and paraphernalia associated with prior use.

Fewer theoretical explanations for cocaine abuse exist than is the case for heroin addiction. This likely reflects the increased contemporary emphasis on empirical findings in explaining cocaine abuse compared to the case for heroin addiction twenty years ago. The primary theoretical explanation of cocaine abuse in the literature focuses on the self-medication hypothesis (Khantzian, 1985), although more classic psychoanalytic explanations persist (for example, Schiffer, 1988).

There is agreement in the literature as to the symptoms that accompany abstinence from cocaine (Gawin and Kleber, 1986a; Kleber and Gawin, 1987). There is less agreement, however, as to whether or not these symptoms constitute an actual physiologically based abstinence or withdrawal syndrome (see, for example, Brower and Paredes, 1987; Satel et al., 1991).

As is the case with opiates, tolerance develops with repeated administration of cocaine. This is particularly the case with respect to cocaine's euphoric and other subjective effects (Ambre et al., 1988; Fischman, 1984). Acute tolerance, that is, tolerance developing over the course of a single administration, also occurs. Dopamine depletion, with resultant postsynaptic receptor supersensitivity, has been proposed as the basis for symptoms seen on discontinuation of cocaine use (Gold and Dackis, 1984).

4

Characteristics and Behavioral Patterns of Cocaine Abusers

Personal Characteristics

Sex and Sex-Related Differences

More men than women use cocaine. In various studies the ratios of male to female users have been 72.6% to 28.4% (Means et al., 1989), 63.3% to 36.7% (Weiss et al., 1986), 78% to 22% (Helfrich et al., 1983), and 82% to 18% (Dougherty and Lesswing, 1989). In the 1992 DAWN study, the rates of emergency room cocaine mentions for males and females per 100,000 population were 72.3 and 32.6, respectively, which corresponds to a ratio of 68.9% to 32.6% (SAMHSA, 1994c). Cocaine addicts presenting for treatment in the study reported by Ziedonis et al. (1994) were predominantly male, among both whites (74%) and African Americans (61%). Lillie-Blanton, Anthony, and Schuster (1993) found males, but not females, to have smoked crack at a higher rate than their representation in a population sample drawn from the 1988 National Household Survey on Drug Abuse (NHSDA). De Leon (1993) noted, however, that among the increasing number of women admitted to therapeutic communities, most were cocaine and/or crack users.

When dependence, not use, is examined, minimal gender differences have been observed for lifetime prevalence rates among cocaine users, a pattern similar to that found for users of analgesics, hallucinogens, inhalants, tobacco, and heroin. Male users of alcohol and cannabis, however, were somewhat more likely than female users to have become dependent, while females were somewhat more likely to have become dependent on sedatives and/or hypnotics. The greatest gender difference appeared with respect to the use of psychedelic drugs (LSD, peyote, mescaline): here 14.1% of male drug users versus 7.2% of females had developed dependence (Anthony, Warner, and Kessler, 1994).

Female cocaine abusers in general differ from males in having started any drug use earlier (Kosten, Gawin, Kosten, and Rounsaville, 1993; Griffin et al., 1989), but cocaine use slightly later (Jones, Lewis, and Shorty, 1993); in being more likely to use cocaine in freebase form than intranasally (Kosten et al., 1993); and in having abused heroin for a longer period of time (Kosten et al., 1993). Females also have been found to have poorer premorbid histories with respect to employment, self-support, and depressive symptomatology (Ellinwood, Smith, and Vaillant, 1966; Griffin et al., 1989); higher rates of a family history of drug dependence (Miller et al., 1989), more severe drug problems at intake (Kosten et al., 1993); and poorer psychological functioning (Griffin et al., 1989). With respect to psychopathology, females have higher rates of current depression and lower rates of Axis I disorders in general, and of antisocial personality disorder in particular (Griffin et al., 1989), as well as higher rates of phobia and lower rates of attention deficit disorder (Rounsaville, Anton, et al., 1991).

Age

AGE AT FIRST ILLICIT DRUG USE

The teen years are typically the time when first use of any illicit drug most frequently takes place. Reported ages at first use range from 17 years (Kang et al., 1991) to 16 years (Means et al., 1989) to 19.1 years (Weiss et al., 1986). Age at first use of any drug of abuse (including licit drugs) for the subjects in the study by Griffin et al. (1989) was 15.6 years for females and 18.5 years for males. Age at first use can vary widely, as evidenced by the range of 11 to 39 years of age reported by Kang et al. (1991). In the Veterans Administration sample studied by Khalsa, Anglin, et al. (1993), mean ages at first use were 18 for marijuana and glue; 18 to 20 for hallucinogens, amphetamines, and "downers"; and 21 to 25 for crystal methamphetamine, heroin, tranquilizers (for example, Valium), and PCP.

Age at first use of cocaine varies greatly, ranging from 12 to 45 years, with a mean of about 22 years of age (Griffin et al., 1989; Kang et al., 1991; Khalsa, Paredes, and Anglin, 1993; Kleinman et al., 1990; Means et al., 1989; Miller, Gold, and Mahler, 1991). Cocaine is typically not the first illicit drug abused by individuals in the United States; that distinction, according to the NADR study, belongs to marijuana, with rates of 66% for white males, 63% for Hispanic males, and 55% for African

American males. A similar pattern (but lower rates) of first use exists for women, with 55% of white females, 50% of Hispanic females, and 45% of African American females having used marijuana as their first illicit drug. By contrast, cocaine was reported as a first drug of abuse for men by only 3% of whites, 5% of Hispanics, and 6% of African Americans. Among women, cocaine was the first drug used by 6% of whites and 9% of both Hispanics and African Americans (Jones, Lewis, and Shorty, 1993). The NADR study sample, of course, comprised injection drug users not in treatment, a "hard-core" group with respect to drug abuse. In this group, age at first use of cocaine when cocaine was the first drug used, was 20.0 years for white males, 20.3 for Hispanic males, and 22.5 for African American males. For females, the ages at first use were slightly later than for males, at 21.8, 21.2, and 22.6 years of age, respectively (Jones, Lewis, and Shorty, 1993).[1]

Among crack cocaine users studied by Weatherby et al. (1992) in Miami, users of both alcohol and marijuana began at a median age of 15, and progressed to noninjected powdered cocaine at 17, noninjected heroin at 19, and crack cocaine at 21 years of age. Where injection use was reported, heroin use began at age 19, and cocaine and speedball injection at age 20. In this study, initiation of crack cocaine use appeared to be a function of the appearance of cocaine in Miami. For older crack users (25–29), the median age at first use of crack was 23, while for those aged 18 to 24, the age at first use was 18. In another Miami-based study, age at first cocaine use in a sample with a median age of 25.1 years was found to be 16 (Pottieger et al., 1992). Snorting of cocaine was the only route used by 82% of the sample at the time of first use, with another 8% using only crack, 6% using both (but no additional forms), and only 4% having initial use experience with another form of cocaine. At the time of the interview, cocaine had been snorted by 93%, 94% had used crack, 45% had tried freebase cocaine, and 21% had injected cocaine intravenously. Also at the time of the interview, 71% were primarily crack users, with this form of usage accounting for at least 75% of their total usage over the preceding 90 days. By this definition, 17% were using cocaine primarily by snorting and 4% by intravenous injection; 8% had mixed patterns of usage.

Most of the subjects in a study by Boyd and Mieczkowski (1990) reported that they had been under 30 when they first tried crack cocaine. Twenty-four percent were between 15 and 19 at age of first use, another 24% were aged 26 to 30, 10% were between ages 31 and 35, and 7% were over 35 years of age. The mean age at first use was just under 26 years, and no differences were found in age at first use between males and females. This sample, which was 93% African American, reported later onset of crack use (3.5 years overall and 4.5 years for African American females) than was the case for the NADR sample. This difference may reflect a difference in sampling, in that the NADR study focused on injection drug users not in treatment. Khalsa, Paredes, and Anglin (1993) found age at first use of cocaine to be related to pattern of progression of drug use. Those subjects in their Veterans Administration cocaine abuser sample who had begun cocaine use at a later age took less time to try the drug again, reported the highest total consumption of cocaine, tended to have a pattern of alternating periods of abstinence and severe use, and allowed more time to pass before entering treatment. By contrast, those users with the lowest total cocaine consumption tended to have started cocaine use at an earlier age, to have had more continuous use and fewer periods of abstinence, and to have entered treatment earlier. Thus, they had a slower rate of progression of cocaine abuse.

AGE AND COCAINE DEPENDENCE

When age is considered in regard to the development of cocaine dependence, cocaine is seen to be most addictive among the young. Data from the NHSDA suggest that crack smokers are significantly younger (mean age, 24 years) than nonsmokers (mean age, 28 years [Lillie-Blanton, Anthony, and Schuster, 1993]). In the National Comorbidity Study (Anthony, Warner, and Kessler, 1994), dependence was present among almost 25% of the group aged 15 to 24. By contrast, only 15% of those aged 25 to 44 had developed dependence. The figure for the younger group may even underestimate the eventual total, since the persons in this group had many years remaining during which they would be at risk for developing dependence. It is of interest to note that earlier use in the Anthony, Warner, and Kessler study was related to higher levels of dependence, whereas Khalsa, Paredes, and Anglin (1993) found later onset of cocaine use to be related to greater severity of abuse. It is difficult to explain this difference.

AGE AT TREATMENT ENTRY

Treatment entry typically occurs in the late twenties, although age at admission can vary substantially. In the study by Dougherty and Lesswing (1989), the average age at admission to an inpatient unit in New York was 27.8 years. In the study by Ziedonis et al. (1994), age at treatment entry ranged from 27 years for whites to 29 years for African Americans. Other reported ages at treatment entry have been 29.9 years (range, 20–65 years; Means et al., 1989), 29.7 years (Weiss et al., 1986), and 29.0 years (Helfrich et al., 1983). The average age of cocaine abusers entering treatment in Veterans Administration settings is considerably higher. Khalsa, Paredes, and Anglin (1993), for example, reported the mean age of male entrants into a VA medical center to be 37. These subjects had started their cocaine careers at an average age of 24 years. In a study by Griffin et al. (1989), women were found to have entered their first treatment earlier than men (24.6 versus 29.1 years).

Race and Ethnicity

Cocaine abusers admitted to treatment are predominately white. In several studies the reported ethnic breakdowns have been white 93.3%, African American 3.3%, Hispanic 3.3% (Weiss et al., 1986); white 83%, African American 12%, Hispanic 4%, and other 4% (Rawson et al., 1993); white treatment sample 58.5% (outreach sample 12.7%), African American treatment sample 25.6% (outreach sample 82.7%), Hispanic treatment sample 14.4% (outreach sample 4.2%), and other treatment sample 1.5% (outreach sample 0.4%; McCoy, Rivers, and Chitwood, 1993); white 64%, other 36% (Rounsaville, Anton, et al., 1991); white 70.4%, African American 28.4%, and Hispanic 1.2% (Means et al., 1989); white 61%, African American 37%, Hispanic 1%, American Indian 1% (Dougherty and Lesswing, 1989); white 50%, African American or Hispanic 50% (Carroll, Ball, and Rounsaville, 1993); white 26.0%, African American 66.0%, Hispanic 7.0%, and other 1.0% (Khalsa, Paredes, and Anglin, 1993); and white 100% (Higgins et al., 1993b). These contrasting statistics are presented to illustrate the very large differences in the racial and ethnic composition of various studies. Since there is a high likelihood of association between race and ethnicity on the one hand and social status or competence and cultural variables on the other, attention needs to be paid to the influence such differences may have on dependent variables, including response to treatment.

Holding constant social and environmental risk factors which may influence association between crack cocaine smoking and race or ethnic group, Lillie-Blanton, Anthony, and Schuster (1993) found 28.3% of crack cocaine smokers to be African Americans, 29% Hispanic Americans, and 42.8% white Americans, proportions about equal to representation of these ethnic groups in this nationally based stratified sample. Rates of crack smoking in excess of those expected for racial or ethnic groups on the basis of population estimates did occur, however, for teens aged 15 to 19, where African Americans reported smoking crack significantly less than white Americans.

Means et al. (1989) suggested that much of what we know about the characteristics of cocaine abusers in outpatient treatment programs is based on clinical experience with what may be unrepresentative samples of whites of upper-middle socioeconomic status, a group that may differ in many ways from other samples. It needs to be emphasized that though useful both in a descriptive sense and with respect to increasing our understanding of the role of personal variables and demography in drug abuse, racial or ethnic group comparisons may be at times misleading, in large part, as Lillie-Blanton, Anthony, and Schuster noted, because of their failure to have intrinsic explanatory power. This was demonstrated by a reanalysis of data from the 1988 NHSDA, which provided evidence that, given similar social and economic conditions, crack use was not a simple function of ethnic-specific variables. The reanalysis, conducted by Lillie-Blanton, Anthony, and Schuster (1993) focused on widely disseminated findings from the NHSDA showing that the rate of use of crack cocaine was twice as high for African Americans and Hispanic Americans as for white Americans. Since the analysis did not take into account underlying community-level or macrosocial differences across racial or ethnic groups, a poststratification procedure was employed which held constant social and environmental factors that might vary from neighborhood to neighborhood. Measured by this procedure, crack use was found *not* to vary from neighborhood to neighborhood for African Americans or for Hispanic Americans when compared with white Americans. Lillie-Blanton, Anthony, and Schuster (1993) suggested that this study pointed out the need to identify neighborhood social characteristics which may be potentially modifiable determinants of drug use. The authors themselves note several limitations of this study, including the use of self-report data, the absence of persons not residing in households, the small size of the sample, and the lack of any attempt to study cultural factors that may vary within or between racial or ethnic groups.

Commenting on Lillie-Blanton, Anthony, and Schuster (1993), other writers have also raised concerns regarding the limitations of racial and ethnic data emerging from the NHSDA with respect to understanding the demographic correlates of drug abuse. Adebimpe (1993) noted the need to consider the possibility that socioeconomic and demographic factors may be potentially confounded by racial and ethnic status. Consideration of this point would help avoid misinterpretation of data such as that presented by Lillie-Blanton, Anthony, and Schuster. Adebimpe also remarked that, given the stronger association between socioeconomic status and drug abuse than between race or ethnicity and drug abuse, it was surprising that the former was not considered an integral aspect of data to be collected in many statistical reports. Directly replying to Lillie-Blanton, Anthony, and Schuster (1993), Gfroerer et al. (1993) suggested that whereas geographic areas with high concentrations of Hispanics and African Americans, as a result of having been oversampled in the NHSDA, had a greater probability of being identified as having at least one crack cocaine abuser, the bias introduced by this fact was known and controlled for by the use of appropriate weighting. When data from the entire NHSDA sample, including neighborhood and personal characteristics, were included as predictors of current drug abuse in multiple regression models, race and/or ethnicity was found not to be a significant predictor of cocaine or other drug use.

Abuse of Other Drugs

As we have seen, most cocaine users are heavy users of other drugs, including heroin, tobacco, alcohol, and marijuana. In the Khalsa, Paredes, and Anglin (1993) study of male cocaine users, use of other drugs was reported as follows: marijuana (82%); amphetamines (32%); hallucinogens (21%); barbiturates (21%); PCP (17%); methamphetamine (18%); and heroin (16%). In the Kleinman et al. (1990) study, marijuana was the first drug abused in addition to cocaine (79% had used marijuana three or more times weekly for a period of at least one month), followed by a relatively low incidence of use of other drugs: amphetamines (used by 16% three times a week or more for at least a month); hallucinogens (15% three times a week or more for at least a month); and barbiturates, other sedatives, heroin, other opiates, inhalants, quaaludes, or phencyclidine (10% three times a week or more for at least a month). Problem drinking was reported for 22% of the sample. Dougherty and Lesswing (1989) found 72% of a sample admitted for inpatient treatment to be addicted to or abusing other substances, including alcohol (37%), alcohol and marijuana (10%), marijuana alone (11%), and multiple drugs (14%). Compared to primary users of heroin or other drugs, however, primary cocaine users among admissions to a therapeutic community less frequently qualified for a diagnosis of alcohol, amphetamine, and marijuana abuse or dependence, while primary heroin abusers more frequently qualified for a diagnosis of barbiturate and amphetamine abuse or dependence, and primary users of the category "other drugs" more frequently qualified for a diagnosis of hallucinogen abuse. A diagnosis of alcohol abuse or dependence was least common among primary cocaine abusers (34.1%) than among either primary opiate (44%) or "other drug" (54%) abusers. Overall, primary cocaine abusers had a lower prevalence of other drug diagnoses as compared to primary heroin or "other drug" abusers (De Leon, 1993). At the same time, however, cocaine abuse was prominent among all categories of drug abusers. More than half of primary opiate users received a diagnosis of cocaine abuse, as well as 79% of primary "other drug" abusers. Havassy, Wasserman and Hall (1993) found that of the first 80 subjects evaluated in an ongoing study who met DSM-III-R criteria for cocaine dependence, 59% met criteria for lifetime alcohol dependence and 56% for lifetime cannabis dependence, while 38% met the criteria for dependence on both substances.

Variables Contributing to the Development of Cocaine Abuse

Social Deviance

Social deviance is highly characteristic of cocaine users, with such behavior usually preceding the onset of drug use. Khalsa, Paredes and Anglin (1993) found a high rate of social deviance among their sample of male cocaine users, with such deviance becoming more pronounced as the users reached adulthood. Common deviant behaviors included stealing and shoplifting. Twelve such behaviors occurred with high frequency before the onset of cocaine use, yet only four (carrying drugs for others, buying stolen goods, threatening with a weapon, and selling drugs) were more common after the onset of cocaine use.

Familial Predisposition

The role of familial and genetic factors in cocaine abuse has, until recently, received relatively little attention. Those studies that have been conducted imply the possibility of a relatively greater prevalence of affective and substance abuse disorders in families of cocaine abusers, thus suggesting the importance of such factors. In the study by Weiss et al. (1988), for example, there was a greater prevalence of affective disorders among family members of hospitalized cocaine abusers who had affective disorders than among family members of patients dependent on other substances. Specifically, first-degree relatives of cocaine abusers had a higher rate of affective disorders than first-degree relatives of those patients dependent on opiates and central nervous system depressants (10.0% versus 7.4%). This finding appears to have been due to higher rates of disorders among female relatives of cocaine abusers in comparison to female relatives of users of other drugs (15.4% versus 10.5%). In the study by Nunes, Quitkin, and Klein (1989), a trend toward a greater amount of familial depression in severely depressed cocaine abusers than in other patients (67% versus 11%) was noted, although these findings were based on a small number of cases.

Alcohol and cannabis dependence were found to be more prevalent in families of probands (the patient or other family member who brings the family under study) with cocaine dependence (Miller et al., 1989). Some 51% of subjects diagnosed as being cocaine-dependent had at least one first- or second-degree relative with a diagnosis of alcohol dependence; this was also the case for 51% of probands with a diagnosis of cocaine and alcohol dependence, 64% for probands with cocaine and marijuana dependence, and 52% for probands with diagnoses of cocaine, alcohol, and marijuana dependence. In all diagnostic categories, females tended to have a greater family history of alcohol dependence.

Studies which have focused on other drugs of abuse have suggested the likelihood of familial transmission. For example, Croughan (1985), after reviewing nine studies of narcotic addicts, found somewhat higher rates of alcohol and narcotic addiction among relatives of addicts than among the general population. Rounsaville, Kosten, et al. (1991) found relatives of opiate addicts seeking treatment to have high rates of alcoholism, drug misuse, depression, and antisocial personality disorder. Noting that such studies have typically focused on first-degree relatives (that is, parents, children, and full siblings), Luthar and Rounsaville (1993), focusing specifically on the children or siblings of drug abusers, studied drug use and psychopathology among cocaine-abusing opioid-addicted probands. Siblings of cocaine abusers were found to have higher than expected vulnerability to developing drug misuse, alcoholism, and antisocial personality disorder. Such vulnerability was not limited to the specific comorbid disorder manifested by the proband relative; proband siblings were vulnerable to a wide variety of disorders. Furthermore, while major depression was related to various other disorders among siblings, a comorbid major psychiatric disorder was strongly associated with substance abuse among siblings, even after possible confounding factors were taken into account. Additionally, from a temporal perspective, drug misuse was found generally to precede other comorbid disorders, including comorbid alcoholism and major depression, a finding consistent with that of an earlier study (Luthar et al., 1992).

Psychodynamic Variables

Relatively little recent literature has attempted to explain cocaine abuse from a psychodynamic viewpoint, other than that by Khantzian, an advocate of the psychoanalytic position. More, although earlier, literature exists with respect to narcotic drugs (see Platt, 1986, pp. 126–130). In one of these few early articles, Milkman and Frosch (1973) suggested that stimulant users preferentially sought drugs such as amphetamines and cocaine to assist in augmenting or bolstering characteristic modes of adaptation. Amphetamine abusers were seen as utilizing "a variety of compensatory maneuvers to maintain a posture of active confrontation with the environment" (p. 242).

In a series of articles from a psychoanalytic position, Khantzian and his associates have presented the view that certain psychological factors play a significant role in predisposing individuals to use of and dependence on drugs. While Khantzian's earlier papers focused on opiate addiction (Khantzian, 1972, 1974; Khantzian, Mack, and Schatzberg, 1974), subsequent ones focused on cocaine addiction (Khantzian and Khantzian, 1984). In general, Khantzian has proposed that the goal of drug use is not a search for euphoria so much as a drive to obtain relief from dysphoria associated with painful drives and affects. The choice of drug is thus predetermined, as it represents the personality pattern and painful affect states with which the individual is attempting to cope. Such drives may be either internal (that is, these painful emotional states) or external (that is, unmanageable realities). Cocaine's appeal to users is seen by Khantzian as lying in its energizing and euphorigenic qualities, which "help to overcome fatigue and depletion states associated with depression and dysthymia" (Khantzian and Khantzian, 1984, p. 757), a view derived from Radó (1933), as well as in the ability of cocaine and other stimulants to increase assertiveness, self-esteem, and frustration tolerance, and to relieve boredom and emptiness (Wieder and Kaplan, 1969). Self-selection of a specific drug or drugs is reflective of the drug's pharmacological properties, with a choice of a preferred drug emerging after experimentation (Khantzian, 1981; Khantzian and Khantzian, 1984). In the case of cocaine, factors affecting the choice of this drug include preexisting chronic depression or dysthymic disorder; cocaine abstinence depression; the hyperactivity/restlessness/emotional lability syndrome or attention deficit disorder; and cyclothymic or bipolar illness. Whereas Khantzian suggests that most addicts prefer a single drug to treat a specific affective disturbance, today's use of multiple substances by many complicates our understanding of the specific affective state being addressed by the individual addict.

Homelessness

Homelessness can easily become a problem for the cocaine abuser. He or she may lose his or her employment, drain family resources, experience rancor within his or her family, and ultimately leave home because of either loss of a residence for economic reasons or ejection by the family. Wallace (1990a) found homelessness to characterize 18.7% of her sample of crack cocaine addicts. Of those asked to leave the household, 51.1% became homeless. Some were shocked into entering treatment as a result, whereas others continued to use crack cocaine. Although 45.7% used shelters, 23.9% spent time on the streets, averaging one to one and a half months.

Cocaine abuse was found to be more common among homeless African Americans than among non-homeless African Americans in the general population, and to be directly related to duration of homelessness and the availability of financial resources with which to purchase drugs (Milburn and Booth, 1992). Homeless drug injectors in another study reported that cocaine and similar drugs helped them to control the overwhelming sense of fear and panic that often accompanied their feelings of despair and self-destruction (Popkin et al., 1993).

Employment

It is relatively common among cocaine abusers presenting for treatment to be employed, although this fact may be more reflective of the use of convenience samples of middle- to upper-middle-class study populations than of the actual employment rates of cocaine abusers as a whole. In the study by Means et al. (1989), 67.9% of persons admitted to treatment were employed. This figure was similar to that for other studies (again possibly reflecting a bias in selection of research samples based on convenience). For example, the percentages employed in two more recent studies were 79% (Arndt et al., 1994) and 42% (Higgins et al., 1993a). Employment rates among subjects in community-based studies are generally lower. Wallace (1990a) reported that only 13.9% of her study subjects were currently employed, while 30.4% were unemployed, 29.1% had been unemployed for over one year, and 22.2% were unemployed but had been employed within the past year. Similarly, Magura et al. (1991) reported 16% employment.[2] Marlowe et al. (1995) reported an employment rate of 10%. Khalsa, Paredes and Anglin (1993) found that almost all the males (99%) in their study of cocaine users had experienced significant periods of employment throughout their adult life. Time spent employed was stable, although the proportion of time spent working began to decrease about three years before treatment entry, as cocaine use increased. Thus, 82% of subjects had been employed 3 to 6 years before treatment, though this figure fell to 70% during the 6 months prior to treatment entry and 43% at the time of admission.

Surprisingly, loss of employment as a result of crack use, while not a rare occurrence, is less common than might be expected. Wallace (1990a) found that 29.4% of the patients in her study had experienced crack-related loss of employment. Chronic use of cocaine results in patterns of lateness, absenteeism, and falling asleep at work, leading to dismissal by employers.

The results of the study by Marlowe et al. (1995) suggest that there may be two entirely different populations of cocaine abusers. One consists of patients attending outpatient clinics or inpatient units that draw substantially on private patients, among whom drug abuse is a deviant behavior, and the other, representing inner-city populations of low socioeconomic status, among whom cocaine use is relatively commonplace, and therefore less associated with deviancy. This point of view is also supported by studies which have found African American substance abusers (primarily opiate addicts) to have less psychopathology than comparable white substance abusers (Platt et al., 1989).

Cocaine Abuse and Crime

Crime among Cocaine Abusers in Treatment

A very large percentage of crime has been found to be related to cocaine use (see Chapter 1). For those in treatment, this relationship also holds. Criminal activities of cocaine-using methadone patients are similar to those of street heroin addicts. Furthermore, among opiate addicts in methadone maintenance treatment, increased involvement in criminal activity appears to be related to increased cocaine abuse (Hunt et al., 1985–86; Hunt et al., 1984). It seems likely that it is the high cost of cocaine which leads some methadone maintenance treatment patients back into criminal activity. Strug et al. (1985) found that cocaine use among such patients was related to both property crime and drug dealing. Because of the more frequent need for cocaine than for heroin, co-caine users may commit crimes more often or involve themselves in higher-paying crimes. Hunt et al. (1985–86) suggested that when the frequency of cocaine use by patients in methadone maintenance treatment exceeded one or two times a week, the cocaine user with limited income was likely to experience increased involvement in property and drug-dealing crimes. Although increased cocaine costs may result in increased criminal activity, however, particularly among abusers with marginal income, it is usually also part of a general lifestyle of drug dealing, drug using, and other illegal activity.

Cocaine users among opioid patients in methadone maintenance treatment who demonstrated increased cocaine use over two to two and a half years of follow-up were found by Kosten, Rounsaville, and Kleber (1988) to have *fewer* legal problems than cocaine users in other types of drug abuse treatment programs. The authors attributed this finding to the seeking of illicit opioids along with cocaine by non-methadone patients, whose need for enough funds to obtain both drugs resulted in more illegal activities.

There appears to be a relationship between cocaine use and criminal activity both before and after admission to methadone maintenance treatment. Nurco et al. (1988) studied this relationship in heroin addicts and found annual numbers of days of cocaine abuse often to be associated with high crime rates across a number of categories of crime. These relationships were greater for African American addicts than for white addicts in Baltimore but not in New York. While this finding was based on small cohorts, and reflected some statistical weaknesses (as shown by a large number of significance tests and inconsistency across the two cities studied), it was concordant with earlier studies which found the number of days involved in crime to be associated with cocaine abuse in methadone maintenance treatment patients in both Baltimore and New York (Chambers, Taylor, and Moffet, 1972; Shaffer et al., 1985). In the study by Chambers, Taylor, and Moffet, cocaine use among persons in methadone maintenance treatment was found to be significantly related to continuation of criminal activity. Some 28.1% of patients in treatment who continued to use cocaine were involved in criminal activities, compared to 9.9% of "non-cheaters."

Aggressive and Violent Behavior

Aggressive behavior has been identified as being associated with cocaine intoxication (De Leon, 1993; Giannini, Miller, et al., 1993; Miller, Gold, and Mahler, 1991), although such a view is not universally accepted (Carr and Meyers, 1988). Cocaine-related violence may range from minor psychological transgressions to major physical acts, including murder and rape. Specifically, Miller, Gold, and Mahler (1991) found the following behavioral effects to be associated with addictive cocaine use: suspiciousness and/or paranoia (84%), anger (42%), violent crimes (42%), violence (32%), and increased physical strength (32%). Among the types of violent crimes associated with addictive cocaine use were verbal arguments (33%), violent arguments (25%), physical fights (23%), armed robbery (22%), robbery (14%), spouse abuse (7%), attempted murder (1%), child abuse (1%), rape (1%), and murder (<1%). Finally, the temporal relationship between last use and the commission of a violent act ranged from immediate (13%), to a few hours later (17%), to days later during acute withdrawal (19%).

In a study of cocaine freebase abusers admitted to a treatment center in the Bahamas, violent behavior before and during hospitalization was found to be concentrated among psychotic patients, with violence playing a role in over half of admissions for this group (Manschreck et al., 1988). In a study by Bunt et al. (1990), however, the presence of outwardly directed violence was found not to differ between cocaine-addicted and schizophrenic patients admitted to a psychiatric inpatient unit. In both groups violence was present for approximately 20% of the patients. When routes of cocaine administration were examined in relation to violence in an outpatient treatment sample by Giannini, Miller, et al. (1993), freebasing and/or crack smoking and use of intravenous routes of administration resulted in the highest levels of violence, and did not differ in intensity of violence. Both were associated with more violence than cocaine use by nasal inhalation. Thus, the level of increased violence was not consistently associated with a prediction of "intensity" of route of cocaine administration (freebasing/crack smoking > intravenous use > nasal insufflation), as hypothesized from intensity of toxic effects.

Crack smoking appears to have a higher likelihood of associated violence than use of other forms of cocaine. When crack smokers presenting at a hospital emergency room in New York City were compared with freebase smokers, intravenous users, and intranasal users, significantly more thoughts and acts of violence were found in the crack group. Interestingly, the presence or absence of psychosis did not relate to the presence of violence or violent ideation. Giannini, Miller, et al. (1993) found use of crack (and freebase) cocaine to be associated with more violence than use of cocaine by nasal inhalation. Intravenous cocaine use, however, was associated with the same amount of violence as crack and/or freebase use. Possible reasons advanced by Honer, Gewirtz, and Turey (1987) for this finding included the faster rise in plasma cocaine concentration associated with crack use, as well as a higher total dose or frequency of crack use, although differences in socioeconomic background of crack users, as well as personality characteristics and expectations of intoxication on the part of those preferring crack, may also account for these findings.

While illicit drugs have been implicated in violence in general, and homicide in particular (Molotsky, 1988; Wolff, 1988), cocaine (Harruff et al., 1988) and crack cocaine (Krajicek, 1988; Tardiff et al., 1994) have been singled out as being associated with a particularly high rate of homicide. Goldstein et al. (1989) identified 26% of homicides which took place in New York City in 1988 as crack-related. Territorial disputes between rival dealers seem to have been most common. Goldstein and associates attributed this high level of violence to the emergent popularity of crack combined with an unstable distribution system and resultant rivalries for control of high profits.

Another stimulant, amphetamine, has been shown to have a biphasic relationship to violence, with an increase in aggressive behavior at low doses and no increase or a slightly lower frequency or intensity at high doses, although this relationship has yet to be established for cocaine (Cherek et al., 1986). Licata et al. (1993) noted that three models explaining the relationship between cocaine and violence exist in the literature: the *psychopharmacological model,* which views aggression as a direct consequence of cocaine ingestion; the *systemic model,* which emphasizes the traditionally violent interactions resulting from the manufacture and distribution of an expensive and illicit commodity; and the *economic-compulsive model,* which views violence as instrumental behavior in support of habitual drug use. The results of one laboratory investigation appear to provide support for the pharmacological interpretation, and suggest that a single dose of cocaine may *directly* result in an increase in aggression, rather than indirectly affecting aggression through increasing toxic paranoia. This study of 30 undergraduates receiving either a placebo, low-dose cocaine (1 mg/kg), or high-dose cocaine (2 mg/kg) found that aggression, as defined by the intensity of electric shocks administered to an increasingly aggressive fictitious opponent during a competitive reaction-time task, was greatest in the high-dose cocaine condition, regardless of level of provocation (Licata et al., 1993).

Usefulness of Self-Reports of Cocaine Abuse

Self-reports of drug use, many of which are used here, are an important, if not essential, element in evaluating treatment outcomes for both clinical and research purposes. There are a number of reasons for this usefulness, including economy and ease of obtaining data, compared to blood and urine sampling; provision of information for periods when other sources of information are not available, as when the patient is not in contact with the clinician or researcher; capturing of information not otherwise available, such as frequency and patterns of use; and efficiency in covering extended periods of time. Yet, self-reports may be inaccurate owing to the subject's inability to remember the relevant details, or because of deliberate distortion resulting from the demand characteristics of the situation (Ehrman and Robbins, 1994).

As is the case with other drugs of abuse, the rates indicated by admission of use of cocaine may underestimate actual use. Substantial underreporting of cocaine and marijuana use was confirmed by Fendrich and Vaughn (1994) in the National Longitudinal Survey of Youth. Underreporting was particularly evident among those interviewed by telephone, minority respondents, and those with low levels of education. Similarly (and also in concert with other drugs of abuse), the numbers admitting to cocaine use are often smaller than findings of cocaine metabolites by other means. McNagny and Parker (1992) found that 39% of 415 patients entering an inner-city walk-in clinic who were enrolled in a study on sexually transmitted diseases, and whose urine was tested for cocaine without their explicit consent, had cocaine metabolites in their urine. Only 45.6% of those with cocaine-positive urine (18% of the entire sample) admitted to cocaine use within one week prior to clinic entry. This report has been criticized on several bases, one of the most significant being that respondents were not informed that their urine specimens were being screened for drug use (Watters et al., 1992). Thus, these findings may not generalize to studies in which investigators are explicit about their interest in drug-using behavior. Watters et al. presented data indicating that drug users explicitly informed of the purpose of the study (that is, an interest in their drug-using and related behaviors) would be more accurate in reporting their drug use. Their study showed an 86.3% agreement between self-report and urinalysis results for cocaine, and 84.9% for heroin.

Reports of drug use have been obtained from relatives and significant others as well as from abusers themselves, although Rounsaville, Wilber, et al. (1981) and Carroll et al. (1993), among others, have questioned the likelihood of obtaining accurate assessments of drug use from this source, since such estimates often underreport actual use. In one study of opiate addicts, good agreement was found between addicts and informants with respect to estimates of current opiate use, employment, and legal pressures, but not with respect to severity of the addict's social, employment, and psychological problems, and in the more detailed aspects of drug use (Rounsaville, Kleber, et al., 1981).

Self-reported cocaine use in methadone maintenance patients has been found to be more accurate than self-reported opiate use (Magura et al., 1987). This differential was attributed to the more severe penalties for opiate use than for use of other drugs, since opiate use contradicts the raison d'être of such programs. Thus, the imposition of sanctions for such use, including discharge from the program, being more immediate and severe inhibits respondents from complete honesty.

The Time-Line (TL) system, developed for use in alcohol studies (O'Farrell and Langenbucher, 1987; Sobell et al., 1979), and which requires the subject to keep a daily diary of substance use, was found to be both valid and reliable for measuring use of cocaine and heroin by patients in methadone maintenance treatment (Ehrman and Robbins, 1994).

Conclusions

More men than women use cocaine, but levels of dependence are equal for both genders. Generally, a male-to-female ratio for cocaine use of from 3:2 to 3:1 has been found, with women being more likely than men to have poor premorbid histories (Griffin et al., 1989; Jones, Lewis, and Shorty, 1993; Kosten et al., 1993).

Cocaine use generally starts in the early twenties (Khalsa, Anglin, et al., 1993; Kleinman et al., 1990), following initial illicit drug use in the late teen years (Kang et al., 1991; Khalsa, Anglin, et al., 1993). Cocaine is a highly addictive drug among young people, with crack dependence present at a high level by the age of 24 (Lillie-Blanton, Anthony, and Schuster, 1993).

Treatment entry for the majority of cocaine abusers typically occurs in the late twenties (Dougherty and Lesswing, 1989; Ziedonis et al., 1994). Cocaine is usually not the first drug of abuse for most cocaine users; among injection drug users, cocaine abuse starts later and dependence occurs later than for opiates. Age at treatment entry may be significantly higher in specialized samples, such as those seeking treatment in Veterans Administration settings (Khalsa, Anglin, et al., 1993).

Racial and ethnic differences among cocaine abusers may be less relevant than sociocultural differences in understanding cocaine abuse. Given similar social and economic conditions, rates of cocaine abuse are more dependent on environmental variables (Lillie-Blanton, Anthony, and Schuster, 1993) than on racial and/or ethnic variables.

Cocaine abusers are heavy users of other drugs. High rates of marijuana, heroin, and alcohol use are present in almost all samples which have been studied (Khalsa, Anglin, et al., 1993; Kleinman et al., 1990).

Many factors appear to contribute to cocaine abuse, although their respective roles have not yet been delineated. Among these are social deviance (for example, stealing, shoplifting, weapons offenses, and so on) and familial histories of affective disorder (Khalsa, Anglin, et al., 1993; Miller et al., 1989; Weiss et al., 1988).

Correlates of cocaine abuse include homelessness and criminal activity (Hunt et al., 1985–86; Strug et al., 1985; Wallace, 1990a). High rates of employment have been reported in many studies (Arndt et al., 1994; Higgins et al., 1993a; Means et al., 1989), but this is likely an artifact of convenience samples studied in inpatient environments, where many patients are likely to have insurance coverage, or of the demographics of the location where the study was conducted. Other community-based studies have found that cocaine abusers tend to be poor, isolated, and devoid of resources (Marlowe et al., 1995). Homelessness is common among crack cocaine addicts, and is not infrequently a consequence of crack abuse (Wallace, 1990a).

Criminal behavior is common in the cocaine-abusing population. This behavior resembles that of heroin addicts, and appears to be related to level of involvement in cocaine abuse (Hunt et al., 1984, 1985–86). Because of the more frequent need for cocaine compared with heroin, cocaine users may commit crimes more often than heroin users or involve themselves in higher-paying crimes (Hunt et al., 1985–86).

Violent behavior, including homicide, appears to be closely associated with cocaine abuse (De Leon, 1993; Giannini, Miller, et al., 1993; Miller, Gold, and Mahler, 1991), particularly with crack smoking (Honer, Gewirtz, and Turley, 1987), although such a view is not universally accepted (Carr and Meyers, 1988). Violence may be present, especially when the cocaine abuser is also psychotic (Manschreck et al., 1988).

III

Psychopathological and Medical Aspects

5

Cocaine Abuse, Psychopathology, and Personality Disorders

Psychopathology

Substance abusers in general, whether in treatment or in the community, have been shown to have higher rates of psychiatric symptomatology and psychopathology than those who are not drug abusers. Until recently, such findings have been developed primarily on alcohol-, heroin-, or polydrug-abusing or addicted populations, and only the most recent studies report findings with primarily cocaine-addicted populations.[1] In one of the earliest of this group of studies, Helfrich et al. (1983) found 99% of 136 cocaine-abusing patients seeking treatment to be psychologically impaired. Some 85% presented with symptoms in 4 or more of 8 symptom groups, with a mean of 5 symptom clusters, and 43% showed major psychological symptoms. They concluded that this sample "exhibited significant and serious psychological distress" (p. 347).

Other studies have reported similar findings, although at lower levels. For example, Halikas et al. (1994), employing the Diagnostic Interview Scale (DIS), found 62% of 207 cocaine abusers seeking outpatient treatment to meet diagnostic criteria for a current psychiatric disorder, while 73% met lifetime criteria for a psychiatric disorder other than substance abuse. Most common were antisocial personality (40%), anxiety (37%), and affective (28%) disorders. Rates of both current and lifetime disorders were higher for women than for men, and anxiety, though not affective disorders, was found to precede regular cocaine use. According to one study (Gold, Washton, and Dackis, 1985) of callers to the National Cocaine Hotline, at least 65% reported symptoms such as depression (83%), anxiety (83%), irritability (87%), sleep problems

(82%), chronic fatigue (76%), apathy and laziness (66%), paranoia (65%), and difficulty concentrating (65%), and at least half reported symptoms such as panic attacks (50%), lack of sexual interest (53%), memory problems (57%), and severe headaches (60%). Although a number of these symptoms may result from cocaine use, other studies suggest that many of these complaints may be present as premorbid characteristics of cocaine users (for example, Chitwood and Morningstar, 1985; Rounsaville, Anton, et al., 1991).

Chitwood and Morningstar (1985) compared treatment-seeking ($N =$ 95) and community ($N = 75$) samples of cocaine abusers and found a higher level of long-term depression in the treatment-seeking group (34%) than in the community sample (11%), as well as higher levels of adverse consequences (that is, job loss, marital breakups, and cocaine overdose) attributed to drug use. Griffin et al. (1989) examined 129 consecutive admissions to a private psychiatric hospital who were diagnosed with cocaine abuse and found the following rates of DSM-III disorders: bipolar/cyclothymic disorders (males, 18.9%; females, 17.7%), major depression (males, 4.2%; females, 23.5%), other Axis I disorders (males, 16.9%; females, 5.9%), and antisocial personality disorder (males, 22.1%; females, 0%). Thus, substantial depressive symptomatology was present in both sexes, although women showed a higher incidence of major depression. Only males received an Axis II diagnosis of antisocial personality disorder. Nearly half of the sample received another Axis I diagnosis in addition to that of substance abuse.

In a group of 298 cocaine abusers seeking inpatient ($N = 149$) or outpatient ($N = 149$) treatment, Rounsaville, Anton, et al. (1991) found current rates for the presence of any psychiatric disorder, in addition to substance abuse, to be 55.7%, while the lifetime prevalence rate was 73.5%. The major categories into which these diagnoses fell, for current and lifetime diagnoses, respectively, were: major depression (4.7% and 30.5%); any affective disorder (44.3% and 60.7%); any anxiety disorder (15.8% and 20.8%); attention deficit disorder (0% and 34.9%); alcoholism (28.9% and 61.7%); any disorder with a hypomanic element (19.9% and 11.1%); and personality disorders (7.7% and 7.7%). When the restrictive Research Diagnostic Criteria for antisocial personality disorder were replaced by those in DSM-III-R, the rate of adult antisocial personality disorder was 32.9%. Significant differences were found to exist between male and females only in the prevalence of phobia (males lower), alcoholism (males higher), and attention deficit disorder (males higher). Psychiatrically impaired cocaine abusers tended to present with more than one type of psychiatric disorder. When the sample was scored for depressive, manic, schizophrenic, and personality disorders, Research Diagnostic Disorder criteria were met for zero categories of disorders by 26.5%, one category of disorder by 30.2%, two categories of disorders by 20.5%, and three or more categories of disorders by 22.8%. In general, rates of disorders present among cocaine abusers seeking treatment were higher than for either in-treatment or community samples.

These findings indicate that cocaine abusers seeking treatment show generally high rates of psychological distress and psychopathology.[2] This should not be totally surprising, since personal distress is a major factor in motivating substance abusers to seek treatment (Oppenheimer, Sheehan, and Taylor, 1988; Rosenbaum, 1982; Smith et al. 1992). Nonetheless, the presence of a high level of psychopathology is not by itself the only variable involved in motivating addicts to seek treatment. When treatment-seeking cocaine addicts were compared with a community sample of untreated cocaine addicts, both samples were found to be similar with respect to severity and chronicity of cocaine use, the employment of self-control strategies to cope with such use, and the overall rates of current and lifetime psychopathology (Carroll and Rounsaville, 1992). The untreated addicts actually reported more concurrent drug and alcohol use, as well as fewer negative consequences of such use, less subjective distress, lower rates of participation in adult social roles, more adequate current social functioning, greater past legal involvement and current involvement in illegal activities, and lower rates of attention deficit disorder and current major depression. On the basis of these findings, a number of which were contrary to expectation, the authors suggested that the treatment seekers may have had amplified perceptions of the negative consequences of cocaine use, and thus felt more pressure to enter treatment. Treatment seeking was found in this study not to be influenced by either lack of control over drug use (for example, a greater frequency of binges and an inability to sustain brief periods of abstinence), the employment of self-control strategies, or higher rates of psychiatric disorders.

Finally, racial, ethnic, and gender differences may exist with respect to the presence of psychiatric comorbidity in cocaine abusers, paralleling findings with opiate abusers (Platt et al., 1989; Steer et al., 1989). In a study of psychiatric comorbidity in African American and white cocaine addicts, Ziedonis and associates (1994) found 55.7% to meet Research Diagnostic Criteria for lifetime psychiatric diagnoses. While African Americans and whites did not differ in overall psychiatric comorbidity, whites had significantly higher rates of DSM-III-R lifetime major depression (45% versus 30%); both Research Diagnostic Criteria

(RDC) and DSM-III-R alcohol dependence (RDC, 86% versus 55%; DSM-III-R, 79% versus 38%); DSM-III-R attention deficit disorder (39% versus 27%); and RDC conduct disorder (53% versus 35%). African Americans, by contrast, were more likely to meet the criteria for a current RDC phobic disorder (17% versus 9%). Whites also had a significantly higher rate of suicidal gestures or attempts (27% versus 13%). When males and females were compared, women had a significantly higher rate of RDC current phobia (21% versus 10%), a lower rate of RDC current alcohol dependence (23% versus 36%), and a higher rate of DSM-III-R childhood attention deficit disorder (25% versus 39%). Male African Americans demonstrated a trend toward a lower rate of RDC major depression (20% versus 36%), as well as a significantly higher RDC lifetime rate of alcohol dependence (70% versus 31%).

Not all studies, however, have found high rates of psychopathology among cocaine abusers. Newcomb, Bentler, and Fahy (1987), in a longitudinal study of 739 young adults aged 19 to 24 years, found only modest correlations between level of psychopathology and level of cocaine use in a sample of "relatively normal young adults" (p. 1183). Positive associations were found for males between cocaine use and low energy and interest, anxious mood, impaired cognitive functions, hostility, sleep disturbance, negative affect, impaired motivation, a lack of purpose in life, and psychotic proneness. For women, frequent cocaine use was associated with low energy and interest, depressed mood, appetite disturbance, anxious mood, impaired cognitive functions, somatic symptoms, hostility, and psychotic proneness. No significant differences emerged between pairs of correlations for males and females. When level of cocaine use by category of psychopathology was examined, no significant differences emerged regarding frequency of use or abuse. More males with an anxiety disorder reported cocaine use (versus males with no disorder), while females with a phobia disorder were significantly less likely to have used cocaine compared with the no diagnosis group. On the basis of these findings, Newcomb, Bentler, and Fahy concluded that "the severe negative psychopathological consequences associated with cocaine use reported in the literature may be the result of highly selected samples" (p. 1182). These authors also noted, however, that it may have been too early to observe such consequences, as a period of four years of cocaine use generally precedes the emergence of severe negative consequences (Clayton, 1985).

On the basis of deviance theory, Schottenfeld, Carroll, and Rounsaville (1993) have suggested that when use of a specific drug is considered particularly deviant in the population, users of the drug are deviant in other respects, and thus high rates of psychopathology can be expected among its users. (This is the "drug-specificity hypothesis of psychopathology.") It follows that a finding of less psychopathology in cocaine abusers should be expected, since the use of this drug is more widespread in the general population than, for instance, opioid abuse. But the pharmacologic properties of cocaine would lead one to expect high rates of psychopathology among cocaine abusers. According to these authors, Schottenfeld, Carroll, and Rounsaville, the latter would be consistent with Gawin and Ellinwood's (1988) finding that prolonged use of stimulants, including amphetamine or cocaine, can result in paranoid states, prolonged anhedonia, and affective disturbances. Additionally, these authors point out that the use of cocaine to self-medicate underlying psychiatric disorders (see, for example, Khantzian and Khantzian, 1984) would also predict greater psychopathology among cocaine abusers. As noted earlier, Khantzian and Khantzian suggested that cocaine was used for a number of self-medicating purposes: to alleviate fatigue, depletion, depression, boredom, or emptiness; to increase assertiveness, self-esteem, and/or frustration tolerance; or to bolster a hyperactive lifestyle and an exaggerated need for self-sufficiency. Schottenfeld and colleagues observed, however, that one reason for high rates of psychopathology in treatment-seeking cocaine abusers might be that cocaine abusers with comorbid psychopathology are more likely to seek treatment than those without psychopathology, leading to an increased prevalence of psychopathology in treatment seekers. This, however, was shown not to be the case in a study by Carroll and Rounsaville (1992), in which untreated cocaine abusers and treatment-seeking cocaine abusers were found to have comparable rates of current and lifetime psychiatric disorders.

Clinical (AXIS I) Disorders

Affective Disorders and Depression

An overrepresentation of affective disorders among cocaine abusers has been found in a number of studies (for example, Gawin and Kleber, 1986a; Kosten, Rounsaville, and Kleber, 1988; Rounsaville, Anton, et al., 1991), although this has not been a universal finding (Bunt et al., 1990). Gawin and Kleber (1986a) found that 54% of their sample of chronic cocaine abusers had a DSM-III Axis I disorder in addition to a cocaine abuse disorder. Depressive disorders were present in 33% of the sample, with the most common being dysthymic disorder (20%) and major depression with melancholia (13%). Cyclothymic disorder was present in 17% of the sample. These findings are similar to those obtained by Weiss et al. (1986), who compared a sample of 30 cocaine abusers hospitalized in 1980–1982 with groups of 91 opioid users and 33 central nervous system depressant users, and found that 53.3% of the cocaine users met DSM-III criteria for the presence of an affective disorder, in contrast with 21.8% of opiate and central nervous system depressant users. Among the cocaine users, unipolar depression was present in 30% of the entire sample, while bipolar and cyclothymic disorders accounted for 23%. In another study, 63% of a sample of 30 outpatient cocaine abusers met DSM-III-R lifetime criteria for an affective disorder, with onset preceding substance dependency. Of the overall sample, 30% met criteria for bipolar spectrum disorders, and 33% met criteria for unipolar depression (Nunes, Quitkin, and Klein, 1989).

In a follow-up to their earlier study, Weiss et al. (1988) examined another group of 149 hospitalized cocaine abusers in 1982–1986, comparing them with 230 opioid addicts and 63 patients dependent on central nervous system depressants. This study found a slightly larger number of affective disorders in the cocaine abusers compared with the other patients (26.8% versus 20.1%), although cyclothymic disorders were present at a significantly higher rate (11.4% versus 2.7%) in the cocaine abuser group. Between the first and second studies, however, the rate of affective disorders among the cocaine abusers declined from 50.0% to 21.0%. This trend was most evident in males, in whom the rate of affective illness declined from 14.3% to 2.3%, while no equivalent changes occurred in either the opioid or central nervous system depressant abuser groups. Weiss et al. (1988) concluded that, between the two periods of data collection, and with the more widespread abuse of cocaine, concurrent affective disorder had become a much less important risk factor for the development of cocaine abuse.

In the study by Kleinman et al. (1990), 28% of subjects were found to have a current depressive syndrome, while 12% had had a major depressive episode at some time during their life. An additional 6% had a dysthymic diagnosis at the time of their interview, while another 1% had a depressive illness not otherwise specified. Thus, 47% of cocaine abusers in this study had an Axis I depressive disorder, and 70% had a dual diagnosis (that is, substance abuse and one other Axis I disorder). The presence of a depressive disorder was associated with a greater likelihood of having used crack or freebase, as opposed to intranasal use, in the previous thirty days. Furthermore, as years of cocaine use increased, the likelihood of having a depressive disorder also increased.

The presence of an Axis I disorder was also associated with having started to use tobacco, marijuana, and cocaine at an early age.

Anthony and Trinkoff (1989), reporting on the findings of the epidemiologic catchment area (ECA) study,[3] noted the presence of a lifetime history of major depression in 14% of males with a diagnosis of drug abuse or dependence, compared with 4% among those without such diagnoses. Similarly, lifetime antisocial personality disorder was present in 38% of males with a drug abuse diagnosis compared to 10% of males without such a diagnosis. Specifically with respect to cocaine use, frequency of use was related to the presence of high levels of depression. Among men aged 18 to 44 years who had used cocaine five times or less, a lifetime diagnosis of major depression was present in 7.6% of cases; among men who had used cocaine more than five times (but not daily), the prevalence of a lifetime diagnosis of major depression was 11.0%; among men with a history of cocaine use for two weeks or more (but who did not meet DSM-III criteria for cocaine abuse), this figure was 14.6%; and among men with a history of cocaine abuse, it was 25.8%. Thus, for men, a lifetime diagnosis of major depression was most prevalent among the heaviest users of cocaine. Similar patterns of association were found with respect to relationships between cocaine use and a current or lifetime diagnosis of panic disorder. For example, among men who had used cocaine five times or less, this prevalence was 1.7%; for those who had used cocaine five times or more (but not daily), it was 2.4%; for men who had used cocaine daily for two weeks or more, 2.3%; and for men who had a history of cocaine abuse, 15.3%.

Cocaine abusers have been found to have high rates of clinical depression. For example, Gawin and Kleber (1986a) found 33% of their sample to have had a diagnosable DSM-III depressive disorder; while Rounsaville, Anton, et al. (1991) found that 44.3% of their subjects met Research Diagnostic Criteria for some current mood disorder. In the latter study, 60.7% met Research Diagnostic Criteria for a lifetime mood disorder, with 30.7% having had at least one episode of major depression, although many of these disorders were of a chronic minor nature (for example, intermittent depressive personality or intermittent hyperthymic personality). By contrast, Marlowe et al. (1995), using the Structural Clinical Interview for the DSM-III-R (SCID) with a sample of 100 consecutive admissions to an outpatient stimulant abuse treatment clinic attended primarily by minority patients (91% African American, 8% white, 1% Hispanic), found affective and anxiety disorders present in only 10% of the cases they examined, a level not very different from that which would be expected in nonpsychiatric settings, particularly in the inner-city, low socioeconomic status population they studied. While 91% of the sample received at least one lifetime DSM-III-R diagnosis in addition to a diagnosis of cocaine abuse or dependence, affective disorders were relatively uncommon (major depression or dysthymia, current, 8%; lifetime, 10%). Similarly, anxiety disorders were also relatively uncommon (current, 8%; lifetime, 8%). Most patients (73%) received Axis II diagnoses, with over one-third receiving more than one personality disorder diagnosis. Cluster B disorders ("dramatic/emotional") were the most common, present in 53% of the sample, with antisocial (23%), borderline (23%), paranoid (21%), and narcissistic (17%) personality being the most common of these. These findings suggest that contemporary urban cocaine abusers may be quite different from earlier samples of cocaine abusers, which were drawn from university-based and inpatient treatment settings. The characteristics of this sample are likely reflective of an inner-city, lower socioeconomic status population, in which substance abuse is relatively commonplace and therefore less strongly associated with deviance. Furthermore, the common features among this sample (that is, affective lability, cognitive rigidity, restricted problem solving, impaired perspective taking, impulsiveness, and paranoid ideation), may be amenable to appropriate intervention involving focused collateral programs (Marlowe et al., 1995).

Finally, while the presence of depression is generally associated with poor treatment outcomes in non–cocaine-abusing opioid addicts in methadone maintenance treatment (Rounsaville et al., 1986; Ziedonis and Kosten, 1991), the presence of depression may serve as a predictor of both positive and negative outcome in pharmacotherapy for cocaine abusers. In a study of cocaine-abusing methadone patients, Ziedonis and Kosten found depression to predict poor treatment outcome with relapse prevention therapy alone, and to predict a good outcome in the case of treatment with medication (amantadine or desipramine).

DO AFFECTIVE DISORDERS PRECIPITATE COCAINE USE?

Depressive symptoms may be an important trigger of cocaine use as well as a consequence of such use. Kosten, Rounsaville, and Kleber (1987) found heroin addicts who were depressed at treatment entry were more likely still to be using cocaine two and a half years later. Furthermore, the presence of depressive symptoms at admission is a significant predictor of continued cocaine use during treatment (Magura et al., 1991). Some 50% of the cocaine-using patients in methadone maintenance treatment in the Magura et al. study reported that their cocaine use increased when they felt "down" or depressed. Not surprisingly, cocaine use does not alleviate depressive symptomatology. In the same study, 82% of the patients also reported that "after using coke, I feel lower than ever" (p. 43). Another study found that anxiety disorders (with the exception of generalized anxiety disorder), antisocial personality disorder, and history of childhood attention deficit disorder preceded initiation of cocaine abuse, while the onset of affective disorders and alcoholism followed the onset of cocaine abuse (Rounsaville, Anton, et al., 1991). Halikas et al. (1994) found that the onset of psychiatric disorders generally preceded the onset of cocaine (or other substance) abuse, with this finding being most pronounced for anxiety disorders, in that anxiety disorders preceded the onset of cocaine abuse for 92.1% of patients, and preceded any substance abuse disorder for 76.6% of subjects. Affective disorders, by contrast, were more likely to follow regular drug use (64.9% of subjects), but to precede a diagnosis of cocaine abuse (92.1%).

AFFECTIVE DISORDER FOLLOWING COCAINE USE

Depression may be a consequence of cocaine use, being most intense during the period immediately following a period of cocaine use. In this regard, Gawin and Kleber (1986a) found that cocaine abusers exhibited a uniform transient major depressive–like symptomatology for a clearly defined period of time (approximately 48 hours). Following this, and assuming continued abstinence, an anhedonic dysphoric state appeared in almost all severe users. In some users a superimposed Axis I–like psychiatric syndrome appeared. Thus, according to Gawin and Kleber, the diagnosis of a major depressive or bipolar disorder requires deferment until the "crash" and its symptoms have passed, or until corroborating evidence is available.

Thus, it is not clear whether depressive symptomatology is a consequence of cocaine use, precipitated by withdrawal of the drug, as suggested by Gawin and Kleber (1986b), or whether, alternatively, cocaine is used to alleviate the symptoms of a premorbid disorder, in particular depression and other affective disorders (Gawin and Kleber, 1986a; Khantzian, 1985; Magura et al., 1991) or to enhance or prolong the elevated mood states which are symptomatic of their cyclical mood disorders (Gawin and Ellinwood, 1988; Rounsaville, Anton, et al., 1991). Likely both explanations are valid.

Attention Deficit Hyperactivity Disorder (ADHD)

Noting earlier work (for example, Khantzian, 1975, 1979; Wurmser, 1974) which had identified the presence of depression, anergia, boredom, low self-esteem, and hyperactive lifestyle in cocaine and stimulant addiction, Khantzian et al. (1984) observed that these features and qualities were also associated with adult forms of attention deficit disorders (see, for example, Huessy et al., 1979; Wender, 1979). More recently, findings from a number of studies have suggested that children with attention deficit hyperactivity disorder may be at increased risk for developing substance abuse disorders (Eyre, Rounsaville, and Kleber, 1982; Horton et al., 1987). Rates of childhood attention deficit disorder found in adult cocaine abusers diagnosed with residual attention deficit disorder can range as high as 34.9% (Rounsaville, Anton, et al., 1991). Self-medication for the symptoms of ADHD may play a role in cocaine use for some individuals with the disorder. In this regard, Weiss et al. (1988) found that those patients in their study who had a diagnosis of ADHD reported temporary improvement of their inattentiveness and impulsiveness during their early use of cocaine.

In the study by Rounsaville, Anton, et al. (1991), more than one-third of the sample had diagnoses of attention deficit disorder either in childhood or persisting into adulthood. This rate, although possibly accounted for by the use of less restrictive diagnostic criteria than were employed previously, is substantially higher than that obtained in previous studies (for example, Gawin and Kleber, 1986a, 1/30 subjects; Weiss et al., 1986, 1/30; Weiss et al., 1988, 7/147). Rounsaville, Anton, et al. (1991) suggested that the cocaine users in their study may have been self-medicating their attention deficit disorder with cocaine.

Carroll and Rounsaville (1993) found that 35% of 298 cocaine abusers seeking treatment met DSM-III-R criteria for childhood attention deficit hyperactivity disorder. The majority were males (78%), met the Research Diagnostic Criteria for conduct disorder (93%) and antisocial personality disorder (47%), and had a history of conduct disorder in first-degree relatives (parents and siblings). When compared with those cocaine abusers without ADHD, cocaine abusers with ADHD tended to be younger and reported more severe substance abuse, earlier onset of cocaine abuse, more frequent and intense cocaine use, preference for intranasal rather than freebase or intravenous use of cocaine, higher rates of alcoholism, and more previous treatment. The authors concluded that there may be more cocaine abusers with a history of ADHD than previously thought; that these persons may differ in significant ways from those without ADHD; and that the poorer outcomes for patients with ADHD emphasizes the need for identification and treatment of residual symptoms of ADHD in cocaine abusers.

Personality (AXIS II) Disorders

Personality disorders have been found to be common among drug abusers in general (see, for example, Nace, Davis, and Gaspari, 1991), opiate abusers (see Platt, 1986, 1995a, for reviews), and alcohol abusers (Hesselbrock, Meyer, and Keener, 1985; Powell et al., 1982; Ross, Glaser, and Germanson, 1988) in particular. This finding has also been confirmed for cocaine abusers, with the common finding in this population of an Axis II diagnosis of borderline or narcissistic personality disorder (Dougherty and Lesswing, 1989; Resnick and Resnick, 1984; Weiss et al., 1986; Yates et al., 1989).

In the Kleinman et al. (1990) study, 58% of subjects were found to have at least one DSM-III-R Axis II disorder, and 40% were found to have two or more such disorders. No particular Axis II disorder predominated, with antisocial (21%), passive-aggressive (21%), borderline (18%), and self-defeating (18%) personality all being represented approximately equally. The authors suggested that these differences in prevalence of antisocial personality disorder may reflect differences in socioeconomic status of the various study samples. Rates of 73% (Marlowe et al., 1995), 74% (Weiss et al., 1993), and 90% (Weiss et al., 1986) have been reported in various studies of cocaine abusers for the presence of at least one Axis II disorder. Weiss and Mirin (1986) found that 90% of the cocaine abusers in their study had a DSM-III Axis II diagnosis, with narcissistic and borderline personality disorder most common. Antisoscial personality disorder was present in only one case. In the Weiss et al. (1986) study, antisocial, borderline, histrionic, and paranoid personality disorders were most common, with all diagnoses being represented except for schizoid personality disorder. In the Marlowe et al. (1995) study, the most commonly diagnosed Axis II disorders were in the DSM-III-R Cluster B (dramatic/emotional) disorder group, with antisocial, borderline, paranoid, and narcissistic personality disorder diagnosed most often. About one-third of cocaine abusers received more than one personality disorder diagnosis, and 60.8% of those diagnosed with antisocial personality disorder also received diagnoses of paranoid or narcissistic personality disorder. This overlap was seen by Marlowe et al. (1995) as reflecting consistent features across much of the sample which may be amenable to collateral interventions (for example, affective lability, cognitive rigidity, restricted problem-solving repertoire, impaired perspective-taking ability, impulsivity, and paranoid ideation).

In particular, as noted by Weiss et al. (1986), it may be difficult to distinguish between personality traits and drug-related behaviors. Thus, the question whether diagnoses of personality disorders remain stable across periods of both abstinence and drug abuse needed to be addressed. This was attempted by Weiss et al. (1993) in a sample of predominantly white hospitalized cocaine abusers. These investigators found a high prevalence rate of Axis II disorders in this group (74% meet diagnostic criteria for at least one Axis II disorder). Furthermore, such personality disorders appeared to be relatively stable, being present during periods of both abstinence and drug use (76% of the patients who received at least one Axis II diagnosis also met criteria for a personality disorder both while abusing substances and when drug-free). Overall, 69% of Axis II diagnoses were present both when drugs were abused and when patients were drug-free.

This study suffers from a number of methodological problems. These include a highly selective sample of cocaine abusers (for example, predominantly white [88%] and employed [70%]); the tendency of the instrument used in this study, the Structured Clinical Interview for DSM-III-R (SCID-II), to overdiagnose personality disorder; the problem of validity of self-report of drug-dependent patients, particularly when being questioned about past psychiatric symptomatology; and the fact that some may not have had sufficiently long drug-free periods in the recent past to recall the experience of being drug-free. It should be noted, however, that this study did not confirm the notion that addiction may itself play a causative role in the development of personality disorders, as has been suggested in the case of alcoholism by Bean-Bayog (1986). Weiss et al. (1993) noted that personality disorders may play a more prominent role in the development of addiction in drug abusers than in alcoholics, as had been suggested by Vaillant (1985).

The presence of drug dependence does not uniformly affect all aspects of an individual's functioning. Weiss et al. (1993) found that recovery in some areas of functioning may occur independently of recovery in other areas. McLellan and associates (1981) obtained similar findings, for both alcoholics and opiate addicts, in that both before and after treatment there was little relationship between severity of the substance abuse problem and severity of problems in other areas of functioning. One exception to this general rule was that improvement in psychological functioning was clearly related to improvement in most other areas, including substance abuse. McLellan et al. suggested that this finding indicated the importance of psychologically oriented therapy in substance abuse treatment.

In the study by Rounsaville, Anton, et al. (1991), cocaine abusers had substantially lower rates of antisocial personality disorder than opiate abusers (7.7% versus 26.5%; 32.9% versus 54.1% without the adult drug abuse exclusion). This finding was explained in terms of cocaine's attractiveness to a wider and less criminally involved cross-section of the general population. Although the distinction between antisocial and non-antisocial personality may not be sufficiently sensitive for certain clinical and research purposes (Cacciola et al., 1994), the presence of antisocial personality disorder still has been found to be a significant prognostic factor in medication outcome studies. Leal, Ziedonis, and Kosten (1994) found antisocial personality disorder to be associated with poorer rates of treatment retention, a response to desipramine, and continued cocaine use. Similarly, in the studies by Rounsaville and Kleber (1984) and Woody et al. (1985), opiate addicts with antisocial personality disorder did worse at follow-up after discharge than did opiate addicts with other diagnoses. The presence of depression, however, did result in a more favorable outcome.

Finally, it should be mentioned that cocaine abusers have been found to have a high rate of diagnosed pathological gambling disorders. Steinberg, Kosten, and Rounsaville (1992) found a 15% rate of pathological gambling in a sample of 298 treatment-seeking cocaine abusers, a figure 10 times the rate found in community samples. Cocaine addicts diagnosed with pathological gambling also had higher rates of attention deficit disorder, alcoholism, and polydrug abuse, as well as more legal problems and higher levels of sensation-seeking behavior.

Psychopathology in Cocaine Abusers versus Abusers of Other Drugs

Alcoholics

It is not clear whether abusers of multiple drugs present more overall psychopathology than abusers of cocaine alone. Weiss et al. (1988) found 37.6% of cocaine abusers in their study to have another Axis I diagnosis present in addition to substance abuse, compared with 38.2% of a group of opioid and depressant users. Similarly, affective disorders were found not to be substantially more prevalent among cocaine users (26.8% of cocaine abusers also had an affective disorder, compared with 20.1% of opioid and depressant abusers).

In general, patients who abuse alcohol in addition to other substances are likely to be more severely psychiatrically impaired than those who abuse one substance (Ross, Glaser, and Germanson, 1988). The question whether cocaine-dependent and cocaine plus alcohol–dependent individuals differ along psychopathological dimensions, thus requiring different treatment courses, was examined by Cunningham et al. (1993). In a study of 144 male inpatients, these investigators found that patients dependent on both cocaine and alcohol showed significantly more symptoms of depression and anxiety and were more likely to have antisocial and avoidant personality disorders than those dependent on cocaine alone. The authors concluded that patients with addictions to both alcohol and cocaine require increased assistance with anxiety and depressive symptomatology, and that, as suggested by Kosten (1991), it is necessary to examine the functional aspects of combined drug use in order to understand the treatment needs of combined drug abusers, since each drug may be used for a specific purpose, as when alcohol is used to attenuate the anxiety associated with the cocaine crash.

Opioid Abusers

When compared with opioid-dependent patients, cocaine-dependent admissions to a Veterans Administration drug treatment unit were found by Malow et al. (1989) to have a lower rate of DSM-III-R personality disorder diagnoses (31% versus 79%). The cocaine-dependent group also had lower rates of borderline (6% versus 35%) and adult antisocial (12% versus 21%) features as well as lower levels of subjective stress. Cocaine-dependent patients in this sample also had a comparatively lower prevalence of self-reported affective disturbance, while the opioid-dependent sample was characterized by higher levels of inappropriate anger, chronic boredom, affective instability, inconsistent work history, and social nonconformity. The authors concluded that cocaine abusers were less maladjusted than opiate abusers. They attributed this difference to the larger number of persons with less pathology attracted to cocaine, which has wider social acceptance than heroin, as well as to earlier treatment entry by cocaine users.

In a later study, cocaine and opioid users were found to have similar patterns of psychopathology on the Minnesota Multiphasic Personality Inventory (MMPI) but to have less psychopathology than speedball users. Cocaine users were, however, more likely than opiate or speedball users to leave a thirty-day inpatient drug treatment program against medical advice, and to be younger, nonwhite, and to have lower IQ scores (Dolan et al., 1991). The authors suggest that the relative youth of cocaine users may reflect the drug's recently enhanced popularity compared to opiates, as well as the more acute debilitating effects of cocaine in comparison to opioids. The debilitating effects of cocaine on cognitive functioning (see, for example, Manschreck et al., 1990) were also proposed as the reason for lower intellectual performance.

Rounsaville, Anton, et al. (1991) found their sample of cocaine users entering treatment to be highly similar to opiate users demographically. When contrasted with the community on the presence of diagnosable DSM-III disorders, both the opiate- and cocaine-using samples had similar rates of any psychiatric disorder, major depression, any affective disorder, phobias, any anxiety disorder, alcoholism, and antisocial personality disorder, all of which were higher than rates in the general community sample. Both opiate and cocaine abusers had lower rates of schizophrenic disorders than in the community. Though similar in this comparison, the opiate and cocaine abuser samples differed from each other with respect to major depression, antisocial personality disorder, mania or hypomania, alcoholism, and a history of childhood attention deficit disorder, all of which were substantially less frequent among cocaine abusers. More frequent were elevated levels of mania. As is the case with opioid addicts, depression in cocaine abusers tended to occur only after the onset of drug abuse, although severity of depression in chronic cocaine abusers (typically rebound disorders) appears to be higher than in the case of opiate abusers. The lifetime prevalence of a depressive disorder was found to increase from 30.5% to 58.7% when depressive episodes occurring during periods of cocaine use were included. Ziedonis et al. (1994) observed that, compared with opiate addicts (Kosten, Rounsaville, and Kleber, 1985), cocaine addicts had lower rates of depression and antisocial personality disorder and higher rates of alcoholism and phobia, leading them to conclude that "self-medication may be of limited utility in explaining rates of dual diagnosis" (p. 48).

Calsyn and Saxon (1990) evaluated 100 consecutively admitted males entering Veterans Administration outpatient treatment for drug abuse on the Millon Clinical Multiaxial Inventory, and found rates of affective disorders to be significantly higher in the primary cocaine-abusing group (58%) than in the primary opiate-abusing group (41%). While the two groups did not differ with respect to psychotic symptomatology (11% versus 8%), Axis II disorders were present at rates of 97% and 90% in the cocaine- and opiate-abusing groups, respectively. The authors concluded that the two groups were highly similar in degree and type of psychopathology, with both exhibiting severe psychiatric illness.

Similarity between primary cocaine abusers and primary opiate or other drug abusers among admissions to therapeutic communities during 1985–1987 has also been found with respect to either current or life-time psychiatric diagnosis. The overwhelming majority of both groups received both lifetime substance abuse and psychiatric diagnosis (primary cocaine abusers, 76.1%; total sample, 78.3%), while smaller numbers received a substance abuse diagnosis only (primary cocaine abusers, 15.2%; total sample, 14.7%) or a psychiatric diagnosis only (primary cocaine abusers, 5.7%; total sample, 4.2%). With respect to current substance abuse and psychiatric diagnoses, 33.9% of primary cocaine abusers and 33.7% of the total sample received dual diagnoses, while almost identical numbers of primary cocaine abusers and the total sample received a substance abuse diagnosis only (32.2% versus 33.7%). With respect to having received a psychiatric diagnosis only, De Leon (1993) found little difference between the primary cocaine abuser group (11.7%) and the total sample (12.3%). The most common psychiatric diagnoses for cocaine users were antisocial personality disorder (present in 42.9% of admissions with a primary cocaine diagnosis), psychosexual dysfunction (42.3%), generalized anxiety disorder (31.7%), phobic disorders (25.9%), and all affective disorders (30.9%). Both lifetime and current psychiatric diagnoses generally did not differ by primary drug, with the exception of dual disorders, which were more frequently present in primary opiate abusers than in primary cocaine or other drug abusers; schizophrenia, which was more frequent among primary other drug users; and phobias, which were least frequent among primary cocaine abusers and most frequent in the other group.

Cocaine and Other Substance Abuse in Psychiatric Patients

In general, histories of substance abuse are likely to be present in psychiatric patients diagnosed with schizophrenia (McLellan, Druley, and Carson, 1978; Schneier and Siris, 1987; Siris et al., 1988). In a study of predominantly schizophrenic psychiatric patients in a community mental health center partial hospitalization unit, Cohen and Henkin (1993) found 65% of patients currently using illicit drugs, although only 18% reported their use as being heavy (that is, more than 10 drug use days in the previous 30). The most commonly used drugs in this sample were marijuana, alcohol, crack cocaine, and cocaine, with alcohol-crack and alcohol-marijuana being the most common combinations.

Several studies (for example, Miller and Tanenbaum, 1989; Weller et al., 1988) have demonstrated substance abuse histories in a substantial proportion of psychiatric inpatients admitted with diagnoses of schizophrenia. Dixon et al. (1991) found that 35% of newly admitted schizophrenics had recently used drugs to such an extent that their functioning was impaired. Almost 50% had experienced some impairment in their lifetime. Cocaine was among the most commonly abused drugs in this study, reflecting a preference for stimulants, cannabis, and hallucinogens over alcohol and sedative-hypnotics. This finding is consistent with other reports that rates of *recent* use of cocaine and other stimulants are higher in patients hospitalized with schizophrenia than in patients hospitalized with other psychiatric diagnoses (Richard, Liskow, and Perry, 1985). This last finding is also consistent with findings that stimulant abuse is more prevalent among schizophrenics than among non-patient controls (Breakey et al., 1974; Richard, Liskow, and Perry, 1985).

In general, cocaine-abusing male schizophrenic patients, when contrasted with nonusers, are likely to be characterized by a history of more hospitalizations, a higher occurrence of paranoid subtypes, and a greater likelihood of being depressed at the time of the interview (Brady et al., 1990). Sevy et al. (1990) confirmed the presence of a greater likelihood of depression among hospitalized schizophrenics with a history of cocaine abuse. Khantzian (1985) has suggested that the high incidence of substance abuse found among persons with schizophrenia and other psychiatric disorders is reflective of misguided attempts at self-medication. Cocaine-using schizophrenics not only have significantly higher hospitalization rates than other substance-using or non-using patients, but also have higher rates of suicidal ideation after cocaine use compared with their own non–cocaine-associated hospitalizations or those of other groups. During hospitalization they receive higher doses of neuroleptics. In general, cocaine use by schizophrenics is usually associated with a poorer illness course (Seibyl et al., 1993). Sevy et al. (1990), however, compared hospitalized schizophrenics with and without a history of cocaine abuse and found that aside from memory problems (conceptual encoding and verbal memory), only greater depression and lower levels of socialization differentiated the two groups.

Reviewing the literature on the acute effects of drug abuse in schizophrenia, Dixon et al. (1990) noted that the evidence has been contradictory on the effects of stimulants on psychosis. Several experimental studies have demonstrated that amphetamines induce psychosis and worsen symptoms (for example, Angrist, Rotrosen, and Gershon, 1980; Janowsky and Davis, 1976), while others have found no effects or even improvements in negative symptoms (for example, Cesarec and Nyman, 1985; van Kammen et al., 1982). When other recent studies are considered, it seems likely that stimulants negatively affect schizophrenia. A clinical study by Brady et al. (1990), conducted with dually diagnosed patients (a DSM-III-R diagnosis of schizoaffective or schizophreniform psychosis plus a lifetime DSM-III-R diagnosis of drug or alcohol abuse or dependence), found that a majority felt that cocaine (as well as cannabis and alcohol) decreased depression, but that cocaine (but not alcohol and cannabis) increased anxiety. The results of this study led the investigators to conclude that cocaine use may worsen the course of schizophrenia and contribute to relapse. This conclusion is consistent with that of Richard, Liskow, and Perry (1985), who found among relapsing schizophrenic patients a high rate of stimulant use prior to relapse, which they believed likely contributed to relapse, and which was unrelated to the regular use of maintenance neuroleptic drugs. Furthermore, Brady et al. (1990) suggested that cocaine, which can produce paranoid symptoms in nonpsychotic individuals, can increase the expression of such symptoms, and may be used by some schizophrenics to self-medicate depressive symptoms, although its use could also precipitate such symptoms.

Cocaine and/or crack use complicates the diagnosis and treatment of other disorders in psychiatric patients (Weiss et al. 1986). In addition, the diagnosis of cocaine abuse, as well as other substance abuse in psychiatric patients, has been demonstrated to be frequently missed. In a cohort of 54 patients, only 1 diagnosis of cocaine abuse or dependence was made at the emergency room level, while 6 were made at the state hospital level. In contrast, 25 were made by a research team (Ananth et al., 1989). Such a high rate of failure in making an accurate diagnosis likely depends on an understanding of the interaction of observable symptoms, cocaine abuse patterns, and underlying psychiatric disorders, since presenting symptoms may vary according to the pattern, quantity, and frequency of crack use, as well as environmental stressors, the nature of psychopathology, and the extent to which it is present (Bunt et al., 1990).

Yet, despite the difficulties present in making a diagnosis of cocaine abuse, the prevalence of such abuse in psychiatric patients has been reported to be quite high. For example, Galanter, Castaneda, and Ferman (1988), after reviewing the literature, concluded that as many as half of all patients seen in emergency rooms are substance abusers, and that substance abuse complicates the presenting symptomatology of as many as one-third of general psychiatric patients. Richard, Liskow, and Perry (1985) found schizophrenic and schizoaffective patients in the Veterans Administration sample they studied to have been more likely to have used stimulants, including cocaine, in the prior six months than nonschizophrenics. This finding was maintained even after those patients with primary substance abuse diagnoses were eliminated from the analysis. The matching of stimulant users with non-users on the basis of age did, however, eliminate this difference. It is possible that this result is due to the inclusion of more character-disordered patients, with their greater likelihood of substance abuse.

Another study found that, among schizophrenic and schizoaffective patients, 13% had a history of cocaine abuse, and another 13% a history of amphetamine abuse (Siris et al., 1988). After reviewing the literature on psychoactive substance abuse in schizophrenia, Schneier and Siris (1987) concluded that schizophrenics used cocaine and amphetamine, as well as cannabis, hallucinogens, inhalants, caffeine, and tobacco, significantly more than other psychiatric patients and nonpatients. (Schizophrenics, however, used alcohol, opiates, and sedative-hypnotics as often as or less frequently than comparison groups.) These findings were confirmed in a more recent study of 40 cocaine-dependent psychiatric inpatients predominantly of low socioeconomic status admitted to a metropolitan hospital because of psychiatric symptoms (Bunt et al., 1990). In this study psychiatric cluster B personality disorders (43%) were identified as the most common disorders present. Of the 17 patients with such disorders, 11 fulfilled criteria for antisocial personality disorder, 6 for borderline personality disorder, and 2 for schizotypal personality disorder. Schizophrenic disorders (33%) and affective disorders (13%) were the second and third most common disorders present. When compared to schizophrenic patients, those patients with cluster B personality disorders used cocaine more frequently and in greater quantities, and had begun crack use at an earlier age.

Finally, as a number of writers have observed, the expression of psychiatric symptomatology in relation to periods of cocaine intoxication may vary widely as a function of drug use parameters (for example, dose, intensity, and frequency of cocaine binges), the social context, and existing premorbid psychopathology (Bunt et al., 1990; Gawin and Kleber, 1986a; Siegel, 1982a).

Psychostimulants appear to be preferentially abused by schizophrenic patients (McLellan and Druley, 1977; Richard, Liskow, and Perry, 1985; Schneier and Siris, 1987). Furthermore, the treatment of cocaine-abusing schizophrenic patients presents special problems, including the difficulty of treating either schizophrenia or stimulant abuse by itself, as well as addressing rapidly changing patterns of drug abuse (Siris, 1990). Among the possible interventions suggested by Siris (1990) for these patients are *maintenance neuroleptic medications* to treat psychotic exacerbations triggered by use of substances of abuse as well as to reduce the potential euphoric and/or psychotogenic effects of abused substances, although such use may foster cocaine use to override undesired neuroleptic effects; *anti-Parkinsonian medications* such as amantadine and bromocriptine to reduce neuroleptic side effects such as neuroleptic-induced akinesia, although these drugs may themselves be abused; *antidepressant medications* such as the tricyclics, and possibly lithium carbonate, to reduce dysphoria and craving (use of monoamine oxidase [MAO] inhibitors is contraindicated owing to the potential for a hypertensive crisis or other complication should a substance of abuse be used); and *psychosocial interventions and hospitalization* for detoxification and management of acute psychosis.

A number of pharmacologic interventions for schizophrenic cocaine-abusing patients have also been recommended by Schottenfeld, Carroll, and Rounsaville (1993). They suggest that, first, where cocaine is used to counter side effects of a neuroleptic, a modification of the dosage of the neuroleptic or a change in the neuroleptic itself may be needed; second, where psychotic symptoms are exacerbated by the use of cocaine, either an increase in the dose of the neuroleptic or a change to another neuroleptic is needed; third, where side effects of the neuroleptic are present, and cocaine may be used to counter them, the use of adjunctive anticholinergic agents or amantadine is called for; and finally, where cocaine is used to counter anhedonia, anergia, or postpsychotic depression, the use of antidepressants is indicated. The authors also suggest that the antidepressants imipramine (Tofranil) and clozapine (Clozaril) may be potentially useful in the treatment of cocaine abuse, the former to treat postpsychotic depression, and the latter because of its low incidence of neuroleptic side effects. They also recommend the use of psychosocial interventions in the treatment of cocaine abuse in patients with comorbid psychiatric diagnoses, particularly when affective instability, rejection sensitivity, and borderline or antisocial personality disorder are present. Cocaine Anonymous and other self-help groups, as well as intensive daily treatment, may provide the level and consistency of support such patients need.

Direct Psychiatric Complications of Cocaine Abuse

Acute Presentation of Psychiatric Problems

The range of psychiatric states produced by cocaine use is diverse, and may include euphoria, dysphoria, paranoid psychosis, violent agitation, and severe depression. In many cases the cocaine user seeking medical attention first presents with psychiatric symptomatology or with syndromes mimicking psychiatric illness (Estroff and Gold, 1986; Post, 1975). A number of people, all attempting to maintain physical control over the patient, may frequently accompany the patient to the emergency room.

As has been noted, the cocaine-intoxicated patient may present with apparent overt psychosis, often an excited delirium characterized by confusion and agitation, delusions, hallucinations, and other paranoid ideation (Schrank, 1993). Bunt et al. (1990) found that cocaine-dependent psychiatric patients showed a high frequency of symptoms of depression, suicidal ideation, paranoia, anxiety, auditory hallucinations, and loose associations. Grandiose and bizarre delusions were only infrequently present, while olfactory and gustatory hallucinations were not found in any patients, and tactile hallucinations occurred in only one case. The relative frequency of psychiatric complications of cocaine abuse is suggested by the Lowenstein et al. (1987b) study at San Francisco General Hospital, in which 75 of 996 emergency room visits and 279 hospital admissions were for psychiatric complications. These included agitation, anxiety, or depression ($N = 33$), psychosis and paranoia ($N = 24$), and suicidal ideation ($N = 18$).

Psychotic states are described by Wetli (1993) as being of sudden onset and involving paranoia, followed by violent activity directed toward objects (particularly glass, such as windows and mirrors). Because of the intense fear of the police which may accompany these behaviors, this state had been labeled the "bull horrors" by users (Wilson, cited by Post, 1975), although this term is used infrequently if at all at present. Often, clothing will be stripped off, and the patient will run through the street shouting and screaming. Attempts at restraint may result in a violent struggle during which the patient appears to experience enormous increase in strength. Rather than indicating incredible strength on the part of the patient, however this may be reflective of an indifference to pain, the result of a marked diminution of pain sensation (Schrank, 1993). At such times cocaine-intoxicated patients represent a risk to health workers in the emergency room. The onset of such states appears to be unrelated to either the amount of cocaine used, blood level of cocaine, route of administration, or frequency of use (Wetli and Fishbain, 1985). Psychiatric symptoms associated with cocaine abuse may, however, be the result of cocaine-induced decreases in cerebral blood flow (Miller et al., 1992).

Acute psychological effects of cocaine intoxication have frequently been cited in the clinical literature. These include acute anxiety states; severe panic attacks; paranoia; acting-out, including assault and harm to self and others; terror and fear of impending death; and hypersomnolence.

Cocaine-induced panic disorder is common in chronic cocaine users. One report indicates that up to 83% of callers to the 800-COCAINE line reported panic attacks as a common adverse effect of cocaine use. The frequency of such attacks appears to be a function of route of cocaine administration, with 64% of freebasers, 57% of injection users, and 42% of inhalers having experienced a panic attack (Washton and Gold, 1984). The frequency of cocaine-induced panic has led to suggestions that it be included as a psychiatric entity (Louie, Lannon, and Ketter, 1989), and it has frequently been found in chronic users of cocaine (Aronson and Craig, 1986; Louie, Lannon, and Ketter, 1989; Pohl, Balon, and Yeragani, 1987), although one retrospective study of emergency room visits and hospital admissions for cocaine-related disorders failed to confirm a relationship between chronicity of use and complications (Lowenstein et al., 1987b). Furthermore, a case report exists of the development of panic disorder following use of a small amount of cocaine (Geracioti and Post, 1991). Conversely, one study reported that 25% of patients with panic disorder had a history of substantial cocaine use (Louie, Lannon, and Ketter, 1989).

Cocaine-induced panic disorder may reflect an underlying dysregulation in noradrenergic function, and may be particularly likely to occur soon after discontinuation of cocaine (McDougle et al., 1994). It has been associated with a history of depressive spells and heavy drinking, and with no use of marijuana during a period of follow-up (Anthony, Tien, and Petronis, 1989).[4] Panic disorder may not appear until after many years of cocaine use, suggesting that it is produced through a kindling mechanism (Louie, Lannon, and Ketter, 1989).[5] It may then persist for months or years, first in association with cocaine use, and then even with complete abstinence from cocaine (Geracioti and Post, 1991; Post et al., 1987). It has also been suggested that drug-induced panic disorders, including those induced by cocaine, are produced by a different mechanism than are "classic" panic disorders, possibly the pharmacological kindling of epileptiform activity in the limbic system (Abraham, 1989; Louie, Lannon, and Ketter, 1989). It may well be that there is more than one mechanism underlying the development of panic disorders in response to cocaine abuse.

Cocaine Psychosis

Cocaine psychosis may occur following prolonged use of cocaine. Paranoid delusions, hallucinations (including those of a visual, auditory, and olfactory nature), and disturbances of sensation (particularly of touch, including "cocaine bugs") may be present in this state, as well as mania (characterized by hyperactivity and distractibility) and delirium, including disorientation and confusion (Brown, 1989).[6] Psychiatric conditions resulting from cocaine use may also be superimposed on pre-existing conditions, resulting in their exacerbation. This may be of particular concern during manic episodes (Dackis et al., 1985–86). Post (1975) described a model of cocaine psychosis which consisted of an orderly progression of clinical syndromes (euphoria, dysphoria, paranoid psychosis) dependent on dosage, chronicity, and genetic and experiential predisposition. In general, cocaine-induced psychosis has been of two forms: confusional psychoses associated with high-dose use of cocaine, and insidious-onset psychoses with affective, paranoid, or schizophreniform features (Manschreck et al., 1988).

In a study of patients with freebase cocaine disorders admitted to a Bahamian psychiatric center, Manschreck et al. (1988) found confusion and Schneiderian symptoms (symptoms specific for a diagnosis of schizophrenia, for example, certain delusions and hallucinations) to be characteristic of these admissions (confusion was present in 42% of cases, delusions in 93%, hallucinations in 83%, and disturbed thinking in 48%), while formication was somewhat infrequent, occurring in 23% of admissions. Cocaine-induced psychosis was also found to share many of the characteristics of acute paranoid schizophrenia in a study of 55 consecutive cocaine-abuser admissions to an inpatient treatment setting for treatment of that psychosis (Brady et al., 1991). Fifty-three percent of this group reported having experienced transient cocaine-induced psychosis. The presence of a psychosis was found to be related to a greater use of cocaine during the past year and to a longer duration of cocaine use. More males than females were found to have developed cocaine psychosis, and 90% developed paranoid delusions directly related to cocaine use. Symptoms present during active cocaine-induced psychosis include hallucinations of any type (96%), auditory hallucinations (83%), visual hallucinations (38%), and tactile hallucinations (21%). Transient behavioral stereotypies (for example, picking and scratching, repeated searching for drugs, including the common behavior of picking through the piling of a rug) were present in 27% of cases.

Lesko et al. (1982) reported on the course of a medically supervised patient suffering from cocaine psychosis resulting from long-term use of the drug. The patient was a psychologically normal individual who was suffering from oral stomatitis, secondary to bone marrow transplant for aplastic anemia. On day 16 of treatment with a topical application of a solution of dyclonine hydrochloride and 3 ml of 10% cocaine every four hours, the patient's pulse rose from 80 to 140 per minute, and nausea, vomiting, headaches, insomnia, chills, and fever were present. Over the next 18 hours he had hallucinations of ants on his clothes, on his food, on hospital personnel, and in his room, saw "shadows" of his mother, and hallucinated having witnessed a cardiac arrest in an adjoining room. Euphoric mood was present, accompanied with irritability and pressured speech. Hyperactivity, jerking muscular movements, twitching of the head and extremities, and fine tremor were also present. After withdrawal of the drug and administration of 10 mg of diazepam, the patient slept for 10 hours, during which his reflexes returned to normal. Although his hallucinations faded over the next 24 hours, increasing suspiciousness, guardedness, and paranoia appeared, disappearing after 60 hours. It is of course possible that the combination of medications this patient was receiving, which included 60 mg daily of prednisone and 2 mg every four hours of levorphanal tartrate, may have contributed to his psychiatric symptomatology.

Intervention in the emergency setting, according to Schrank (1993), typically involves a rapid assessment for a compromised airway or ventilation, trauma, or neurologic deficit. The checking of vital signs (pulse rate and quality, pupillary reflexes, and skin temperature) should not await the more thorough examination which should take place following sedation. Where restraints are required to minimize injury, care should be taken to avoid the risk of extremity ischemia, respiratory compromise, or inhibition of heat loss. Parenteral sedation, typically diazepam or another benzodiazepine, should be initiated, the patient started on an intravenous infusion of isotonic fluids, and then ideally maintained in a quiet environment. Typically, the postsedation course is several hours of deep sleep, followed by gradual awakening, with little recall of preceding events (Schrank, 1993).

Effects of Cocaine Abuse on Memory and Cognition

Salutary effects of cocaine on the performance of normal (non–sleep-deprived) subjects does not appear to have been empirically documented before a study conducted by Higgins et al. (1990), which demonstrated a small (4%) but consistent dose-dependent increment in performance in non–sleep-deprived individuals. This increment was similar to that obtained in other studies for amphetamine (Weiss and Laties, 1962).

Cocaine, at different times, both enhanced and decreased performance on a digit symbol substitution test, though no effect was found on acquisition of new material.

Cocaine abuse has deleterious effects on memory and performance. Both acute and chronic use of cocaine may result in neuropsychological impairment. Strickland et al. (1993) examined a group of long-term cocaine users without symptoms of stroke or transient ischemic attacks who had been drug-free for six months, and found brain perfusion deficits, as well as associated deficits in attention, concentration, learning, memory, and other functions.[7] A study by Berry et al. (1993) found impairments in memory, visuospatial abilities, and concentration to persist in hospitalized cocaine abusers during the acute phase of withdrawal, independent of withdrawal-related depression. Furthermore, many of these effects persisted beyond two weeks after termination of cocaine use. The effects of cocaine may be longer-lasting for motor, as compared to sensory, functioning (Roberts and Bauer, 1993). Ardila, Rosselli, and Strumwasser (1991) found the performance of chronic crack abusers on a basic neuropsychological battery to be lower than expected on the basis of age and educational background. Such deficits were directly related to lifetime amount of cocaine used.

Neuropsychological impairment may result from the transient hypertension produced by cocaine, as well as from the overstimulation of dopaminergic pathways and their consequent hypoexcitability when cocaine is discontinued (O'Malley and Gawin, 1990), although other, currently unidentified mechanisms may also be operative. It has yet to be demonstrated conclusively, however, that abuse of cocaine and other stimulants so disrupts the dopaminergic system so as to result in a long-term impairment of the ability to experience reward (Reed and Grant, 1990). Also, it is possible that adverse consequences from cocaine use may not appear for several years (Gawin and Ellinwood, 1988).

The importance of cognitive and performance deficits during cocaine withdrawal was noted by Herning et al. (1990), who observed that cognitive impairments (for example, attentional problems or memory loss) may hinder effective psychiatric treatment, and poor job performance may put the withdrawing cocaine user and the public at risk of accidents.

Some performance decrements may be transitory in nature; others may be more permanent. For example, brief decrements were shown in performance on a maze task, while persistently poor performance on the Paced Auditory Serial Addition Test was found in patients treated for freebase cocaine abuse (Melamed and Bleiberg, 1986). Some cognitive alterations may result from sleep loss and depression in patients withdrawing from cocaine (Baxter, 1983; Gawin and Kleber, 1986a).

At the information-processing level, stimulants disrupt stimulus evaluation (Herning et al., 1985) as well as response selection and response execution (Frowein, 1981). Reporting preliminary data from a study of cognitive information processing and performance in cocaine abusers before and during treatment, Herning et al. (1990) found specific cognitive impairments at two stages in the processing of stimulus information. These included a delay in stimulus evaluation on the first day of treatment, as well as a slowed reaction time on the Sternberg Memory Task, which lasted for the duration of testing. Three major explanations for these findings were suggested: a long-term readjustment in neurotransmitter systems; the unmasking of a residual-function neurological alteration produced by cocaine use; or the identification of a preexisting constitutional cognitive alteration. Herning et al. (1990) suggested that the second of these three explanations was the most likely, and that this factor contributed to relapse.

The possible cognitive impairment produced by heavy cocaine use was also investigated in studies by Melamed and Bleiberg (1986) and Volkow et al. (1988). Using Positron-Emission Tomography (PET), Volkow et al. (1988) found deranged cerebral blood flow in the prefrontal cortexes of chronic cocaine abusers. Continued relative decreased cerebral blood flow persisted after ten days of withdrawal. This finding was interpreted as resulting from vasospasm in cerebral arteries which had been chronically exposed to the sympathomimetic actions of cocaine. As noted by Herning et al. (1990), however, both of these studies were limited to the first ten days of abstinence and had no control groups.

There are several reports in the clinical literature of memory loss associated with stimulant abuse. Memory impairment has been demonstrated with amphetamine abuse, at least with respect to word storage and retrieval and short-term memory for sentences and detailed events (Conners, et al., 1969; Schiorring, 1981). Amphetamines, however, appear to enhance human memory consolidation (Soetens, D'Hooge, and Hueting, 1993), and use of amphetamines has also been demonstrated to enhance performance of many nonverbal intellectual capacities, particularly in children, including maze performance, spatial relations, visual memory, and auditory synthesis (Hurst et al., 1969; Rapoport et al., 1978). Additionally, both amphetamines and cocaine enhance avoidance learning and memory in rats (Janak and Martinez, 1992).

Few rigorous studies exist, however, which have evaluated the neuropsychological consequences of *chronic* cocaine use. One study

(Manschreck et al., 1990), in which abstinent severe freebase cocaine abusers on an inpatient unit in the Bahamas were evaluated, found some decrement on measures of short-term auditory recall, but no differences from normal subjects on a wide range of other tasks. In fact, on a task of visuospatial learning and recall (maze tracing), abstinent cocaine abusers did better than controls. O'Malley and his colleagues appear to have conducted what may have been the first controlled studies in this area. In the first of two studies, O'Malley et al. (1988, 1992) compared 20 recently abstinent cocaine abusers with 20 matched controls on a number of neuropsychological measures. The results indicated a poorer performance by the recently abstinent cocaine abusers on the arithmetic subtest of the WAIS-R, Story Memory (a measure of verbal forgetting), the Halstead Category test, the Symbol Digit Modalities test, and the summary score of the Neuropsychological Screening Exam (NSE). Scores on the last two measures were in the mildly impaired range; 50% of the cocaine abusers scored in the impaired range on the summary index of the NSE versus 15% of the controls. Surprisingly, however, the cocaine abusers had higher oral fluency scores. O'Malley and Gawin (1990) concluded that these findings suggested an association between recent abstinence from cocaine and problems in concentration, memory, and nonverbal problem solving and abstracting ability.

A second study (O'Malley et al., 1989) employed a more extensive neuropsychological screening battery. A sample of 25 outpatients who had achieved an average of 135 days of abstinence was compared with a sample of demographically matched normal controls. None of the subjects had a lifetime or current history of drug or alcohol abuse other than cocaine or stimulant abuse. The cocaine abusers were found to perform more poorly than controls on measures of complex cognitive motor skills, simple motor skills, and overall summary scores. Measures of specific tasks suggested poorer performance by the cocaine abusers on a number of tests, including those of spatial relations, grooved pegboard, and grip strength. Memory, especially retention of nonverbal material, was also poorer in the cocaine abuser group. With the exception of grip strength and spatial relations, the cocaine abusers' scores were all within the normal ranges, however. It was concluded that processes involving vigilance, memory, and motor functioning may be most affected by cocaine abuse. Furthermore, neuropsychological performance was related to amount and recency of cocaine use.

Spencer (1990), in commenting on the research aspects of studying the residual effects of abused drugs on behavior, suggested several issues which require attention: the need to separate transient from longer-term effects; the need to track performance in children who have stopped abusing drugs in order to evaluate the effects of such use (the drug alone or in combination with other drugs) on cognitive, social, and emotional development; the need to evaluate the components of behavior which are affected adversely by drug use; and the need to evaluate individual differences with respect to residual drug effects in order to explain vulnerability to the development of substance abuse habits. Noting the need first to establish the existence of residual drug effects, Spencer observed that it remains to be clarified whether long-term drug abuse produces irreversible brain damage or more subtle reversible brain dysfunction. Such knowledge will contribute to the ability, through the evaluation of a patient's strengths and weaknesses, to develop effective treatment planning strategies. It is clear, however, that such development requires a new technology for assessing and indexing deficits resulting from long-term substance abuse.

A thoughtful review of the conceptual and methodological issues facing researchers investigating the long-term neurobehavioral consequences of substance abuse has been provided by Reed and Grant (1990). *Conceptual issues* include the problems inherent in defining central nervous system events which can be measured only indirectly; the need to understand the natural history of drug-related brain disorder; the need to understand whether recovery from drug-induced central nervous system effects is partial, permanent, or temporary; the need to develop an appropriate nosology of subclinical and reversible neurobehavioral disorders associated with substance abuse; and the need to determine the effect of coexisting factors which may influence the relationship between pre–substance abuse status and outcome, as well as the outcomes of different patterns of substance abuse.

Measurement considerations for neurobehavioral strategies used to study central nervous system effects of drugs, the importance of which, while obvious, are often insufficiently acknowledged. These include attention to issues such as the need for measurements to demonstrate construct, concurrent, and predictive validity; possess reliability in order to reflect change accurately; possess sensitivity and specificity sufficient to detect both strong and weak signals while ignoring system "noise"; employ neuropsychiatric tests that can provide broad measurement across a wide spectrum of intellectual abilities; develop appropriate normative samples against which information on brain-behavior relationships can be evaluated; and standardize methods of administration.

Confounds and cofactors not related to measurement, but which may influence neuropsychological function, include age and education, both of which are likely to influence whether or not any substance is abused; the abuse of multiple substances, which makes it difficult to separate the effects of any single substance from those of others as well as from effects of their interaction; quantification of drug use behaviors more precisely than through a dichotomy; the type of preparation and route of administration, as well as the presence of adulterants; indirect (biosocial) measures of immersion in drug use in addition to amount and frequency of the drug consumed during a specific period of time; the influence on neuropsychological functioning of premorbid and concurrent medical risk, some of which may result from involvement in the drug abuse lifestyle; and selective attrition from studies, particularly resulting from cofactors such as education and intelligence. In summarizing these issues, Reed and Grant (1990) note that "ignoring the need to account for these sources of variance would leave us with a confusion of contradictory findings and an inadequate increase in sorely needed knowledge" (p. 35).

More generally, although a large number of published studies have reported adverse physical effects of cocaine abuse, there are two general problems which prevent a clear interpretation of such findings. The first relates to the absence of appropriate baseline data which would allow for the development of estimates of the relative incidence and prevalence of these problems. For example, does a report of x cases in a practice represent $x/100$ cases or $x/10,000$ cases? It is not always easy to draw such conclusions from the data which are presented.

Second, the literature suffers from a number of methodological problems. Mayes et al. (1992) have outlined them in the case of the effects of prenatal exposure to cocaine. Their list of issues is applicable to other areas in which the health complications of cocaine abuse are presently or potentially evident. It includes the following: poorly defined or highly selective study samples and resultant inability to generalize to larger populations; poorly defined methodologies for identification of women who have used cocaine during pregnancy, since self-report underestimates cocaine use, and positive urine assays at the time of birth can accurately reflect cocaine use only during the prior four days; a lack of effective measurement of the timing, intensity, and duration of cocaine use during pregnancy; the inability to determine the effects of cocaine use during pregnancy apart from those attributable to other negative influences, including drugs of abuse (alcohol, heroin, marijuana, tobacco), poor health behaviors (inadequate nutrition, poor prenatal care), and the presence of sexually transmitted diseases; the difficulty of untangling the effects of intrauterine cocaine from other potentially confounding negative influences of cocaine on the infant's family and community and on parenting behaviors (for example, poverty, violence, abandonment, homelessness, multiple short-term foster placements, and inadequate or abusive parenting); and the need to identify the specific functions in children which are likely to be compromised by exposure to cocaine, and the effects of cocaine on the systems which may regulate them, particularly the neurotransmitter and autonomic nervous system. In the absence of such information, mislabeling prenatally cocaine-exposed children as damaged carries with it significant medical and psychosocial risks for these children. Such risks include lowered expectations and resultant lack of commitment to allocate resources for remediation, increased difficulties in locating adoptive homes, and biasing of further research reports.

Conclusions

Cocaine abusers have been found to possess high rates of psychopathology. Depending on the sample studied, about three-quarters of cocaine abusers presenting for treatment have a diagnosable lifetime psychiatric disorder; approximately half present with a current psychiatric disorder (Halikas et al., 1994; Helfrich et al., 1983; Rounsaville, Anton, et al., 1991). It is likely, as is the case with opiate abusers (see, for example, Oppenheimer, Sheehan, and Taylor, 1988; Smith et al., 1992), that the distress associated with the presence of such disorders is a motivating element in seeking treatment. Cocaine abusers who seek treatment may also have an amplified perception of the negative consequences of cocaine abuse (Carroll and Rounsaville, 1992). Where cocaine abusers have not been found to possess significant psychopathology, they have not sought treatment, raising the question whether high rates of psychopathology are sampling artifacts (Newcomb et al., 1987).

Cocaine abusers have generally been found to have high rates of affective disorders in general, and clinical depression in particular (see, for example, Anthony and Trinkoff, 1989; Gawin and Kleber, 1986a; Kleinman et al., 1990; Weiss et al., 1986). At the same time, only a relatively small proportion of such users have been found to have bipolar or cyclothymic disorders (see, for example, Gawin and Kleber, 1986a; Weiss et al., 1986). It is not clear whether depression is a consequence of cocaine use, precipitated by the drug (Gawin and Kleber, 1986a; Rawson et al., 1986), or whether, alternatively, cocaine is used to alleviate the symptoms of a premorbid depressive disorder (Khantzian, 1985; Magura et al., 1991). Likely, both sequences may be found.

It is notable that the literature is relatively sparse on the issue of personality traits of the cocaine abuser. By contrast, for many years the heroin addiction literature reflected a widespread search for the "addictive personality" (see, for example, Platt, 1986, chap. 8). Perhaps this reflects a lesson learned. It is probable, however, that cocaine is selected by some drug users because of specific effects. Such effects may be desired by the user in order to self-medicate psychiatric symptoms or aversive states (depression, boredom, fatigue), or because of specific needs (to bolster a certain lifestyle or to increase self-esteem; Schottenfeld, Carroll, and Rounsaville, 1993).

Psychiatric functioning is related to outcome among substance abusers, with poor functioning predictive of poorer outcome (McLellan et al., 1983). In particular, the presence of depression has been associated with poor treatment outcomes among both opiate (Kosten, Rounsaville, and Kleber, 1986, 1987; Rounsaville et al., 1986) and cocaine abusers, unless medication is employed, in which case depression is associated with better outcomes (Ziedonis and Kosten, 1991).

The presence of dual diagnosis represents a complicating factor both with respect to treatment and with respect to prognosis for recovery. Much of the knowledge on this issue, however, has derived from studies of opiate addicts (Platt, 1986, 1995a). In a comparison of hospitalized cocaine abusers with a similar group of patients dependent on opiates or central nervous system depressants, Weiss et al. (1986) found a significantly higher prevalence of affective disorders among the cocaine abusers than among abusers of opiates and central nervous system depressants. This finding was present despite the similarity in demography and current symptomatology between the two groups. The most frequent diagnoses were major depression, found in 20% of chronic cocaine abusers, cyclothymic disorder (16.7%), bipolar disorder (6.7%), and atypical depression (10.0%). Thus, over half of the cocaine abusers in this study received another Axis I diagnosis beside substance abuse. Axis II diagnoses, primarily borderline and narcissistic disorders, were present in 90.0% of the cocaine abusers. Weiss et al. (1986) concluded that a careful diagnostic search for other psychiatric disorders, particularly affective disorders, was necessary in evaluating and treating cocaine abusers.

The presence of attention deficit and hyperactivity disorder (ADHD) may predispose individuals to cocaine abuse (Eyre, Rounsaville, and Kleber, 1982; Horton et al., 1987). High rates of ADHD have been found among cocaine abusers (Carroll and Rounsaville, 1993; Rounsaville, Anton et al., 1991), and the suggestion has been made that cocaine abusers with ADHD may be self-medicating their symptoms (Khantzian et al., 1984).

Psychopathy and other Axis II disorders are a very common finding among cocaine abusers, with rates of prevalence approaching 75% to 90% in several studies. A wide range of such disorders is generally seen, including antisocial, passive-aggressive, borderline, histrionic, paranoid, and self-defeating personality (Marlowe et al., 1995; Weiss et al., 1986, 1993). It has been suggested that such characteristics are relatively stable across periods of both cocaine use and abstinence (Weiss et al., 1993).

When compared with abusers of opiates or cocaine-opiate combinations, cocaine abusers appear to be similar demographically (Calsyn and Saxon, 1990; Rounsaville, Anton, et al., 1991) and to possess less psychopathology (Malow et al., 1989). While the former finding may possibly be reflective of the particular clinical settings in which patients were seen, the latter may be reflective of the more widespread and socially acceptable use of cocaine.

Many cocaine abusers are also abusers of other drugs, in accord with poly-drug abuse being the predominant pattern among American substance abusers (Flaherty, Kotranski, and Fox, 1984). Alcohol, opiates, and other substances are commonly used by cocaine abusers (Cunningham et al., 1993; Malow et al., 1989; Ross, Glaser, and Germanson, 1988). Use of alcohol in particular, in addition to cocaine, appears to be associated with more severe psychiatric impairment (Ross, Glaser, and Germanson, 1988). As Carroll et al. (1993) have suggested, this finding supports the importance of detecting and treating concurrent alcoholism in cocaine abusers, since the cessation of cocaine use in the presence of alcoholism is extremely unlikely.

Cocaine and other drug abuse is a common finding in psychiatric patients diagnosed with schizophrenia (Dixon et al., 1991; McLellan, Woody, and O'Brien, 1978; Schneier and Siris, 1987; Siris et al., 1988). Lifetime and current impairment rates owing to substance abuse in this population are in the range of 35% to 50% (Galanter, Castaneda, and Ferman, 1988; Miller and Tannenbaum, 1989; Weller et al., 1988). Such substance abuse is associated with worse histories, a higher likelihood of current depression and suicide, a poorer response to treatment, and a poorer prognosis (Brady et al., 1990; Seibyl et al., 1993; Sevy et al., 1990). Cocaine and other stimulants appear to be preferentially abused by schizophrenic patients (McLellan and Druley, 1977; Richard, Liskow, and Perry, 1985). Although there is some conflicting evidence on the issue (Cesarec and Nyman, 1985; van Kammen et al., 1982), recent studies indicate that the use of stimulants negatively impacts the course of schizophrenia (Brady et al., 1990; Richard, Liskow, and Perry, 1985). The use of cocaine and other stimulants also complicates the course and treatment of other psychiatric disorders as well as making their diagnosis more difficult (Ananth et al., 1989).

The initial presentation of cocaine abuse in the emergency setting typically involves either real or apparent psychiatric symptoms (Estroff and Gold, 1986), often of sudden onset (Wetli, 1993). This presentation may be highly varied owing to the wide range of psychiatric symptoms which may be present (Bunt et al., 1990). Anxiety, panic, depression, psychosis, paranoia, and suicidal ideation are among the most common symptoms (Lowenstein et al., 1987b). Cocaine psychosis, either of insidious onset or resulting from high-dose cocaine use, may be present (Lesko et al., 1982; Manschreck et al., 1988).

Cocaine may adversely affect memory and cognition; it does not appear to provide significant improvement in performance. Many neuropsychological effects of cocaine are reversible following termination of cocaine use (Bleiberg, 1986), while others may persist (Berry et al., 1993; Roberts and Bauer, 1993). Neuropsychological impairment may be a function of amount and recency of use (O'Malley et al., 1992). Little evidence exists regarding the effects of chronic use.

Cocaine is likely to have a small and largely immediate salutary effect on performance (Higgins et al., 1990) as well as a larger deleterious effect with chronic use (Berry et al., 1993; Strickland et al., 1993). It is not yet clear how much of the decrements seen with cocaine use is reversible with abstinence (O'Malley et al., 1988, 1992; Spencer, 1990).

6

Medical and Related Consequences of Cocaine Abuse

Until relatively recently, cocaine was not universally considered a dangerous drug, although observers were aware of serious and unpredictable reactions to its use, including psychotic behavior, hyperthermia, convulsions, respiratory arrest, and sudden death. Absence of an apparent "physical" dependency contributed to this perception (Wetli, 1993). Not so long ago Grinspoon and Bakalar (1980), writing about cocaine in the *Comprehensive Textbook of Psychiatry,* commented that "if it is used no more than two or three times a week, cocaine creates no serious problems" (p. 1621). Cocaine, however, should be considered a dangerous drug. The most severe complications, including death, can occur anytime, even with the first use of cocaine (Brown et al., 1992).

Medical examiner data for the United States indicated that, in 1991, cocaine was implicated in 46.2% of drug abuse–related deaths in metropolitan areas, versus 36.3% for alcohol in combination with other drugs and 36% for heroin and/or morphine (NIDA, 1992). In 1992 the figure for cocaine remained stable at 47.2% of drug abuse–related deaths in metropolitan areas versus 38.9% for alcohol in combination with other drugs and 40.1% for heroin and/or morphine (SAMHSA, 1994b).[1] During 1991, in emergency rooms surveyed by DAWN, cocaine (with 25.7% of mentions) was exceeded only by alcohol in combination with other drugs (30.9%) as the most frequently mentioned drug. This figure was far in excess of that for heroin (9.1% of mentions; SAMHSA, 1994a). The figures for emergency room mentions increased significantly for both categories of abuse between 1991 and 1992, with cocaine accounting for 27.6% of all mentions and alcohol in combination with other drugs (including cocaine) accounting for 32.7% in 1992. (It should be noted, however, that these figures do not include indirect consequences of drug use such as drug-related homicide or suicide.)

Despite the suggestion that infrequent use of cocaine ("if used no more than two or three times per week") "creates no serious problems," or that use of cocaine at low doses does not appear to carry with it a very high risk of severe medical complications (see, for example, Brody, Slovis, and Wrenn, 1990; Washton and Stone-Washton, 1990), the *potential* of significant medical, as well as of personal and social, complications always exists. This is particularly true given individual differences in tolerance and preexisting medical conditions, and any individual's lack of knowledge about such factors. Thus, *any* use carries with it a potentially high risk. In this regard Maranto's (1985) reference to cocaine intoxication as "pharmacological Russian roulette" is indeed warranted.

In general, use of cocaine at high doses or during binges produces an exaggeration of the drug's subjective and behavioral effects. In addition, such use may trigger a number of acute psychological and physical responses, and some of the latter are potentially fatal. For example, cocaine use appears to carry with it many possible cardiovascular complications (Karch and Billingham, 1988), as well as those risks associated with injection use of any drug (Platt, 1986). The latter group includes local and distant abscesses caused by bacterial organisms, either at the site of injection or at points where the bacteria have been carried by the bloodstream; pulmonary and circulatory thromboses caused by particles of injected foreign matter; infectious diseases (hepatitis, HIV) resulting from sharing of needles with other users; kidney infections; and others. Extensive discussions of these risks and complications can be found in Platt (1986).

Presentation of Cocaine-Related Medical Problems

The presentation of medical problems associated with cocaine abuse may vary widely, since the clinical manifestations of cocaine use may include any of a range of symptoms and systems: malnutrition; exhaustion; neurologic symptoms (seizures, headache, syncope, transient ischemic attack); psychiatric manifestations (altered mental status, suicide attempts); cardiovascular symptoms (cardiac arrest, chest pain, palpitations, dyspnea); and venous; musculoskeletal; dermatological (hives); gastrointestinal (abdominal pain); pulmonary; infectious; obstetric; and neonatal complications (Derlet and Albertson, 1989a;

Goldfrank and Hoffman, 1993). In a sample of 233 consecutive admissions of 216 cocaine-using persons to a hospital medical emergency service, complaints were primarily cardiopulmonary (56.2%), neurologic (39.1%), and psychiatric (35.8%). Over 57% of patients presented with complaints involving more than one organ system. The cardiopulmonary complaints tended to be chest pain (present in 39.5% of patients), shortness of breath (21.9%), and palpitations (20.6%). These events only rarely reflected ischemia. Other frequent complaints included anxiety (21.9%), dizziness (12.9%), and headache (12.0%). Altered mental state was seen in 27.4% of patients, with diagnoses ranging from psychosis to coma. Short-term pharmacologic intervention was needed in only 24% of cases, and only 9.9% of patients were admitted. Mortality for this sample was less than 1% (Brody, Slovis, and Wrenn, 1990). These findings were generally consistent with those reported by Derlet and Albertson (1989a), who found the primary presenting complaints to be altered mental status (29.2%), chest pain (15.3%), syncope (13.9%), attempted suicide (9.5%), and palpitations (8.8%).

Cocaine or other drug abuse is not, however, always the presenting problem in drug-abusing patients seen in hospital emergency rooms, despite the fact that the medical problem for which the patient is there may be cocaine-related. Of patients treated in an urban emergency department for major trauma, 42% were tested for drug abuse. Of these, 38% tested positive for cocaine. Of 102 patients who had been injured in motor vehicle accidents, 20% tested positive for cocaine. For those under age 40 who were injured in motor vehicle accidents, 30% tested positive for cocaine. Such findings suggest that cocaine-related trauma may be underreported (Brookoff, Campbell, and Shaw, 1993). In a study of motor vehicle accident fatalities in New York City between 1984 and 1987, recent cocaine use was detected at autopsy in 18.2% of cases, while alcohol and cocaine metabolites were found in 10.0% of cases (Marzuk et al., 1990). These figures represented a substantial increase over the period prior to 1983, when cocaine metabolites were identified in 0.2% of drivers at autopsy (Cimbura et al., 1982). Marzuk et al. (1990) noted, however, that such findings do not establish that those persons with cocaine metabolites present at autopsy were impaired immediately prior to the fatal accident, but show only that use had occurred within the previous forty-eight hours.

It should also be noted that drug addicts in general, and crack addicts in particular, usually report their health status as relatively good, although women are somewhat less likely to do so, as are persons who are HIV-seropositive (McCoy and Miles, 1992). Yet, chronic cocaine abusers have a variety of medical problems, many of which are associated with high-risk practices such as injection drug use or the exchange of sex for drugs. These include common disorders such as venereal disease as well as less common systemic disorders such as bacterial endocarditis. Furthermore, several reports have suggested that the *actual* health status of drug users is substantially poorer than that of the general population. Thus, there is an inconsistency between self-perception of health and the actual facts. McCoy and Miles (1992) note that males, who are more likely than females to be injection drug users, have higher rates of endocarditis, whereas females, who are less likely to inject drugs but who are more likely to be sex partners of injection drug users, are more likely to have sexually transmitted diseases. Other factors accounting for differential reported incidence of specific disorders, according to the same study, are the greater efficiency of transmission of STDs from men to women, a differential presence of asymptomatic gonorrhea, and a less sensitive test response among women.

Acute Cocaine Intoxication

At least four acute, and potentially fatal, intoxication syndromes following cocaine use have been described in the literature:

The first, most common presentation is of sudden onset and is characterized by *headache, cold sweats, rapid pulse, tremors, and nausea, followed by generalized seizures, unconsciousness, and sudden death* unless prompt intervention takes place (DiMaio and Garriott, 1978; Roehrich and Gold, 1991). Dysphoria and hyperthermia may also be present. The primary mechanism resulting in death in this syndrome has been postulated to be respiratory paralysis, secondary to the effects of cocaine on the medulla, although direct toxic effects of cocaine on the heart may also play a role. Death is likely to occur within minutes of the onset of symptoms.

Excited delirium, a less common but also potentially fatal intoxication syndrome with a psychiatric presentation, is characterized by excited, paranoid delirium (typified by fear, panic, shouting, physical violence, hyperactivity, and thrashing about), and is accompanied by panic and uncontrolled behavior, mydriasis, hyperpyrexia, and tachypnea (Fishbain and Wetli, 1981; Roehrich and Gold, 1991; Wetli and Fishbain, 1985). This syndrome appears to be closely related to a third, the *neuroleptic malignant syndrome,* which is characterized by hyperthermia and akinesia, or muscular rigidity, as well as by altered consciousness and autonomic dysfunction, as evidenced by delirium, increased heart rate and blood pressure, and diaphoresis (Delay and Deniker, 1968; Levenson, 1985; Pope, Keck, and McElroy, 1986). Rapid progression and irreversibility are likely unless the patient is hydrated and the body temperature is lowered. This disorder results in death in more than 25% of reported cases (Kosten and Kleber, 1988).

A *variant of the neuroleptic malignant* syndrome has also been described, in which intermittent rigidity, as well as intermittent dystonia alternating with substantial agitation, is present (Kosten and Kleber, 1988). This variant may involve decreased postsynaptic availability of dopamine resulting from either direct receptor blockade by neuroleptics (as has been proposed in classic neuroleptic malignant syndrome) or the *relative* depletion of dopamine in hypothalamic and mesolimbic systems (as has been proposed to be the case in cocaine withdrawal). Whereas the classic neuroleptic malignant syndrome is characterized by hyperpyrexia and muscular rigidity (Levenson, 1985), the variant syndrome, as described by Kosten and Kleber (1988), is characterized by minimal rigidity. These writers suggest that dopamine antagonists, the usually indicated intervention for cocaine overdose, are contraindicated when minimal rigidity is present, and that dopamine agonists may reverse this syndrome.

Cocaine abuse may be difficult to diagnose in the absence of obvious signs of such use. Three clinical presentations have been described by Lehrer and Gold (1987). The first is *slight intoxication,* which may be characterized, on the one hand, by giddiness, a high level of energy, talkativeness, and supreme confidence, or, on the other hand, by anxiety and agitation. Tachycardia, increased respiratory rate, pallor, and dilated pupils may persist following the cessation of subjective symptoms. Some 20 to 30 minutes after use of the drug, irritability and depression may appear.

The second presentation, *overdose,* constitutes a medical emergency. The patient may present with acutely psychotic or manic behavior, including paranoia, panic, agitation, or less frequently grandiosity. Delusional behavior centering on pursuit by unknown persons and assaultive behavior in response to perceived threat may be present, as well as tactile, visual, or auditory hallucinations. Existing psychiatric illnesses may be exacerbated, and suicide risk is high, particularly in cases of preexisting psychiatric illness. Physical signs of overdose may be *neurological* (gross tremor, facial and other muscular twitching, increased deep muscle tendon reflexes, and a positive Babinski sign may precede fullblown seizures), *cardiovascular* (tachycardia and premature ventricular contractions may trigger ventricular fibrillation, or direct toxic effects of cocaine on the myocardium may result in heart failure), or *respiratory* (these include pulmonary edema and respiratory collapse). Hyperthermia, coma, and flaccid paralysis may also be present.

Third, *chronic use* may be reflected in a wide variety of physical problems (sore throat, nasal sores, nosebleeds, sinus problems) and psychiatric problems (anergia, insomnia, depression, mania, psychosis). Lehrer and Gold (1987) note that users of cocaine rarely admit to such use, making diagnosis difficult for the physician. Furthermore, cocaine abuse needs to be ruled out before diagnosis of a number of other disorders (for example, adult onset seizures, impotence, infertility, concentration and memory problems, eating disorders, and so on) can be made.

Overdose

Cocaine overdose can occur regardless of route of administration. Once a relatively rare event, it appears to be increasing in frequency of occurrence (see DAWN data, at the beginning of this chapter). In San Francisco, seizures associated with cocaine overdose increased from 4% of all seizures associated with poisoning and drug intoxication in 1981 to 23% from 1988 to 1989 (Olson et al., 1994). One study (Pottieger et al., 1992) found cocaine overdose very common among a combined sample of 350 street users and 349 users in treatment: 40.3% had had at least one cocaine overdose, 26.6% had had at least two, 17.6% at least three, and 10.3% had overdosed four or more times. These rates were substantially higher for the street sample than the in-treatment sample. This finding was true regardless of route of administration (crack use, snorting, or intravenous injection). As to ever having overdosed, only 11.0% of crack users in the treatment sample had done so, compared to 25.5% in the street sample. For snorters, the figures were 5.2% and 55.8%, and in the case of intravenous use 14.5% and 64%. Thus, substantial differences existed between the treatment and street samples with respect to cocaine overdose. Not surprisingly, the street sample also used cocaine more frequently than the treatment sample (91.1% of the former reported daily use of cocaine, versus 18.3% of the latter), although the treatment sample had used more cocaine over time (55.6% of the treatment sample had used a cumulative total of 720 doses, versus 31.4% of the street sample). The street sample were more likely, however, to use only one form of cocaine (89.7% versus 52.1%). These results suggested to Pottieger et al. (1992) that the street sample engaged in riskier drug use behaviors, apparently accepting such risks as part of their involvement in drug use. By contrast, the treatment sample, perhaps having recognized out-of-control behavior prior to treatment entry, were much more conservative in their risk-taking.

Cocaine overdose was (and remains) always possible with the inhalation of powdered cocaine. The unknown purity of street-purchased cocaine may lead to miscalculations concerning actual potency, and to the use of additional doses. The increasingly common use of crack, however, has resulted in a shift from a powder highly diluted with adulterants (only 15–60% pure) to the highly purified base used for smoking (Gay, 1983). The short duration of action of cocaine and the resultant large number of administrations over an extended period of time, regardless of route of administration, also increase the risk of overdose by error (Pottieger et al., 1992).

The study by Pottieger et al. (1992) examined the possibility that increased use of cocaine might be related to age. They reported that use of crack versus other forms of cocaine was not more frequent among younger users than among older users, and that younger users may use smaller quantities of cocaine. Furthermore, overdosing in males was found to be more common where the novice had not been taught how to use crack by an experienced user (18.2% versus 10.8%), though this relationship was in the opposite direction for females (0.0% versus 10.5%). This study presented no evidence suggesting that overdose of crack occurred earlier in cocaine use careers, or that crack users have a higher overdose risk because of using more cocaine. Finally, overdosing was found to lead to changes in drug use—not to quitting (none quit in the street sample, 14.3% in the treatment sample), but rather to shifting to crack use (33.6% in the street sample and 28.6% in the treatment sample). Overdosing was also very unlikely to drive users into treatment.

Cocaine overdose is dose-related but not dose-specific, with wide variations depending on route of administration and patient characteristics. Oral use of cocaine may result in less toxicity than use by inhalation, injection, and smoking, owing to the rapid hydrolyzation of cocaine in the stomach (Gay, 1982). Use of a series of small doses of cocaine below the seizure threshold (that is, the smallest amount of cocaine which may trigger a seizure) may result in the same symptoms that use of a single large dose may previously have produced. Such a "kindling effect" may be particularly likely to trigger seizures (Post and Kopanda, 1976; Post, Kopanda, and Black 1976; and see Chapter 2).

After reviewing the literature on cocaine-related death, Smart and Anglin (1987) concluded that "death from cocaine, when it does occur, is usually rapid, sometimes unpredictable, and is likely to be reported with greater frequency if popular usage increases" (p. 310). They also reached a number of more specific conclusions about the lethality of cocaine, including the following:

1. The LD_{100} (the level at which a certain dose is likely to be lethal for all subjects, versus LD_{50}, the dose level likely to cause death in 50% of subjects) of cocaine for rats is between 35 and 100 mg/kg, for mice between 75 and 100 mg/kg, and for dogs between 16.5 and 24.4 mg/kg.

2. Route of administration affects the minimum lethal dose in animals, with injections into tissue underlying mucous membranes more likely to be fatal than either intravenous or intraperitoneal injection.

3. The lethality of cocaine can be reduced by barbital and chlorpromazine.

4. The range of postmortem cocaine levels in humans is substantial (1–25 micrograms/ml; note, though, that most studies of cocaine-related death in humans do not provide dose levels or postmortem blood cocaine levels).

5. Death may occur with less than the level achieved with a single large street dose.

6. It is not yet clear whether males or females are more susceptible to the lethal effects of cocaine.

Whereas therapeutically safe doses of cocaine, when used locally in surgical patients, average 0.3 mg/l, postmortem blood cocaine levels as high as 6.2 mg/l have been reported in cases of fatal overdose (Kosten and Kleber, 1988; Mittleman and Wetli, 1984). The lethal dose of cocaine has been considered to be 1.2 grams, but as little as 21 mgs, the size of an average "snort," may be toxic (Nakamura and Noguchi, 1981). Wetli and Fishbain (1985) reported blood concentrations averaging 0.6 mg/l in five cases of fatal overdose, or a level some ten times lower than that seen in fatal cocaine overdoses. The range of postmortem blood concentrations of cocaine has been found to vary widely in other studies as well: postmortem blood levels of cocaine were found to range from 0.11 to 75 mg/dl in the study by DiMaio and Garriott (1978). A detailed review of these studies through 1985 may be found in Smart and Anglin (1987).

In an average-sized individual of 70 kilograms (155 lbs.), the fatal dose of cocaine appears to be approximately 1 gm (Rodriguez, 1989). Gay (1981, 1982) estimated the fatal dose to be 1,400 mg by ingestion for a 70 kg individual and 750 to 800 mg by other routes (subcutaneous, intravenous, or inhalation). Doses of cocaine in the 100–300 mg range and above have been reported to have been safely administered topically to the nasal mucosa (Andriani and Zepernick, 1964; Johns et al., 1977; Pearman, 1979). Death has resulted, however, from less than 25 mg applied directly to the mucous membranes for the purpose of inducing local anesthesia (Gay, 1983; Rodriguez, 1989), although death at this dose level is rare. Jones (1984) reported that a survey of plastic surgeons found 5 fatalities and 34 severe reactions among 108,000 patients given topical cocaine. One common source of cocaine overdose occurs when packages of cocaine which have been swallowed or inserted in the vagina or rectum for the purposes of smuggling rupture (for "body packer syndrome," see Beck and Hale, 1993; Commissaris, 1989; Malbrain et al., 1994; McCarron and Wood, 1983).[2] What must be remembered about cocaine with respect to lethality is its *low* therapeutic ratio and *low* margin of safety (Gay, 1981).

Specific Systematic Complications

Many of the medical consequences of cocaine abuse may result from the effects of cocaine's impact on the cardiovascular system. These complications then affect other systems. Among the actions of cocaine on the vascular system, according to Goldfrank and Hoffman (1993), are *neurologic* (intracerebral hemorrhage, cerebral infarction, seizures, migraine headache, vasculitis, and blindness); *cardiac* (myocardial infarction, myocardial ischemia, coronary vasospasm, arrhythmias, myocarditis, and cardiomyopathy); *great vessel* (aortic dissection and rupture, hypertension); *gastrointestinal* (mesenteric ischemia and infarction, gastrointestinal perforation, hepatic failure, and bowel infarction); *pulmonary* (pulmonary edema and infarction); *musculoskeletal* (rhabdomyolysis); *dermatologic* (local ischemia); *uterine, placental, obstetrical, and neonatal* (abruptio placentae, spontaneous abortion, prematurity, developmental delays, growth retardation, and congenital abnormalities); *genitourinary* (renal and testicular infarction, myoglobinuric renal failure); and *venous* actions (vasculitis, superficial and deep venous thrombosis, and thrombophlebitis).

Cardiovascular System

Adverse vascular consequences of cocaine use are most likely related to the vasoconstrictive effects of the drug. Such effects, which produce a simultaneous increase in cardiac output and peripheral resistance, result in transient hypertension (O'Malley and Gawin, 1990).

Cocaine has specific, potentially life-threatening cardiovascular effects. These effects are not limited to parenteral use of the drug and occur regardless of route of administration (Isner et al., 1986). Cardiovascular problems are very common among cocaine abusers, and may be reflective of myocardial infarction or neurological vascular complications in young, otherwise low-risk cocaine users (Olshaker, 1994). Abnormal electrocardiogram variations have been found in 56% to 84% of patients with cocaine-related chest pain, although there has been a suggestion that such abnormalities may be attributable to "normal" variation (Hollander et al., 1994).

Cardiovascular effects of cocaine are likely due to cocaine's inhibition of norepinephrine reuptake at the nerve terminal. This results in tachycardia, vasoconstriction, and increased systolic blood pressure. Consequences of such changes may include ischemia or acute myocardial infarction resulting from an increased myocardial oxygen demand (Ascher, Stauffer, and Gaasch, 1988; Coleman, Ross, and Naughton, 1982; Weiss, 1986). Coronary artery constriction and spasm may also result directly from cocaine use, and may compromise cardiac functioning, resulting in cardiac crises (Allred and Ewer, 1981; Lam and Goldschlager, 1988; Lange et al., 1989; Rod and Zucker, 1987; Simpson and Edwards, 1986).

Cocaine is itself arrhythmogenic, either directly through toxic effects on cardiac tissue or through its effects on catecholamines. Arrhythmias produced directly by cocaine include sinus tachycardia, ventricular premature contractions, ventricular tachycardia and fibrillation, and asystole. Such cocaine-induced acute cardiac changes may occur in patients in whom there is no apparent predisposition for or prior history of coronary artery disease (Cregler and Mark, 1986a, b; Howard, Hueter, and Davis, 1985; Isner et al., 1986). Thus, the presence of undiagnosed myocardial injury in patients with a history of cocaine abuse should not be an unexpected finding, although the extent to which such damage may be attributable in part to adulterants or cigarette smoking is unknown (Tanenbaum and Miller, 1992). In those persons with underlying coronary artery disease, the use of cocaine represents a serious potential hazard. Other cardiovascular complications may include asystole and ventricular fibrillation (Nanji and Filipenko, 1984), accelerated ventricular rhythm (Benchimol, Bartall, and Desser, 1978), aortic rupture (Barth, Bray, and Roberts, 1986), hypertension (Rappolt, Gay, and Inaba, 1977), vascular headaches (Satel and Gawin, 1989), deep vein thrombosis (Lisse and Davis, 1989), and the acceleration of coronary atherosclerosis (Dressler, Malekzadeh, and Roberts, 1990).

Peng, French, and Pelikan (1989) reported seven cases of congestive heart failure in patients with a history of cocaine abuse, and concluded that long-term abuse of cocaine may have played a role in the development of this problem. The laboratory findings by Abel et al. (1989) of a direct myocardial depressant effect of cocaine provides support for such an interpretation. It has also been suggested that chronic cocaine use may result in irreversible cardiovascular damage (Wetli, 1993). Similarly, Langer, Perry, and Bement (1989) have suggested that chronic cocaine use may result in accelerated atherosclerosis. One explanation for these effects may be that cocaine has the potential to induce arterial damage directly, through biochemical or histopathological changes in the arterial wall, although the exact mechanism for these effects is not known.

Given all the potential cardiac risks associated with the illicit use of cocaine, it is not surprising that the drug is likely to be implicated in sudden death among abusers (Karch and Billingham, 1988). Cardiac fatalities, though relatively rare events, are a well-publicized consequence of cocaine use. They are most likely to occur in patients who have become hyperthermic and whose behavior is agitated. Schrank (1993) reported that, in her own and her colleagues' experience, the prognosis for cocaine-induced cardiac arrest is "dismal."

Central Nervous System

The profound effects of cocaine on the central nervous system are well illustrated by the following statement: "Cocaine is a drug with serious and unpredictable effects on the brain [and] crack is the most toxic of the street drugs abused over the past three decades ... Permanent neurological injury can occur with first-time use" (Miller et al., 1993, p. 129).

Cocaine abuse has been associated with a number of significant neurologic complications, including subarachnoid hemorrhage, cerebral infarction, cerebral ischemia, intraparenchymal hemorrhage, seizures, cerebral vasculitis, cerebral arterial spasm, anterior spinal artery syndrome, lateral medullary syndrome, partial motor seizures, and death (Cregler and Mark, 1986a, b; Kaye and Fainstat, 1987; Krendel et al., 1990; Levine et al., 1990; Lichtenfield, Rubin, and Feldman, 1984; Mody et al., 1988; Morrow and McQuillen, 1993). The relative frequency of neurologic complaints is not high, although their potential seriousness is. In the study by Lowenstein et al. (1987a) of 996 emergency room visits and 279 hospital admissions with complications of cocaine abuse at San Francisco General Hospital, 57 cases presented with neurological complications. These included one or more seizures ($N = 29$), focal neurological symptoms or signs ($N = 12$), including transient sensory and motor complaints ($N = 3$), and blurriness or loss of vision ($N = 2$), headache ($N = 10$), and transient loss of consciousness ($N = 6$). Neurologic complications seen in the case study report by Mody et al. (1988) were primarily associated with acute use of cocaine (79%) rather than chronic use (21%). Many subtle cocaine-related neurological complications, previously undiagnosed, may now begin to be identified as a result of positron emission tomography (PET) technology (Tumeh et al., 1990).

CONVULSIONS AND SEIZURES

In at least one study (Lowenstein et al., 1987a), convulsions and seizures represented the most common complications of cocaine use. The appearance of convulsions and seizures may be in part a function of cocaine's lowering of the seizure threshold (Jonsson, O'Meara, and Young, 1983; Ritchie and Greene, 1990). Seizure may also be secondary to central nervous system–induced cardiac events (Mittleman and Wetli, 1984), or it may in part be the result of cocaine-induced high fevers (Roberts, Quattrocchi, and Howland, 1984). Seizures, however, are not necessarily a prerequisite to, or accompaniment of, other toxic effects of cocaine, including cardiac toxicity (Isner et al., 1986).

Unlike the case for amphetamines, where seizures are more likely to result from repeated use, seizures may occur at the first use of cocaine (Van Dyke and Byck, 1982). Seizures may also occur with use of even small quantities of cocaine (Alldredge, Lowenstein, and Simon, 1989). Cocaine-induced tonic-clonic seizures generally occur within minutes of administration of the drug through intravenous, nasal, or inhalation routes; the time of onset following oral use is less predictable (Schrank, 1993). Seizures resulting from cocaine use appear to occur with equal frequency regardless of route (Alldredge, Lowenstein, and Simon, 1989; Holland et al., 1992). In the case of cocaine overdose, generalized seizures, usually rapid in their onset, may not appear for as long as an hour after use, and may result in respiratory collapse and death (Wetli and Wright, 1979).

Cocaine-induced seizures are typically isolated and of limited duration, and are unlikely to result in residual damage. Repeated seizures, however, carry the risk of respiratory arrest, thus requiring aggressive management which consists of administration of diazepam or other benzodiazepines in addition to the maintenance of an open airway. Administration of phenytoin or phenobarbital should be considered if diazepam proves ineffective. Neuromuscular blockade or general anesthesia may also be needed, and complications resulting from hyperthermia, rhabdomyolysis, respiratory and lactic acidoses, hypoglycemia, electrolyte disturbances, and trauma require rapid management. Once stabilization has been achieved, evaluation for central nervous system hemorrhage, stroke, trauma, and the presence of other drugs of abuse should be initiated immediately. In the event of uncomplicated seizure, some preventive education about the risks of cocaine use should be provided (Schrank, 1993).

Children and adolescents may present neurologic manifestations secondary to passive intoxication as a result of having been in rooms where crack cocaine was being smoked. In a study of 41 children aged 2 months to 18 years with documented exposure to cocaine, Mott, Packer, and Soldin (1994) found evidence of seizures ($N = 7$), blunting of pain (6), delirium (4), dizziness (1), drooling (1), and ataxia (1). While the difficulties of determining the neurological effects of cocaine were acknowledged, two major drug-related patterns were observed: seizures and blunting of pain in each child of less than 5 years of age; and in children over age 11, delirium, dizziness, drooling, and lethargy. The authors concluded that cocaine exposure is common in children, as are neurologic manifestations of such exposure; that passive inhalation of cocaine is associated with both focal and generalized seizures with evidence of structural brain injury; that in children predisposed to seizures, exposure to cocaine lowers the seizure threshold; that in children over 8 years of age, manifestations of cocaine exposure are similar to those seen in adults; and that adolescents exposed to cocaine experience higher than normal rates of trauma and motor vehicle accidents. As a result of these findings, the authors recommended urine toxicological screens in the event of all first-time seizures, as well as first-time febrile seizures. The importance of this recommendation is underlined by the finding that 5.4% of young children presenting at an urban pediatric emergency room were found to test positive for benzoylecgonine (Rosenberg et al., 1991).

Other central nervous system effects which may be precipitated by cocaine, and which often cease after discontinuation of cocaine use, include tics, persistent mechanical repetition of speech or movement, ataxia, and disturbed gait (Estroff and Gold, 1987). Cerebral atrophy has also been identified as a possible complication of cocaine use. Habitual cocaine users, compared with first-time users and headache patients, have been found to have a significantly higher rate of atrophy, primarily of the frontal lobes, suggesting not only that cerebral atrophy develops in chronic cocaine abusers, but also that its severity is a function of the duration of abuse (Pascual-Leone, Dhuna, and Anderson, 1991). These findings are consistent with those obtained in another study (Tumeh et al., 1990), although the mechanisms for this atrophy, other than possibly being the result of ischemia, were unclear. Finally, since cocaine has a direct effect on the temperature-regulating centers of the central nervous system, hyperpyrexia may occur, together with peripheral vasoconstriction, resulting in a decrease in rate of heat loss, and thus hyperpyrexia, which can lead to possible seizures and death (Kosten and Kleber, 1988; Levenson, 1985).

STROKE

Cerebrovascular accidents (strokes) have been observed in temporal association with cocaine use (Brust and Richter, 1977; Klonoff, Andrews, and Obana, 1989; Lichtenfeld, Rubin, and Feldman, 1984; Petty et al., 1990; Schrank, 1993; Schwartz and Cohen, 1984; Wojak and Flamm, 1987), sometimes within minutes of intranasal administration (Brown et al. 1992; Cregler and Mark, 1986b). Strokes related to cocaine abuse have increased markedly in the United States since the early 1980s, while the overall number of strokes has decreased by 50% (Klonoff, Andrews, and Obana, 1989). Stroke is likely to be observed as a consequence of cocaine abuse in young adults, a group that normally has a relatively low expected incidence of strokes. Among drugs of abuse, cocaine may account for a significant proportion of such cases. Kaku and Lowenstein (1989) examined 65 cases of stroke which occurred in persons under age 50 "in the setting of recreational drug use" (p. 162), and found cocaine abuse implicated in 31 cases, heroin in 26, amphetamine in 15, Ritalin in 5, and PCP in 2 cases.

Reviewing the findings of a number of studies, Brown et al. (1992) found ischemic manifestations, intraparenchymal hemorrhage, and subarachnoid hemorrhage to be the most common central nervous system manifestations of cocaine abuse, with hemorrhage occurring at about twice the rate of ischemias. When hemorrhage was present, approximately half of patients were found to have a preexisting vascular abnormality. Levine et al. (1990) found cerebrovascular events associated with crack cocaine use in 28 cases to be primarily cerebral infarction in the areas supplied by the middle cerebral artery ($N = 10$), anterior cerebral artery ($N = 3$), and vertebrobasilar arteries ($N = 4$), and hemorrhage, either subarachnoid ($N = 5$) or intraparenchymal ($N = 4$). Acute neurological symptoms occurred immediately or within one hour after using cocaine in 64% of cases, with 45% of patients having severe headache as an early symptom.

Nervous system hemorrhagic ischemic complications of cocaine use have been seen at times as secondary to complications of the cardiovascular system, such as myocardial infarction, acute coronary artery thrombosis, cardiac arrhythmias, asystole, or respiratory arrest (Brown et al., 1992). The absence of traditional risk factors for stroke led Daras, Tuchman, and Marks (1991) to suggest the possibility that multiple overlapping mechanisms may account for cocaine-related infarcts. Among those identified in their study were vasospasm, sudden onset of hypertension, myocardial infarction with cardiac arrhythmias, increased platelet aggregation, and hypotension. Additionally, embolisms resulting from impurities in injected street cocaine (for example, talc, sugar, mannitol) have been seen as possibly affecting the central nervous system through decreased perfusion or the creation of embolisms. Although intracranial hemorrhage resulting from the use of cocaine usually occurs within seconds, or sometimes minutes, of cocaine use, it may also lag behind use by as much as twelve hours, though explaining the mechanism(s) underlying such long delays of hemorrhage is problematic (Brown et al., 1992). Stroke may follow administration of cocaine by any route (Klonoff, Andrews, and Obana, 1989). No evidence exists for a relationship between route of administration and type of stroke (Rowbotham and Lowenstein, 1990).

A "remarkable consistency" in findings in brain hemorrhage associated with cocaine has been noted by Miller et al. (1993). At least 50% of patients demonstrated an underlying abnormality in cerebral blood vessels, typically arteriovenous malformations and cerebral aneurysms. Where cocaine-induced stroke occurs in patients with underlying vascular malformations, the likely explanatory mechanism is the transient elevation of blood pressure that occurs following ingestion of cocaine (Brown et al., 1992; Wojak and Flamm, 1987). Headaches may be present after cocaine use, and their presence may be suggestive of intracranial hemorrhage (Cregler and Mark, 1986b). Subsequent to these sympathetically induced effects, blood pressure is likely to drop as the result of direct toxic effects on the myocardium (Goldfrank and Hoffman, 1993).

Since, as noted earlier, most central nervous system infarctions and hemorrhages attributable to cocaine generally occur in young patients who otherwise have a low prevalence of stroke (Kaku and Lowenstein, 1989; Rowbotham and Lowenstein, 1990), cocaine use should be considered a possible cause when stroke or intracerebral hemorrhage is seen in patients under age 40 (Brown et al., 1992). Finally, cerebral infarction in infants has been attributed to maternal use of cocaine (Singer et al., 1994). Chasnoff et al. (1986) suggested the need to consider maternal cocaine abuse in the differential diagnosis of neonates with perinatal cerebral infarction.

HEADACHE

Headache has been associated with cocaine abuse in a number of published clinical reports (DiMaio and Garriott, 1978; Goldfrank and Hoffman, 1993; Lowenstein et al., 1987a; Roehrich and Gold, 1991; Satel and Gawin, 1989; Washton, Gold, and Pottash, 1984). Cocaine-related headache is directly related to level of cocaine use, with 22% of low-, 58% of medium-, and 79% of high-use individuals reporting headaches (Chitwood, 1985). Headaches appear always to precede cerebrovascular accidents, although patients with vascular headaches triggered by cocaine *without* subsequent neurologic diagnoses are unlikely to be admitted to a hospital and thus are generally absent from studies (Lipton, Choy-Kwong, and Solomon, 1989).

There have, however, been conflicting reports in the literature concerning the relationship between cocaine and migraine headaches. Dhopesh, Maany, and Herring (1991) noted that this inconsistency is long-standing. For example, they cite a case report that the relief of migraine through self-medication with cocaine freebase led to the development of a full-blown cocaine dependency disorder (Brower, 1988), while other reports suggest that migraine headaches resulting from cocaine use have led some patients to stop their abuse of the drug (Satel and Gawin, 1989). In a survey of inpatient polysubstance abusers, Dhopesh, Maany, and Herring (1991) found that cocaine could trigger headaches several hours after use. Cocaine, however, was more likely to relieve migraine-like headaches in chronic headache sufferers than in those who suffered only occasional headaches. This combination of immediate headache relief followed by onset of headache several hours later suggested to the researchers that these effects were the result of the immediate vasoconstrictive effects of cocaine, followed by vasodilation during the withdrawal period.

Mechanisms Underlying Central Nervous System Complications

Many of the central nervous system effects noted so far are likely caused by the increased blood pressure and tachycardia resulting from adrenergic effects triggered by the administration of cocaine, although cerebral vasoconstriction may also play a role (Caplan, Hier, and Banks, 1982; Lichtenfeld, Rubin, and Feldman, 1984). Predisposing vascular lesions, such as aneurysms or arteriovenous malformations, may account for a significant percentage of cocaine-related strokes (Green et al., 1990; Klonoff, Andrews, and Obana, 1989). In this regard, Miller et al. (1993) noted what they considered a remarkable consistency in brain hemorrhage associated with cocaine. At least 50% of patients demonstrated predisposing vascular lesions.

Thus, the evidence supports the observation of Miller et al. (1993) that "cocaine is a drug with serious and unpredictable effects on the brain." Furthermore, with respect to crack, they note that "crack is the most toxic of the street drugs abused over the past three decades ... [P]ermanent neurological damage can result even with first time use" (p. 129). While infrequent use is indeed less dangerous, it is clearly not risk-free.

Respiratory System

Signs of cocaine use found in the nasal air passages include chronic irritation and rhinitis, rhinorrhea, stuffiness, atrophy of the nasal mucosa, madarosis, ulceration, necrosis, and perforation of the nasal septum.[3] Many of these effects are the result of cocaine's vasoconstrictive effects secondary to sympathetic nervous system activation and irritation of the respiratory mucosa (Meisels and Loke, 1993). A study of 336 recovering adolescent cocaine abusers found the presence of nasal symptoms to be related to frequency of cocaine inhalation, with frequent abusers generally reporting more symptoms, including nasal crusts or scabs, "sinus problems," recurrent nosebleeds, or combinations of these (Schwartz et al., 1989). Cessation of use often results in vascular dilation and rhinorrhea (Estroff and Gold, 1986).

In extreme cases, or where use is prolonged, significant structural damage to the nasal cavity may occur, including disintegration of the nasal cartilage and loss of the structural integrity of the nasal cavity (Brown et al., 1992). According to Wetli (1993), this damage may result from one or more of three mechanisms: intermittent vasoconstrictive effects of cocaine, which limit the supply of oxygen and nutrients to the affected areas; the dissociation of cocaine hydrochloride into a weak base and a strong acid; and direct toxic effects of cocaine on capillary epithelial cells, resulting in capillary destruction and tissue breakdown. Of course, the presence of potentially toxic adulterants may greatly expand the potential mechanisms by which damage can occur (Shannon, 1988). Loss of the sense of smell may also occur, although one study has suggested that olfactory damage is unlikely to be permanent (Gordon et al., 1990), despite earlier reports suggesting this was the case (for example, Schwartz et al., 1989). Aspiration of cocaine into the frontal sinuses can produce infection and inflammation. Decreased carbon monoxide diffusing capacity has been reported by Itkonen, Schnoll, and Glassroth (1984) and Weiss et al. (1981), although findings with respect to this complication were not confirmed in another study (Tashkin et al., 1987).

Inhalation or smoking of powdered cocaine can produce significant respiratory complications, including cough, production of bloody or black sputum, hemoptysis, chest pain, and wheezing and shortness of breath (Khalsa, Tashkin, and Perrochet, 1992). Such complications may also be present in 25% to 60% of cocaine freebase abusers, but relatively few seek medical attention for them (Laposata and Mayo, 1993). Frequently, chest pain is the reason that drives the cocaine user to seek medical attention (Gold, 1992). Similarly, the smoking of crack can cause acute, severe respiratory symptomatology; abnormalities in lung function; and, in some cases, life-threatening lung injury. For example, smoking of freebase cocaine has been reported to result in spontaneous pneumomediastinium and pneumopericardium (Adrouny and Magnusson, 1985; Bush et al., 1984; Shesser, Davis, and Edelstein, 1981). Murray et al. (1988) found that chronic cocaine use resulted in pulmonary artery hypertrophy and hyperplasia in the absence of foreign body microembolization, a high frequency of occult pulmonary hemorrhage, and bronchospasm resulting from inhalation of cocaine. Bailey et al. (1994) have suggested that pulmonary hemorrhage is more common than is believed, and that chronic pulmonary disease (for example, interstitial hemoptysis) may occur in long-term cocaine users.

Heavy, habitual crack smoking was found by Tashkin et al. (1992) to be associated with a number of respiratory problems. These included symptoms of an acute nature, including cough, black sputum, and chest pain; an obstructive ventilatory abnormality involving the large airways; and mild but significant impairment in the carbon monoxide defusing capacity of the lung. These findings were interpreted by the authors as suggesting that heavy, habitual crack smoking results in respiratory tract injury and an abnormality of gas diffusion at the alveolar-capillary level. Inhalation of cocaine can also result in anesthesia and paralysis of the pharynx and larynx, resulting in hoarseness and possibly an aspiration pneumonia (Estroff and Gold, 1986). The term "crack lung" has been coined to describe a condition in which the patient presents with the symptoms of pneumonia in the absence of x-ray confirmation of such a condition and failure to respond to standard treatment (Barden, 1989). The symptoms of oxygen starvation and blood loss in persons with this condition may be fatal (Gold, 1992).

Other respiratory complications of inhalation of freebase or crack cocaine use include pneumothorax, interstitial pneumonitis, and subcutaneous emphysema (Aroesty, Stanley, and Crockett, 1986; O'Donnell et al., 1991; Shesser, Davis, and Edelstein, 1981). Bronchospasm may also be seen in association with the smoking of crack cocaine (Schrank, 1993). In some patients bronchospasm may result in association with an immunoglobulin-E–mediated hypersensitivity reaction (Ettinger and Albin, 1989). Pneumonia is another complication of crack smoking, caused either by acquired organisms or by undiagnosed hypersensitivity reactions. Finally, crack smoking is frequently associated with tracheobronchitis accompanied by severe cough (Delbono, O'Brien, and Murphy, 1989). A moderate level of pulmonary edema is a not uncommon postmortem finding in cocaine-related death (Allred and Ewer, 1981; Schrank, 1993).

The effects of crack inhalation may appear after relatively short use, and may persist after cessation of use (Itkonen, Schnoll, and Glassroth, 1984). Among habitual marijuana users, "moderate" crack cocaine use (lifetime use, 1 to 12 occasions) was found to result in damage to both large and small airways. Such damage was independent of concomitant marijuana use and was synergistic with the effects of tobacco smoking. Cocaine smoking did not appear to affect pulmonary microcirculation, however (Tashkin et al., 1987). One problem in accurately attributing pulmonary complications to cocaine abuse is the fact that many cocaine abusers also smoke tobacco and marijuana (Laposata and Mayo, 1993).

Gastrointestinal System

Cocaine use may cause abdominal pain, typically in the mild-to-moderate range, accompanied by vomiting. These episodes last only a few hours, are accompanied by nonspecific physical signs and negative laboratory findings, and are resolved spontaneously. Such events are likely the result of mild intestinal ischemia resulting from the vasoconstrictive effects of cocaine on the mesenteric vessels. A high rate of gastroduodenal perforation has been found to be associated with crack use (Lee et al., 1990). Ulceration and other signs consistent with pseudomembranous colitis may result secondary to mucosal ischemia

(Brown, Rosenholtz, and Marshall, 1994; Fishel et al., 1985). Focal vasospasm, intravascular thrombosis, or systemic hypotension resulting from cardiac complications of cocaine may also result in bowel insults, including acute mesenteric ischemia (Freudenberger, Cappell, and Hutt, 1990). Severe mesenteric ischemia can lead to bowel infarction, accompanied by elevated white blood cell count, metabolic acidosis, and shock (Schrank, 1993).

As noted in Chapter 2, the oral ingestion of cocaine does not reduce its effectiveness. In fact, highs produced by oral ingestion may be at least as effective, dose for dose, as those produced by inhalation, while the subjective effects may be even greater (Van Dyke et al., 1978). Although oral ingestion is not as common as inhalation or injection use, complications may occur not only as a result of deliberate ingestion, but also as a result of the rupture of swallowed cocaine-filled packages (usually condoms) being smuggled past customs inspection barriers by "body packers" or "mules." In both cases intestinal ischemia may occur, with resultant gangrene, owing to the vasoconstrictive effects of cocaine on bowel vasculature (Cregler and Mark, 1986a). Particularly where large doses are involved, death may result either from complications of gangrene or from the effects of drug overdose. The management of cases in which unruptured ingested packets of cocaine are present has been described by Caruana et al. (1984). Although surgical removal was recommended in the past to avoid massive cocaine poisoning from ruptured packets, improvements in packaging (now including machine packaging) and materials, in addition to frequent refusal of surgeons to intervene, has generally led to a more conservative observational approach (Schrank, 1993). Ingestion may also occur when unpackaged or poorly packaged cocaine is swallowed by an individual desiring to dispose of the drug when facing imminent arrest. Here the risk of cocaine intoxication in higher, although the doses involved may be smaller. Crack cocaine may be less dangerous than the hydrochloride form owing to the limited solubility of crack cocaine (Schrank, 1993).

Genitourinary System

A number of degenerative disorders resulting from cocaine use involve the kidneys. Rhabdomyolysis and myoglobinuria are particularly common among patients presenting at the emergency room with cocaine-related problems. Hypertensive patients may also be at risk for acute tubular necrosis (Schrank, 1993). Two cases of acute renal complications (infarction or failure) following cocaine use have been reported (Kramer and Turner, 1993; Turbat-Herrera, 1994).

Obstetrical and Neonatal Complications

Cocaine use by pregnant women represents a potentially significant threat to the neonate, although the extent of this threat is disputed (Finnegan, 1994; Streissguth and Finnegan, 1996). The prevalence of cocaine use in expectant or nursing mothers ranges from 12% to 15% (see, for example, Chasnoff, Landress, and Barrett, 1990; Galanter et al., 1992; Rowbotham and Lowenstein, 1990). In New York City the rate of illicit drug use during pregnancy has been reported to range from 11% to 20%, most involving cocaine or crack (Chavkin, 1990). The increase between 1980 and 1989 of delivering mothers reporting use of cocaine and/or crack during pregnancy from 1.0 per 1,000 live births to 23 per 1,000 live births (Greenberg et al., 1991) represents a public health problem of major magnitude. In a study by Chasnoff, Landress, and Barrett (1990), the prevalence of cocaine use by pregnant women was not found to differ as a function of medical setting (private office versus public clinics). While overall prevalence of drug use also did not differ as a function of race or ethnicity (white versus African American), African American women were more likely to use cocaine (7.5% versus 1.8%), while white women were more likely to use cannabinoids (14.4% versus 6.0%). A more recent study suggests that rates of cocaine use in pregnant women have begun to decline (Yawn et al., 1994).

Adverse outcomes in pregnancy may occur through both direct effects on the developing fetus and alteration of the normal course of pregnancy. Cocaine has been found to cross the placenta and accumulate in fetal tissues (Shah, May, and Yates, 1980). Thus, direct effects on fetal tissue, as well as indirect effects, are possible. The former may occur through reductions in oxygen delivery to the fetus by catecholamine-mediated vasoconstriction of uterine arteries (Ellis et al., 1993). Furthermore, fetal hypoxia may itself stimulate the release of catecholamines (Cohen et al., 1984; Ellis et al., 1993; Phillippe, 1983). Perinatal complications of cocaine abuse may be equally severe whether the cocaine use is erratic or daily (Burkett et al., 1994). Examples of consequences for the developing fetus through the direct effects of cocaine include increased risk of congenital malformations (including skull defects and congenital heart defects), perinatal mortality, developmental impairments, and even strokes in the infant during birth (Bingol et al., 1987; Chasnoff et al., 1985).

Indirectly, cocaine use may alter the course of pregnancy, resulting in adverse outcomes, including premature detachment of the placenta, or abruptio placentae (Acker et al., 1983; Bingol et al., 1987; Chasnoff, 1985; Chasnoff et al., 1989); uterine rupture (Iriye et al., 1994); placenta previa (Handler et al., 1994); premature onset of labor (Cherukuri et al., 1988; Chouteau, Namerow, and Leppert, 1988; Dinsmoor, Irons, and Christmas, 1994); and vaginal bleeding. Each has been observed immediately after intravenous use of cocaine, and loss of the fetus may result (Bingol et al., 1987). Problems encountered in neonates where maternal cocaine use has been present include small size for gestational age and low birth weight, and decreased head circumference (Bingol et al., 1987; Chasnoff, 1986; Chasnoff et al., 1985, 1989; Cherukuri et al., 1988; Chiu, Vaughn, and Carzoli, 1990; Chouteau, Namerow, and Leppert, 1988; Galanter et al., 1992; Hadeed and Siegel, 1989; Ryan, Ehrlich, and Finnegan, 1987; Woods et al., 1993; Zuckerman et al., 1989), although such findings are not universal (see, for example, Chasnoff, 1985; Madden, Payne and Miller, 1986). Other adverse effects include limb-reduction defects (Hoyme et al., 1990) and genitourinary tract or renal abnormalities (Chasnoff, 1985; Chasnoff and Chisum, 1987; Chasnoff, Chisum, and Kaplan, 1988; Chávez, Mulinare, and Cordero, 1989), including "prune belly syndrome" (a congenital condition in which there is a partial or complete absence of the abdominal muscles; in males this condition is often accompanied by genitourinary anomalies), hypospadias, and hydronephrosis. Cocaine-exposed very low birth weight infants were found to be at higher risk of intraventricular hemorrhage. They are also more likely to be placed outside maternal care, and to have a higher incidence of cognitive and motor delay at follow-up.

Among other consequences of maternal cocaine use during pregnancy are microcephaly, which was reported in two studies as occurring in as many as 21% (Hadeed and Siegel, 1989) and 43% (Fries et al., 1993), respectively, of newborn infants whose mothers had used cocaine during pregnancy (although the latter figure likely includes infants with fetal alcohol syndrome), and retarded intrauterine growth (Cabral, Timperi, and Buchner, 1989). Cerebral lesions, including diffuse atrophy, deep brain cysts, perinatal infarction, and hemorrhages, may also be present in neonates (Chasnoff et al., 1986; Ferriero, Partridge, and Wong, 1988). Brown et al. (1992) have suggested that such effects, in their similarity to those seen in low birth weight infants, may be associated with fetal hypoxia and its effects on the regulation of cerebral blood flow. Cocaine use during pregnancy was found in one study to be the best predictor of the increased incidence of a variety of childbirth outcomes, including abortions and poor prenatal care. After controlling for prematurity, cocaine use was also the best predictor of preterm birth and of low birth weight. Maternal use of cocaine and alcohol in combination also best predicted decreased linear growth, after controlling for prematurity (Singer et al., 1994).

The greater prevalence of medical problems in infants born to cocaine-using mothers may be in part a function of the relatively lower likelihood of such mothers' having had appropriate prenatal care. It may also reflect a diminished ability to care for infants. One study demonstrated that cocaine-addicted mothers generally made fewer prenatal visits to a physician, and reported more depressive symptoms following delivery (Woods et al., 1993). Rates of spontaneous abortion among women who use cocaine during pregnancy also appear to be even higher than those observed among women who use heroin during pregnancy (Chasnoff et al., 1985; Ryan, Ehrlich, and Finnegan, 1987).

It is likely that cocaine has teratogenic effects, and may indeed be a true teratogen, capable of inducing both structural and neurologic injury in the fetus (Gingras et al., 1992). Administration of cocaine at midgestation can result in congenital anomalies in mice (Mahalik, Gautiere, and Mann, 1980) and rats (Webster, Brown-Woodman, and Lipson, 1990), and several studies have found increased rates of such anomalies in infants born to cocaine-exposed women, likely owing to insults to the fetus at different stages of development (Bingol et al., 1987; Dominguez et al., 1991). Brown et al. (1992) noted that evidence exists for a finding of increased rates of central nervous system lesions resulting from in utero use of cocaine, given findings of a prevalence of 12% to 15% cocaine use in expectant or nursing mothers (see, for example, Chasnoff, Landress, and Barrett, 1990; Rowbotham and Lowenstein, 1990). The authors concluded that such findings suggest that cocaine use during pregnancy is common, and that the public health implications of such use are alarming. In an analysis of variables contributing to poor perinatal outcome and cocaine exposure, the single best predictor of outcome was cocaine use (Eyler et al., 1990), even after controlling for socioeconomic status (Hurt, Brodsky, and Giannetta, 1990). Finally, a prospective, controlled study of prenatal cocaine exposure failed to find any congenital anomalies of the developing eye among infants (Stafford et al., 1994).

Some of these adverse outcomes have been attributed to indirect effects on the fetus resulting from cocaine's pharmacological actions, that is, alterations of uterine blood flow, including maternal and fetal vasoconstriction, tachycardia, hypertension, and contraction of the fetus (Bingol et al. 1987; Chasnoff, 1991). Adverse consequences of these effects include growth retardation, microcephaly, and congenital anomalies, all attributable to intrauterine hypoxia and malnutrition secondary to vasoconstriction. Chasnoff (1991) attributes these problems to disruption of fetal development rather than to malformations. Neurobehavioral problems, however, may result from direct toxic effects of cocaine on the developing nervous system. Such effects may present a particularly intractable problem. Unlike other complications, which may be decreased by simple cessation of cocaine use, central nervous system complications may not be reversible by cessation of cocaine abuse.

Infants exposed to cocaine were found by Chasnoff et al. (1985) to have significantly depressed interactional behavior and a poor organizational response to environmental stimuli. The authors concluded that cocaine exerts an effect on the outcome of pregnancy as well as on neonatal neurobehavior. Another report by Chasnoff (1985) also attributed neurobehavioral deficiencies to cocaine use during pregnancy. These findings of adverse effects on mothers and newborns have been disputed, however. Woods et al. (1993) failed to find differences between cocaine-exposed and nonexposed infants with respect to neonatal performance on the Brazelton Scale at birth or one month of age. Furthermore, the teratogenic effect of maternal cocaine administration has been questioned with particular emphasis placed on a lack of replication of findings, as well as on the lack of controls in these studies for other contributing factors such as cigarette smoking, alcohol or other drug consumption, low socioeconomic status, age, sexually transmitted diseases, and so on (Finnegan, 1994; Streissguth and Finnegan, 1996). Final determination of these effects clearly awaits additional study.

Little et al. (1989) compared pregnancy outcomes and health status of infants born to 53 women who had abused cocaine during pregnancy (all had abused the drug during the first trimester, most by intravenous injection, and about three-quarters throughout the pregnancy) with a group of 100 nonexposed mothers and infants. Complications more often present in the cocaine-exposed group included preterm labor, meconium, tachycardia, lower birth weight, and congenital cardiac anomalies. Chiu, Vaughn, and Carzoli (1990) also found cocaine-exposed infants to have a lower mean birth weight (by 378 grams) than their healthy counterparts and to require longer hospital stays. While weight differences at birth may disappear by 6 months of age, stunting of length may persist past this point, despite adequate nourishment (Harsham, Keller, and Disbrow, 1994).

Chasnoff et al. (1989) compared outcomes for women who had used cocaine only during the first trimester of pregnancy, women who had used cocaine throughout their pregnancies, and groups of non-users. Women who had used cocaine throughout pregnancy had an increased rate of preterm delivery, low birth weight infants, and intrauterine growth retardation. Those women who had used cocaine only during the first trimester had rates of complications similar to those for the drug-free group. The incidence of abruptio placentae, however, did not decrease if the woman abstained from cocaine use during the last two trimesters of pregnancy. Thus, improved intrauterine growth was present when cocaine use ceased after the first trimester, suggesting that for those patients who stop drug use, continued normal fetal growth will take place. Also, damage done to placental and uterine vessels during the first trimester of pregnancy appears not to be reversed by cessation of cocaine use during the second and third trimesters. Infants in both cocaine-using groups, however, were significantly impaired with respect to orientation, motor, and regulation behaviors. A study by Kliegman and associates (1994) found that only cocaine use near the time of delivery remained a predictor of prematurity and low birth weight after multivariate analysis. This study raised the question of whether as-yet-unknown socioeconomic or cultural factors, aside from or in addition to the pharmacological properties of cocaine, could have contributed to the duration of gestation or fetal growth.

The results of a three-year longitudinal prospective study of the long-term developmental effects of cocaine exposure in utero were reported by Azuma and Chasnoff (1993). Drug exposure was found to have a direct effect on cognitive ability at 3 years of age; such effects, however, were found to be mediated indirectly by head circumference, home environment, and level of task perseverance.

Yet, not all studies have found adverse effects attributable to perinatal cocaine abuse. For example, a study by Madden, Payne, and Miller (1986) found no deleterious effects on infants at birth of prenatal cocaine and other drug use (as identified by mothers' positive urine toxicologies). Nonetheless, given that this was a report of unremarkable findings in a small-sample, uncontrolled case study, it does not strongly counter the findings already presented. Likewise, Nair, Rothblum, and Hebel (1994) compared neonates with evidence of fetal exposure to drugs of abuse, including cocaine, and found no effects of such exposure on birth weight, head circumference, length, and Apgar scores, although cocaine and/or opiate–exposed infants had a greater length of hospital stay. Similarly, Beeram and associates (1994) found no effect of intrauterine cocaine exposure on the incidence of respiratory distress syndrome in very low birth weight infants. Intrauterine exposure to cocaine was also not found to influence the prevalence or severity of intraventricular hemorrhage in preterm infants by McLenan et al. (1994). With respect to intellectual development, Barone (1993), employing an uncontrolled case study methodology, found the literacy development of children 1 through 7 years of age who had been prenatally exposed to crack or cocaine to fall within a normal range.

A distinctive phenotype has been described for a "fetal cocaine syndrome" (see, for example, Fries et al., 1993), but definition and evaluation of this syndrome are difficult owing to the high rate of alcohol abuse accompanying cocaine abuse when the latter is present in pregnant women, and the resulting high rates of fetal alcohol syndrome in neonates (Fries et al., 1993), as well as the lack of well-defined symptomatology, since a wide spectrum of physical defects resulting from vasoconstriction, hypertension, and infarcts may result from cocaine use, their expression reflecting timing, patterns, and extent of cocaine abuse during pregnancy (Plessinger and Woods, 1993). Since even a single exposure to cocaine during pregnancy may place an organ system at risk by producing infarction, edema, or necrosis, and repeated exposures are more likely the case than not, identification of specific defects is nearly impossible.

Exposure after birth may also have deleterious effects. In this regard, a case of an infant suffering acute pulmonary edema following passive inhalation of freebase cocaine was reported by Batlle and Wilcox (1993).

Finally, with only one exception (Fritz et al., 1993), there has been very little exploration of the developmental risk factors before age 16 which predispose women to use cocaine during pregnancy, apart from studies of factors which predispose women in general to drug use (for example, Hawkins, Lishner, and Catalano, 1986; Kandel, 1982). Comparing women in an inner-city public hospital who had used cocaine shortly before delivery of their children (as evidenced by the child's positive cocaine test) with a demographically comparable comparison group, Fritz et al. (1993) found higher overall past and present use of a broad range of drugs (including all forms of cocaine), as well as adverse developmental events (inconsistent presence of, mental illness in, and substance abuse by caregivers, physical and/or sexual abuse, school dysfunction, and substance abuse), and lower levels of general adaptive functioning (illegal activity and incarceration, welfare support, low educational attainment, psychiatric hospitalization, and a history of homelessness). Thus, the authors concluded that "women who have poor impulse control and ego function by virtue of early chaotic home experience ... will be particularly susceptible to the destructive influence of drug use. The transmission of child abuse to the next generation is all too likely an outcome if the drug abuse of the new mothers is left untreated" (p. 195).

Maternal cocaine use may result in vasculitis in the form of placentitis or chorioamnionitis, which adversely affects the maternal-fetal vascular interface by altering the permeability of these barriers to maternal blood. This in turn can allow greater numbers of potentially infected inflammatory cells in this tissue, and thus in the fetus. An inflammatory reaction may also occur in the fetus, making it more susceptible to viral infection. Cocaine may also alter the mother's immunodeficiency and accelerate opportunistic infections such as cytomegalovirus, resulting in placentitis. Moreover, the fetus's developing immune system may be adversely affected (Lyman, 1993).

Rather than leave this section on too pessimistic a note, however, it may be well to consider the concerns which have been raised regarding the studies conducted in this area. Chasnoff (1991), after reviewing the literature on the adverse effects of cocaine use during pregnancy, identified a number of methodological issues in such studies which were of concern. These included: the failure to define adequately the nature and extent of drug use, particularly drug use secondary to cocaine use, at the inception of the study; the failure specifically to identify patterns and timing of drug use, including duration of such use and the time during the pregnancy when the use had taken place; inadequate consideration of the setting within which subjects are recruited, which limits the generalizability of findings; the failure to identify the frequency of drug use and dose, including route of administration, purity (concentration) of the drug, possible contaminants, and other drugs used in addition to cocaine; the failure to consider the effects of other variables in the prenatal environment, including nutrition, previous history, prenatal care, maternal age, race, health, genetic makeup, socioeconomic status, and geographic location, all of which may affect outcome; and the failure to utilize appropriate comparison groups.

Other writers have also commented on the paucity of data allowing definitive conclusions to be drawn on this issue. Hutchings (1993), for example, noted that it is as yet unknown to what extent the teratogenic effects of cocaine also result from concurrent maternal abuse of alcohol and cigarettes. Zuckerman, Mayes, and their associates (Mayes et al., 1992; Zuckerman and Bresnahan, 1991), like Chasnoff (1991) and Hutchings (1993), noted that many of the studies regarding the effects of cocaine on the newborn suffer from poor or absent controls, small number of subjects, and the confounding effects of other variables that contribute to poor outcomes (use of other drugs; biological and sociological cofactors). Thus, inconsistent findings abound, and no prospective, long-term study of the effects of intrauterine cocaine, nonopiate exposure has appeared in the peer-reviewed literature (Mayes et al., 1992).

Immune System

Cocaine use may compromise the immune system, perhaps further complicating the effects of the human immunodeficiency virus (Klein, Newton, and Friedman, 1988). A number of studies in animals (for example, Klein et al., 1993; Lopez and Watson, 1994; Vaz, Lefkowitz, and Lefkowitz, 1993), as well as in humans (for example, Delafuente and DeVane, 1991), have all suggested that cocaine may impair immune functioning. In the study by Klein et al. (1993), cocaine was found moderately but consistently to suppress phytohemagglutinin-induced proliferation of T-cells at drug concentrations found in drug abusers. Another study (Ruiz et al., 1994) found reductions in the total percentage of CD4+ T-cells in cocaine-intoxicated patients, and a direct correlation was established between certain T-cell percentages and cocaine levels. (A T-cell is a lymphocyte which plays a crucial role in cell-mediated immunological responses. The CD4 molecule on the surface of T-cells is the receptor site through which the virus enters the cell.) Thus, cocaine has modulating effects on the immune system, and different immune functions may be affected by different concentrations of the drug. A study by Siddiqui, Brown, and Makuch (1993) found an association between continued cocaine use and declines in CD4+ counts over a four-month period in seropositive injection drug users, but not among a comparable group of noninjectors. The administration of alcohol in combination with cocaine may also impair immune functioning beyond that attributable to cocaine. It is likely that the formation of cocaethylene during the simultaneous consumption of alcohol and cocaine enhances the immunotoxicity of cocaine (Pirozhkov, Watson, and Chen, 1992).

Injection use of cocaine significantly increases the risk of HIV infection. The prevalence of seropositivity for HIV was found to be 35% in daily intravenous cocaine users (Chaisson et al., 1989). This rate exceeded that for monthly (16%) and weekly (18%) users, and non-users (8%). With respect to current intravenous use of drug mixtures (at least once weekly), seropositivity was highest for cocaine alone (28%), followed by use of heroin and cocaine in combination (25%), heroin and cocaine separately (21%), and heroin only (9%). The intravenous use of cocaine by frequency and race indicated that such use was highest for African American injection drug users (47% versus 30% for whites and 37% for Hispanics), and that the higher risk of HIV infection was concentrated in this group and among Hispanics (seropositivity among African American daily users, 60%; Hispanics, 36%; whites, 6%). With respect to other risk factors, reported use of a shooting gallery in the previous year was twice as high among daily cocaine users (31%) as among those who had never used cocaine (15%). The number of persons with whom drug paraphernalia was shared was associated with frequency of cocaine injection (33% of daily cocaine users versus 9% for those who had never used cocaine). Chaisson et al. (1989) concluded that the rapid increase in injection use of cocaine during the three years prior to the study and the more frequent injection of cocaine than other drugs (up to ten times daily), owing to its relatively short duration of action, accounted in part for these high rates of seropositivity. The fact that more frequent injection of cocaine was associated with increased sharing of paraphernalia and use of shooting galleries also increased the risk of exposure to HIV. Similarly, among patients in methadone maintenance treatment, cocaine use has been found to be positively associated with frequency of injection drug use, number of injections, heroin use, and sexual intercourse without condoms (Bux, Lamb, and Iguchi, 1995).

Acute Complications

Hyperthermia

Hyperthermia related to cocaine use may result from sympathetic discharge, excess motor activity, seizures, increased metabolic rate, vasoconstriction, and loss of thermoregulatory control. Often hyperthermia accompanies toxic delirium, when there is a high risk of cardiovascular collapse. A case study of severe hyperthermia secondary to IV drug abuse has been reported (Roberts, Quattrocchi, and Howland, 1984). Complications of hyperthermia include neurologic damage, rhabdomysis, renal failure, coagulopathies, shock, and hepatic failure (Schrank, 1993).

Shock

Profound shock may occur in cocaine users in the absence of a direct cause (for example, arrhythmia, infarction, or hemorrhage). While the underlying mechanism is unclear, it may be the result of volume depletion owing to inadequate oral intake of fluids and increased insensible fluid losses. Atypical central nervous system effects leading to vasodilatation may also play a role (Schrank, 1993).

Complications of Injection Use of Drugs

As was discussed in Chapter 2, there are multiple risks associated with injection use of cocaine, as is the case with other drugs of abuse. These risks include, among others, complications of *infectious diseases,* among which are viral hepatitis, HIV, and staphylococcal-related infections resulting in endocarditis, septicemia, renal disease, and skin lesions; and *emboli* resulting from the injection of inert substances or from bacterial infection, causing stroke, pulmonary complications, and lymphatic complications.

Chronic Complications

Chronic use of cocaine may result in a variety of other medical problems. Cocaine use, for example, has been found to affect blood glucose levels through sensitization to epinephrine, which mobilizes glucose (Cregler and Mark, 1986a), as well as through poor diet and noncompliance with medication regimens; and also the antihypertensive effects of guanethidine and related drugs through sensitization effects on catecholamines (Cohen, 1984). It may cause significant weight loss in persons with eating disorders (Cregler and Mark, 1986a).

Eating Disorders

Persons on a cocaine binge may experience significant weight loss and malnutrition because of losing all interest in activities not directly connected with obtaining the drug (Cregler and Mark, 1986a; Estroff and Gold, 1987). Jonas and Gold (1986) found that 22% of admissions to inpatient treatment met DSM-III criteria for bulimia, 18% met DSM-III criteria for both anorexia nervosa and bulimia, and 2% met DSM-III criteria for anorexia nervosa alone. They did not find support for the hypothesis that cocaine was being used to self-medicate an eating disorder, since no more than 26% of any of the three diagnostic groups felt that cocaine helped address their eating problems. Jonas and Gold thus cautioned wariness in attributing eating disorders to drug abuse alone, and suggested that patients with either an eating or a drug abuse disorder be carefully assessed for the presence of the other problem. Because of poor nutrition secondary to drug abuse, vitamin deficiencies have also been reported (Estroff and Gold, 1987).

The Eyes

Although apparently relatively uncommon, eye-related complications of crack smoking have been the subject of several reports. Cocaine-related chronic mydriasis has been reported by several writers (Siegel, 1978; Tames and Goldenring, 1986), as has a case of unilateral pharmacological mydriasis attributable to exposure to crack cocaine (Zeiter, McHenry and McDermott, 1990). McHenry et al. (1989) reported a case of bilateral corneal epithelial defects attributable to crack smoking, which they labeled "crack eye." It resulted from the irritating effects of alkaloidal crack cocaine smoke, the consequent anesthetization of the corneal surface, and vigorous rubbing of the eye, all of which contributed to a denuding of the corneal epithelium. Two cases of infectious keratitis related to crack use, one of bacterial origin (Strominger, Sachs, and Hersh, 1990) and the other of fungal origin (Zagelbaum, Tannenbaum, and Hersh, 1991), have also been reported. Ravin and Ravin (1979) reported a case in which putting powdered cocaine into the eyes resulted in simultaneous bilateral corneal ulcers and blindness. Sachs, Zagelbaum, and Hersh (1993) introduced the term "crack eye syndrome" to cover a spectrum of eye diseases attributable to crack cocaine use, including microbial keratitis, corneal epithelial defects, and superficial punctate epithelial keratopathy. They attributed these disorders either to a direct toxic effect of crack smoke on the corneal epithelium or to the production of an anesthetic effect leading to decreased corneal sensation, and ultimately to resultant disruption of the normal blink reflex. Chronic exposure keratopathy may then lead to infection. The alkalinity of crack cocaine could also result in a low-grade chemical burn, which would also predispose to infections. Finally, the irritating effects of crack smoke lead users to rub their eyes vigorously, which may, either by itself or in combination with the cited factors, lead to eye damage.

Bilateral amblyopia temporally associated with crack cocaine use, and accompanied by bilateral loss of vision, has also been reported. According to Hoffman and Reimer (1993), this condition most likely resulted from a direct vasoconstrictive effect on the retinal vasculature.

Secondary involvement of the optic nerves as a result of inflammatory lesions of adjacent tissue, including the orbit, meninges, and paranasal sinuses, while rare, has been reported. Newman et al. (1988) described such a case, in which they attributed optic nerve involvement in a compulsive intranasal cocaine abuser to extensive ischemic necrosis of mucosal and bony structures, which led to subsequent involvement of the optic nerve.

Oral Cavity

Oral use of cocaine via direct application to the gums may result in lacerations of the gingival mucosa and, with chronic use, in periodontal disease and loss of teeth (Lee, Mohammadi, and Dixon, 1991). Long-term administration of cocaine may mask dental pain through its local anesthetic action. When the anesthesia wears off, the dental pain may be of such an intensity, or the teeth so badly damaged, that extraction is required (Estroff and Gold, 1986). Bruxism (grinding of teeth) has also been noted as a complication of cocaine intoxication (Cohen, 1984).

Skeletomuscular System

Cocaine abusers are likely to be at risk for rhabdomyolysis, an acute and potentially fatal disease of skeletal muscle, in which muscle cell contents are spilled into the bloodstream (Krohn, Slowman-Kovacs, and Leapman, 1988; Merigian and Roberts, 1987). This disorder may result from tissue ischemia as a consequence of arterial vasoconstriction or as a direct, toxic effect of cocaine on muscle metabolism (Roth et al., 1988). Rhabdomyolysis is a frequent occurrence in agitated patients with excessive motor activity, seizures, hyperthermia, coma, or hypotension (Schrank, 1993). Welch, Todd, and Krause (1991) reported rhabdomyolysis to be present in 24% of patients presenting with cocaine-related complaints. Complications observed in cocaine-associated rhabdomyolysis include acute renal failure, hepatic dysfunction, elevated uric acid levels, metabolic acidosis, and death. Although the pathophysiology resulting in this disorder in cocaine abusers is unknown, cocaine-induced arterial vasoconstriction resulting in ischemia, hypotension, malignant hypothermia, or direct toxic effects on myocytes or muscle metabolism have been suggested as causes (Roth et al., 1988). In the study by Welch, Todd, and Krause (1991), a high proportion of cases of rhabdomyolysis were not predictable from history or physical examination. Thus, laboratory evaluation was recommended as essential in the presence of signs associated with this disease, which include myoglobinuria, nausea, vomiting, myalgias, muscle swelling and tenderness, and weakness (Koffler, Friedler, and Massry, 1976). A classification system for the purpose of predicting the severity of cocaine-associated rhabdomyolysis has been developed by Brody et al. (1990).

Cocaine-Related Mortality

Until recently, the general impression was that death from cocaine use was relatively infrequent, if not "extremely rare" (Lundberg et al., 1977, p. 407). While cocaine use has increased dramatically since the 1970s, it is likely that many cocaine-related deaths were not identified as such until the prevalence of cocaine abuse resulted in attention being given to indirectly related deaths (that is, deaths from causes other than overdose). Even then, all cocaine-related deaths may not be captured (Schuster, 1991). Pollock et al. (1991), for example, found that 75% more cocaine-related deaths in 25 metropolitan areas were reported to DAWN (6,057) than were reported in national vital statistics (3,466) over a six-year period. Among almost 700 medical examiner cases studied in New Jersey during 1986–87, toxicology findings indicated that cocaine alone was the drug most often present, while among intravenous drug users, the combination of cocaine and heroin was most often present (Haberman, French, and Chin, 1993). Among cocaine-related fatalities occurring in New York City between January 1 and November 1, 1986, 38.7% also involved opiates, and 32.6% also involved ethanol. Barbiturates and minor tranquilizers were present in only 2.0% of cases (Tardiff et al., 1989).

Among deaths in New York City where cocaine was present in the body at postmortem, 4.2% were found to have resulted from cocaine overdose (Tardiff et al., 1989). It is likely, however, that cocaine use was a contributor to a large proportion of other causes of death, including homicides, suicides, and automobile accidents, as well as acute cardiac and cerebrovascular events (myocardial infarction, ruptured dissecting aneurysms, cerebral hemorrhage), which are relatively uncommon in younger persons. Furthermore, current death certification practices and constraints imposed by the use of the International Classification of Diseases, Ninth Revision (ICD-9), may result in substantial misclassification (and consequent underreporting) of cocaine-related deaths (Young and Pollock, 1993).

Death may occur after administration of the drug by any route (Mittleman and Wetli, 1984), and may be rapid in onset, in the form of collapse without time for intervention, or it may be preceded by symptoms such as confusion or convulsions (Estroff and Gold, 1986). Conditions attributable to cocaine use and resulting in death may include generalized convulsions, respiratory failure, cardiac arrhythmias, or paralysis of the heart muscle. Multiple drug use is frequently implicated in cocaine-related deaths (Chitwood, 1985; Mittleman and Wetli, 1984; Siegel, 1984). Sudden death may occur following a state of excited delirium resulting from cocaine intoxication. Death may be particularly likely when restraint of patients with agitated delirium is attempted, with resultant minor head injury. An analysis of four such deaths by the Philadelphia Medical Examiner's Office suggested that the actual mechanism in such cases involves a terminal arrhythmia resulting from sympathetic sensitization of the myocardium and the stress of struggle, sometimes superimposed on preexisting natural disease (Mirchandani et al., 1994). Often, such deaths are perceived as being caused by unnecessarily forceful intervention by the police (Wetli, 1993).

Aside from complications of the use of cocaine itself, use of crack cocaine carries with it a not insignificant risk of death from violence related to activities associated with obtaining money for further purchases of drugs (Roehrich and Gold, 1991). Some 37.5% of medical examiner cases in New York City involving cocaine were deaths resulting from homicide (Tardiff et al., 1989). This risk applies to the crime victims as well as to the crack addicts themselves (Wetli, 1993).

The question why some cocaine abusers experience severe ischemic or other complications, including death, while others do not was raised by Devenyi (1989). Observing that a common factor in many of the medical complications of cocaine abuse is the intense vasoconstriction resulting from the inhibitory effects of cocaine on norepinephrine reuptake at noradrenergic nerve endings, Devenyi suggested the possibility of a genetic factor underlying proneness to cocaine toxicity. Such a genetic factor might possibly act through a metabolic pathway involving plasma cholinesterase, an enzyme that plays a role in the metabolism and elimination of cocaine.

Deaths and injuries may also result from automobile and other accidents which occur while the person is cocaine-intoxicated (Cohen, 1984). It is likely that many such events are undetected, and thus underreported. Evidence for such a view comes from a roadside study of reckless drivers in Memphis, Tennessee, in which 59% of persons stopped for reckless driving, who were not apparently impaired by alcohol, tested positive for cocaine and/or marijuana. Of those persons assessed as being moderately or extremely intoxicated who tested positive for marijuana and/or cocaine, 21% tested positive for cocaine only, 45% for marijuana only, and 19% for both. Of those persons assessed as being mildly or not intoxicated, 14% tested positive for marijuana, and none for cocaine or cocaine and marijuana. Initial denial of cocaine use was high (82%), although the number of those admitting to cocaine use rose to 87% after being told of positive test results (Brookoff et al., 1994). In a study conducted in California in 1982–83, cocaine was detected in 11% of 440 drivers aged 15 to 34 who were killed in motor vehicle accidents, although the relationship of cocaine to responsibility for the crash could not be ascertained (Williams et al., 1985).

Suicide has been implicated as a frequent cause of death among cocaine users. In a study of suicides in San Diego, marijuana, alcohol, and cocaine were the most frequently abused substances. Of persons under age 30 who committed suicide, 30% had histories of cocaine abuse (Fowler, Rich, and Young, 1986). Most suicides were polydrug abusers, and alcohol use was closely associated with substance abuse in these cases. Unfortunately, this study did not estimate the prevalence of cocaine use at autopsy. A review of all suicides under the age of 61 in New York City during 1985 (the year when crack became widely available there) found that of 570 cases, cocaine metabolites were detected at autopsy in 105 (21.8%). Using conservative criteria, an estimate of 18.4%, or about one out of five suicides, was arrived at. Ethanol involvement was present in approximately half the cases across all demographic categories. Cocaine involvement was greater for males than for females (24.3% versus 14.5%) and among Hispanics (36.9%), followed by African Americans (23.7%), and whites (12.4%). The largest percentages of cocaine involvement were in persons aged 21 to 30 years (28.8%) and 31 to 40 years (24.8%; Marzuk et al., 1992).

Persistent crack use has been found to be related to suicide among methadone patients (Des Jarlais et al., 1992). The authors of this study interpreted this finding as indicative of the presence of severe depression. Attempted suicide was also found by De Leon (1993) to be significantly higher among crack-abusing admissions to a therapeutic community (26.2% had attempted suicide at least once during their lifetime) than among non–crack cocaine abusers (11.7%) and among abusers of drugs other than cocaine (6.9%). Suicide attempt rates were higher for females than males in this sample, but were not influenced by other demographic variables.

Although suicide is a risk of cocaine intoxication, death may also result indirectly from bizarre behaviors associated with cocaine-induced psychosis. Wetli (1993) cites the examples of cocaine users drowning in a canal or other body of water after running from a domicile, cringing in a closet while a small fire on the stove generated sufficient carbon monoxide to kill them, and being accidentally shot while fending off imaginary attackers.

Conclusions

Current medical knowledge supports a view of cocaine as a dangerous drug with highly unpredictable consequences related to its use. The fact that many of these consequences are life-threatening and can occur regardless of the dose used suggests that earlier views of cocaine as harmless or as placing the user at minimal risk are incorrect and represent a disservice to that part of the population at risk of cocaine abuse.

The presentation of clinical manifestations of cocaine abuse may vary greatly, presenting difficulties in diagnosis. The clinical presentation of cocaine abuse may include any of the following: malnutrition; exhaustion; neurologic symptoms (seizures, headache, syncope, transient ischemic attack); psychiatric manifestations (altered mental status, suicide attempts); cardiovascular symptoms (cardiac arrest, chest pain, palpitations, dyspnea); and venous, musculoskeletal, dermatological (hives), gastrointestinal (abdominal pain), pulmonary (dyspnea), infectious, obstetric, and neonatal complications (Derlet and Albertson, 1989a; Goldfrank and Hoffman, 1993). Cocaine abuse, even if a significant contributor to the presenting problem, may not, however, be the primary complaint.

Several acute, and potentially fatal, syndromes of cocaine intoxication have been described. These include a clinical picture of sudden onset of symptoms, possibly followed by death within minutes. A second is characterized by an excited delirium and florid psychiatric symptomatology, and a third (the neuroleptic malignant syndrome) by hyperthermia, muscular rigidity, and dehydration followed by death (Kosten and Kleber, 1988; Roehrich and Gold, 1991; Wetli and Fishbain, 1985). A fourth syndrome, a variant of the neuroleptic malignant syndrome, in which intermittent rigidity is present together with intermittent dystonia and agitation, has also been described (Kosten and Kleber, 1988).

Cocaine overdose, once relatively infrequent, is becoming a more common event. Among heavy cocaine users it is a common experience, and is independent of route of administration (Pottieger et al., 1992). Shifts in routes of administration from inhalation of powdered cocaine to crack use may in part account for this increase owing to the increased purity of crack.

Relatively little evidence is available as to whether certain physiological abnormalities resulting from cocaine use are reversible on discontinuation of use. In two studies, decreases in myocardial ischemia (Nademanee et al., 1989) and pulmonary symptoms (DelBono, O'Brien, and Murphy, 1989) were found to follow a period of abstinence.

Acute psychiatric complications of cocaine use may be of sudden onset and include a wide variety of symptoms. Euphoria, dysphoria, anxiety, agitation (sometimes violent), panic disorder, paranoid psychosis, and severe depression are among the psychiatric problems which have been described in association with cocaine use. Apparent overt psychosis, often an excited delirium characterized by confusion and agitation, delusions, hallucinations, other paranoid ideation, and suicidal ideation, may also be present (Bunt et al., 1990; Schrank, 1993).

Specific systemic effects of cocaine are varied, and appear to involve every organ system. Some are life-threatening. In particular, cocaine may have life-threatening effects on the cardiovascular system, including the blood vessels which supply the central nervous system. Many of these systemic effects are the result of cocaine's profound vasoconstrictive effects, which may cause a simultaneous increase in cardiac input and both central and peripheral vasoconstriction. Direct central nervous system effects may include the precipitation of convulsions and seizures owing to cocaine's lowering of the seizure threshold.

Many reports concerning physical complications of cocaine abuse are case studies. While valuable in their own right, these require confirmation with larger-scale studies. An overreliance on case studies and small-sample clinical reports has sometimes resulted in conflicting findings.

Maternal cocaine use may have severe adverse effects on the developing fetus. Such effects may be direct (for example, teratogenic effects) or indirect (for example, actions affecting maternal blood flow). Here, as in other areas of cocaine research, there are inconsistent findings, although many of these may be due to the differential effects of cocaine depending on the point in the development of the fetus when cocaine was used, as well as the amount used, and other factors (Fries et al., 1993). Studies in this area also suffer from deficiencies in sampling and design, limiting their generalization value (Chasnoff, 1991; Hutchings, 1993; Mayes et al., 1992).

Lest pessimism prevail regarding the discouraging picture of adverse birth outcomes resulting from cocaine use, Racine, Joyce, and Anderson (1993) demonstrated the effectiveness of prenatal care in significantly improving birth weight among infants of cocaine-abusing mothers. It is clear that more interventions which target this high-risk population are needed.

Injection drug use of cocaine is a major risk factor in the transmission of HIV. Current use of cocaine alone, particularly on a daily basis, has been found to be most closely related to rates of seropositivity, exceeding that found for use of cocaine by other routes, cocaine in combination with heroin, and heroin alone (Chaisson et al., 1989).

Death resulting from cocaine abuse may be indirect, as in automobile or other accidents. Such causes of death may be more common than was previous believed, and thus may represent a much higher than reported rate of cocaine-related mortality (Brookoff et al., 1994; Cohen, 1984; Roehrich and Gold, 1991). Cocaine may also be involved to a greater extent in suicidal behavior than was previously believed (Des Jarlais et al., 1992; Fowler, Rich, and Young, 1986; Wetli, 1993).

7

Cocaine Abuse and Sexual Behavior

Sexual Functioning

Cocaine has been alleged to be an aphrodisiac, enhancing sexual performance (see, for example, Bowser, 1989; Carr and Meyers, 1988; Grinspoon and Bakalar, 1985; Macdonald et al., 1988), although many writers, particularly those with a medical or scientific background, are careful to note that the salutary effects of cocaine on sexual performance are likely to be very short-lived. Such a belief is nonetheless widespread on the part of users (see, for example, Ashley, 1975; Parr, 1976; Wesson, 1982). Where data have been collected on the issue, however, this belief has not been borne out (Feucht, 1993; Weiss and Mirin, 1987). Siegel (1984), for example, found that only 13% of respondents reported heightened sexual stimulation from the use of cocaine. There may in actuality be a physiological basis for the belief, in that increased dopamine activity may be related to increased sexual drive (Buffum, 1982, 1988).

It is more likely that continued cocaine use causes inhibition of sexual interest. Weatherby et al. (1992) found that crack users reported both a decreased desire for sex (57%, versus 36.6% reporting an increased desire) and diminished physical ability to have sex following smoking of crack (56.1%, versus 28.8% reporting increased ability). Both adverse effects were greater in magnitude for males than for females. Chitwood (1985) found that 29% of cocaine abusers overall, and 43% of heavy users, reported a lack of sexual interest as a consequence of cocaine use. Furthermore, this loss of interest was greater for intravenous users than for those who used the inhalation route (38% versus 22%). Macdonald et al. (1988) also found gender-related effects of cocaine on sexual functioning, although some of his findings were in the opposite direction with respect to sex from those reported by Chitwood (1985). For example, 22.4% of women reported that cocaine had a positive effect on their sex lives, while 48.2% reported a negative effect. For males, 40.4% reported a positive effect, while 28.7% reported negative effects. Males were more likely than females to report both positive and negative effects (18.4% versus 5.9%), while women were more likely than men to report no effect (23.5% versus 12.5%). When perceived effects on sex life were examined as a function of route of administration, there was an approximately even split between those who reported positive versus negative effects for both snorters and freebasers. One significant exception was among injection users, who overwhelmingly reported a negative effect on their sex lives (90.9%). In general, negative sexual experiences increased with chronic cocaine use.

Certainly the use of crack cocaine may, at the least, lower inhibitions and provide a context within which increased sexual activity may be acceptable or to some extent expected (Feucht, 1993). Furthermore, by elevating mood and heightening sensory awareness, cocaine can temporarily improve sexual performance. The acute use of cocaine, however, even in low doses, can result in spontaneous ejaculation and orgasm without genital stimulation. Tolerance develops rapidly to the sexually stimulating effects of cocaine. Long-term use by males, particularly at high doses, may result in sexual dysfunctions such as difficulty in maintaining an erection and ejaculating, as well as in frequent periods of diminished libido. Female users may have difficulty in reaching orgasm. For both males and females, aberrant sexual behavior, including compulsive masturbation and multiple-partner marathons, may take place. Cocaine-induced sexual dysfunctions (for example, spontaneous orgasm, decreased libido) may be the result of alterations of the neurotransmitter system, including alterations of dopamine transmission, while the sexual excitement produced by cocaine may be due to amygdaloid stimulation or dopamine's effects on the neurotransmitter system (Cregler and Mark, 1986a; Gold, 1992; Gold and Dackis, 1984; Siegel, 1982b; Smith, Wesson, and Apter-Marsh, 1984).

While cocaine initially enhances sexual behavior, continued use may also result in a complete loss of sexual interest, as well as in priapism and ejaculatory failure (Gay and Sheppard, 1973; Grinspoon and Bakalar, 1985) and gynecomastia (Siegel, 1982b). Although acute exposure to cocaine decreases the motion kinetics of human spermatozoa, cocaine has not been found to affect sperm motility and fertilizing capability (Yelian et al., 1994). In females, cocaine use may result in galactorrhea, amenorrhea, and infertility (Gold, 1992). Finally, it should be mentioned that the practice of direct topical application of cocaine to the genitals, while resulting in the desired effect of prolonging sexual intercourse by decreasing sensation, may have the potentially serious complication of decreasing blood flow to the tissue involved, with resultant ulceration (Weiss and Mirin, 1987).

Compulsive Sexuality and the Treatment Process

As many as 70% of cocaine addicts entering treatment have been reported by Washton (1989b) to be "dually addicted" to cocaine and sex. Cocaine-related compulsive sexuality may contribute to chronic relapse, treatment failure, and perpetuation of high-risk sexual behavior that may foster the spread of acquired immune deficiency syndrome and other sexually transmitted diseases. To Washton (1989b), "undiagnosed and untreated compulsive sexuality is one of the most common, preventable relapse factors in cocaine treatment today" (p. 24).

Drug-related compulsive sexuality must be viewed as a primary problem which is part of a dual addiction to drugs and sex (Washton and Stone-Washton, 1993). This should be the case even where there is no history of such a disorder prior to involvement with cocaine. Compulsive sexuality may continue despite treatment of the cocaine addiction, as well as precipitate powerful cravings for cocaine (and vice versa). Thus, the treatment of the sexual compulsion is a priority. In order to treat it successfully, total drug abstinence must be achieved. The patient is then asked to abstain from all sexual activity for thirty days, during which the clinician can teach the patient how to differentiate between "normal" and compulsive/addictive sex, how to identify relapse triggers, and how to respond to them safely (Washton and Stone-Washton, 1993).

Cocaine and the Spread of Sexually Transmitted Diseases

The widespread use of cocaine, especially crack cocaine, has been identified by a number of writers as having accelerated the spread of AIDS and other sexually transmitted diseases (STDs) through three routes: increased sexual activity resulting from cocaine use, sexual activity with injection drug users, and prostitution. Injection drug use and sex with injection drug users, both of which involve the exchange of bodily fluids, are well-established risk factors for the transmission of the human immunodeficiency virus (HIV).[1] As noted previously, injection use of cocaine is common among injection drug users (IDUs). Fully half of all injection drug users inject on a daily basis, and sharing of injection equipment is common (Magura et al., 1989; Stephens, Feucht, and Gibbs, 1993).

After reviewing the epidemiological literature, Marx and associates (1991) concluded that recent increases in reported rates of syphilis, gonorrhea, chancroid, and sexually transmitted human immunodeficiency virus infection appeared to be related to crack cocaine use. Crack use itself, as well as the practice of exchanging money for sex or drugs, and the use of other drugs or cocaine in other forms, were related to sexually transmitted diseases in a majority of the studies that were reviewed. Typical of the findings were those by Rolfs, Goldberg, and Sharrar (1990), who tested the hypothesis that cocaine-addicted female prostitutes exchanging sex for crack cocaine were responsible for an outbreak of syphilis in metropolitan areas. In a case-control study in sexually transmitted disease clinics in Philadelphia, risk factors for men included having used cocaine in the three months before the interview; having given a woman drugs in exchange for sex; having had sex at a "crack house" or a place where drugs were sold or used; and having had sex with a woman on the day they met. For women, the risk factors included having used cocaine in the three months before the interview and having accepted money or drugs for sex. For men, intravenous use of cocaine was more strongly related to a diagnosis of syphilis than was non-intravenous use. For women, non-intravenous use of cocaine, primarily inhalation, was most strongly associated with syphilis. For both men and women, cocaine use remained a significant risk factor even after controlling for having sex with a prostitute (for men) and for prostitution (for women). The researchers concluded that both cocaine use and the sexual behaviors associated with it were risk factors for syphilis, although the association between syphilis and cocaine use was not fully explained by contact with prostitutes in the case of men or by prostitution in the case of women.

The link between cocaine use on the one hand, either in its smokeable form or when used by injection, and sexually transmitted diseases on the other is well illustrated by the findings reported by Farley, Hadler, and Gunn (1990). This study found a direct association between cocaine use and syphilis in Connecticut between 1986 and 1988. As syphilis rates rose, the number of women who reported prostitution or illicit drug use also increased. In 1988, 41% of women with syphilis reported having used cocaine, while 19% reported having engaged in prostitution. Similarly, among women charged with possession of illegal drugs or incarcerated for prostitution, use of cocaine was associated with the highest syphilis rates. A study conducted in Detroit and Dallas in 1989–90 found that both male and female crack users, compared with non-crack users, were more likely to report having had four or more sexual partners during the critical period for acquiring or passing on infection, and that for females, crack use was strongly associated with exchanging sex for money or drugs (Greenberg, Schnell, and Conlon, 1992).

In the United States, daily cocaine injection is associated with an increased seroprevalence of HIV infection. In areas of high seroprevalence, daily use of injected cocaine averages 40%, while in areas of low seroprevalence, daily injection use averages 24%. This difference is most evident among Hispanics, for whom 23.1% in the low prevalence areas report daily cocaine injection use versus 50% in the high prevalence areas. For African Americans this difference is 27% and 39.5%, and for whites 19% and 27%, respectively (Siegal, Carlson, and Falck, 1993).

In San Francisco, daily cocaine use has been found to be a strong predictor of HIV infection among African American and Hispanic injection drug users not in treatment. The use of cocaine alone was most strongly associated with HIV seropositivity, the rate exceeding that for cocaine and heroin in combination. There was no such association with the use of heroin alone (Chaisson et al., 1989). A study of 697 medical examiner cases in New Jersey in 1986–87, however, found that cases in which there were toxicology findings of the presence of both cocaine and heroin were most likely to be HIV-positive, followed by cases with cocaine or heroin present alone (Haberman, French, and Chin, 1993). The researchers suggested that this difference reflected different modes of use and differing study populations, in that, first, the San Francisco sample consisted of intravenous drug users who had been enrolled in or who had sought entry into treatment, while the New Jersey sample consisted of unselected deaths investigated by the state medical examiner's office; and second, at the time of the study cocaine injection was very prevalent in San Francisco while smokeable crack was more common in New Jersey.

In a study of risk factors in female crack cocaine abusers associated with acquisition of early syphilis, use of crack within the previous three months was found to be the only specific drug-related risk factor associated with such acquisition. Other risk factors identified included number of drug-using partners, number of partners exchanging sex for drugs and money, and number of partners with whom sex and drugs were shared. Furthermore, women were at higher risk of contracting syphilis than were men who engaged in the same high-risk behaviors. Further, increased rates of syphilis during the time period studied (1987–1990) likely resulted from increases in high-risk behaviors, including sex with numerous partners, drug use, and so on (Finelli, Budd, and Spitalny, 1993). Webber and Hauser (1993) have suggested that the increase in the number of cases of congenital syphilis seen in New York City between 1982 and 1988 was related to cocaine dependence among women.

Among pregnant inner-city women, crack cocaine use has been related to HIV seropositivity. In a study of 80 pregnant women, seropositivity was found to be associated with a history of crack cocaine use, as well as intravenous drug use, and a history of sexually transmitted diseases. After adjusting for the risk factors which were present, a history of crack cocaine use remained significantly associated with HIV infection (Lindsay et al., 1992). A relationship between cocaine use and increased prevalence of syphilis has also been confirmed for parturient women. In a sample of 1,206 pregnant women, the presence of cocaine metabolites was found to be positively associated with positive tests for syphilis (18.7% of patients with positive cocaine screens versus 2.4% for patients with negative urine screens) and for HIV (7.6% of patients with positive cocaine screens versus 1.4% for patients with negative urine screens; Minkoff et al., 1990). Children born to mothers who use crack cocaine are thus likely to be at higher risk for congenital syphilis (as well as other STDs, including HIV infection). Chiu, Vaughn, and Carzoli (1990), for example, reported that nearly 80% of female symptomatic congenital syphilis cases at the University of Florida Medical Center involved a history of maternal cocaine abuse. This finding has been confirmed in other studies. Ricci, Fojaco, and O'Sullivan (1989), in a study conducted in Miami, also found the use of crack cocaine by expectant mothers to be associated with high rates of congenital syphilis. Similar findings were obtained in a study conducted in New York, in which the odds of being exposed to cocaine were found to be 3.9 times greater among mothers of children born with congenital syphilis as compared with case controls (Greenberg et al., 1991).

Sexual Behavior of Injection Drug Users

Sexually active male injection drug users were found to have had a mean of 4.61 (median, 2.0) female sexual partners during the year prior to interview. Sexually active female IDUs were found to have had an average of 5.28 (median, 1.0) male sexual partners during this same period (Wells et al., 1993). Sex partners of injection drug users are at an especially high risk for HIV infection (Deren et al., 1993). This is particularly the case when the sex partners themselves engage in injection drug abuse. While injection drug users in general exceed their sex partners in the frequent and very frequent use of marijuana and alcohol, sex partners of injection drug users have been found to exceed injection drug users in the frequent and very frequent use of crack cocaine. This finding holds true for all categories of gender, age, and race, with the exception of Pacific Islanders (Feucht, Stephens, and Sullivan, 1993). Injection use of cocaine was greater among male and white sex partners, however. Among these injection drug users, nearly two-thirds had used cocaine in the previous six months. Younger sex partners were more likely than older sex partners to have injected cocaine in the previous six months. Daily or more frequent use of injection cocaine was present in less than one-fourth of sex partners. The highest rates of frequent and very frequent injection use were among female and African American sex partners (Feucht, Stephens, and Sullivan, 1993). When compared with injection heroin use, injection use of cocaine alone among sex partners was lower (51.7% for heroin versus 23.5% for cocaine). Feucht and associates suggested that the low percentage of sex partners who had ever injected cocaine probably reflected the many routes by which cocaine can be used. Similarly, use of heroin-cocaine combinations was rare among sex partners.

Crack Smoking and Sexually Transmitted Diseases

Crack smoking is associated with an increased risk of contracting sexually transmitted diseases, including HIV. This increased risk occurs through practices such as sex with multiple partners, the exchange of sex for money or drugs, and the failure to use condoms (Chiasson et al., 1991; Diaz and Chu, 1993; Weatherby et al., 1992). Several reports have also indicated that the presence of both syphilis (Diaz and Chu, 1993; Ricci, Fojaco, and O'Sullivan, 1989; Rolfs, Goldberg, and Sharrar, 1990) and HIV-positivity (Bastien et al., 1990; Hoegsberg et al., 1989; Schoenbaum, Hartel, and Friedland, 1990) are related to a greater likelihood of crack use, although one study (Wolfe et al., 1990) failed to confirm this association. High-risk sexual behavior among crack users appears to continue regardless of HIV status or the presence of AIDS. Diaz and Chu (1993) found that crack users who had been aware of their HIV status for at least five years continued to engage in exchanging sex for drugs or money in the same proportions as crack users who had been aware of their infection for less than five years.

Recent increases in the incidence of sexually transmitted diseases have been attributed in part to increased rates of drug use, in particular crack cocaine use (Marx et al., 1991). In a sample of 1,356 regular crack smokers (defined as having smoked crack at least three days each week in the previous thirty days) and nonsmokers in three cities (Miami, New York, and San Francisco), crack cocaine smokers, regardless of whether they had also injected the drug or not, reported higher rates of high-risk behaviors than those who did not smoke crack (Edlin et al., 1992). Such behaviors included engaging in high-risk sex acts, having numerous sex partners, being likely to have exchanged sex for money, and having had a sexually transmitted disease. Furthermore, such rates were generally higher among non-IDUs than among injectors and higher among men than among women. Condom use, while somewhat more common with paying than with nonpaying partners, was generally rare. Involvement in drug abuse treatment during the previous year was infrequent, with most crack users never having been in such treatment, although a large majority of the sample had visited a medical clinic or hospital emergency room during this time. Edlin and associates concluded that education and prevention efforts were needed to reach this high-risk population, and that institutions such as emergency rooms, medical clinics, high schools, public assistance agencies, and jails, all of which a majority of the sample had contact with, were convenient sites for reaching these persons.

Among crack smokers attending a sexually transmitted disease clinic in New York who denied male-to-male sexual contact, intravenous drug use, and heterosexual contact with an intravenous drug user, seroprevalence was significantly lower than among crack smokers who admitted these risk factors (males, 3.6% versus 12%; females, 4.2% versus 12%). In the group of crack smokers denying such risk factors, the behaviors most closely associated with HIV infection were use of crack and prostitution for women, and history of syphilis and crack use for men. Here again, the findings suggest that the higher rates of sexual behaviors associated with crack use may result in an increased risk of contracting HIV (Chiasson et al., 1991).

Crack Use and Sexual Behavior

In a study of methadone maintenance patients, crack use has been found to be related to two measures of unsafe sexual behavior: having injection drug users among regular sexual partners and engaging in prostitution (Des Jarlais et al., 1992).

There are a number of reasons for the high likelihood of sexual transmission of HIV among injection drug users. Booth, Watters, and Chitwood (1993) include among such reasons the fact that injection drug users represent the primary source for heterosexual and perinatal transmission of HIV to non-injection drug users in the United States (see, for example, Friedland and Klein, 1987); that male injection drug users have more non-injecting sex partners than injecting partners, while the majority of female injection drug users are more likely to have other injectors as sex partners (see, for example, Feucht, Stephens, and Roman, 1990); and that the number of sex partners was the only risk factor for HIV infection identified in a study of female IDUs who had not injected during the past three years (see, for example, Schoenbaum et al., 1989). Furthermore, crack cocaine is seen as playing a particularly key role in the sexual transmission of HIV and other sexually transmitted diseases in that its use is associated with high-risk sexual behaviors (Booth, Watters, and Chitwood, 1993; Chiasson et al., 1991; Chirgwin et al., 1991; Greenberg et al., 1991).

Examining the relationships between high-risk sexual behavior on the one hand and crack and injection drug use on the other, Booth, Watters, and Chitwood (1993) assessed sexual risk behaviors in injection drug users, crack smokers, and injection drug users who smoked crack. They found an increased risk of acquiring HIV through sexual transmission to be associated with crack use, particularly among those who also injected drugs. Crack-smoking injection drug users were more likely to report having had sex with an injector; exchanging sex for money and/or drugs; using drugs before or during sex; and having unprotected intercourse. With respect to drug use, crack users who also injected drugs both injected more than those who only injected and used drugs more frequently. Thus, the authors concluded that persons engaged in crack use were at an increased risk of heterosexual transmission of HIV.

Exchanging sexual favors for drugs and money and having sexual relations under the influence of crack were found to be two of five risk behaviors associated with infection and with transmission of STDs in a study of African American adolescent crack users in Oakland and San Francisco (Fullilove et al., 1990). When these two variables were considered in conjunction with three other possible crack-related factors (self-reported history of an STD, having had more than five sexual partners per year, and not having used a condom in one's last sexual encounter), 73% of the sample reported at least one, and 31% reported three or more such risk factors. This study, while confirming that crack users were "sexual risktakers," did not, however, unambiguously link such increased risk to crack use. In a second study, using crack (as well as having one or more relatives who used drugs) was found to be clearly associated with engaging in one of four STD/HIV risk behaviors (engaging in sexual intercourse while under the influence of drugs or alcohol, exchanging sexual favors for drugs or money, not using a condom in one's most recent sexual contact, and having had five or more sexual partners during the previous year). Non-users living in the same inner-city neighborhoods were not as likely to have engaged in such behaviors (Fullilove et al., 1993).

In the NADR study, the frequency of crack use was found to be positively associated with the number of sex partners reported by injection drug users. Multiple sex partners were reported by 68.4% of daily crack smokers and 57.7% of less frequent users of crack, in contrast with only 38.9% of those who did not smoke crack. These relationships are well illustrated by the fact that daily crack users were three times more likely (33.8%) than injection drug users who did not smoke crack (10.6%) to have had more than five sex partners during the previous six months (Chitwood, 1993).

When Wells et al. (1993) examined the reasons given by male IDUs for using drugs in connection with sex, they reported that drugs helped them relax for sex, enhanced sexual performance, or helped them meet sexual partners. Similarly, these male injection drug users, when compared with men who did not report using drugs to enhance sexual performance, reported greater frequency of anal intercourse, fellatio, and cunnilingus, less relative frequency of vaginal intercourse, more sexual partners, and greater involvement in being paid for sex and paying for sex. Women who reported using drugs to enhance sex reported greater frequency of anal intercourse and more sexual partners.

PROSTITUTION

The need to obtain funds to purchase cocaine may drive women into prostitution as a means of supporting their use (see, for example, Bourgois, 1989; Bowser, 1989; Inciardi, 1990; Inciardi, Lockwood, and Pottieger, 1991; Murphy and Rosenbaum, 1992). Feucht (1993) observed that this situation has created greater competition for customers, thus resulting in unsafe sex practices, such as meeting customers' requests to engage in sex without condoms, as well as in driving older prostitutes from the streets owing to increased competition from newer, younger entrants into the trade (see, for example, Shedlin, 1990). Among the many-faceted relationships found in crack cocaine use and prostitution, according to Feucht (1993), are *addiction to crack,* with the resultant need to secure money for the drug and to engage in more frequent sex-for-money transactions and riskier sex practices (reported by 78.4% of prostitutes interviewed); *utilization of crack as a facilitator of prostitution,* reducing inhibitions and enabling prostitutes to work under very difficult conditions; and *marketplace economics,* in which procurement of crack and procurement of sex are part of the same marketplace process, involving prostitutes as drug couriers, barterers, and small-scale dealers, and giving them common interests with drug dealers.

SEX FOR DRUGS

The need to obtain funds in order to continue taking drugs may result in promiscuous sexual behavior. Cates (cited by Goldsmith, 1988), commenting on the rise in syphilis and sexually transmitted diseases among heterosexuals, related it to the bartering of "sexual services" for crack cocaine and drew the following analogy: "The crack house of today has become what the gay bathhouse was yesterday with regard to all sexually transmitted diseases" (p. 2009).

In a study of crack cocaine users in Miami, Weatherby et al. (1992) found that 76% of female and 48% of male crack users had traded sex for money or drugs, compared to 4% of women and 9% of men who had never used crack. McCoy and Miles (1992) also found such a relationship in Miami, in that significantly more women than men reported having exchanged sex for drugs (33.8% versus 17.2%) or for money (59.5% versus 17%). Furthermore, among men, when frequency of crack use was controlled for, involvement in trading sex for drugs versus sex for money did not relate to level of crack cocaine use, whereas women more frequently engaged in trading sex for money than for drugs, without regard to level of crack use (heavy users, 73.2% versus 44.6%; light users, 47% versus 24%).

The practice of trading sex for crack, in which women may have many sexual partners, places them and their partners at risk of infection with venereal disease or HIV (Chiasson et al., 1991; Sterk, 1988). Additionally, Goldstein, Ouellet, and Fendrich (1992) found that persons engaged in sex-for-drugs transactions use the greatest variety and largest amount of drugs, and use them more frequently. Their study presented a historical review of sex-for-drugs research over the prior two decades, and compared similarities and differences between contemporary and previous prostitution patterns. Among their findings were that many female crack users, though not all, chose to barter sex for crack, as one of a number of ways to satisfy their desire for the drug. Such bartering is usually associated with traditional prostitution as well. The authors concluded that the introduction of crack cocaine affected the drugs-and-prostitution relationship, both directly and indirectly, by lowering the price of sex for street prostitutes while at the same time requiring increased activity to secure supplies of cocaine, which has a shorter duration of action than heroin;[2] by altering the social status of cocaine, which not so long ago was considered a high-status drug; and by increasing the level of social disorganization in illicit street activities as a result of violence stemming from conflicts associated with competition in crack distribution, as well as with prostitution.

In the NADR study, 30.4% of male and 72.1% of female injection drug users reported that they had exchanged sex for drugs and/or money. For both males and females, higher frequencies of crack use were associated with this practice. The exchange of sex for drugs was not accounted for by traditional prostitution behavior. Furthermore, a majority of crack-using female IDUs engaged in traditional prostitution, while a majority of daily crack-using female IDUs exchanged sex for both money and drugs (Chitwood, 1993). Thus, injection drug users and their sexual partners who use crack are more likely than their non-using peers to engage in exchanging sex for drugs or money. Also, crack use, while related to nontraditional prostitution involving the trading of sex for crack or money, was not related to traditional prostitution.

CONDOM USE

The failure to use condoms has clearly been linked to the transmission of HIV and sexually transmitted disease infection. In the NADR study, unprotected sex was the rule rather than the exception. Only 12.4% of those male injection drug users with one sex partner reported any condom use, and an additional 9.7% reported always using one. Among male injection drug users, those with multiple sex partners were more likely than those with one sex partner to report some condom use (29.5%), but only 9.1% reported always using a condom. For males, crack use was not related to condom use. For female injection drug users, 9.7% of those with one partner reported some condom use, and an additional 7.8% reported always using a condom. Furthermore, 47.1% of females with multiple sex partners during the previous six months reported some condom use, with an additional 16.4% reporting always having used a condom. For female injection drug users, daily crack use was marginally positively related to condom use (Chitwood, 1993). The frequency of condom use by sexually active injection drug users in a study by Wells et al. (1993) was found to be very low for vaginal inter-course for both men and women. In the study of sex-for-drugs traders conducted by Weatherby et al. (1992), 38% of male and 4% of female crack users reported never using condoms, while 18% of males and 41% of females said they always used condoms. Among those who did not trade sex for drugs, condom use was less frequent than among traders: 22% always used condoms, while 55% reported never using condoms.

Interventions to Control the Spread of AIDS

As of the mid-1990s, AIDS was a uniformly fatal disease, with a life ex-pectancy of less than two years after the onset of the first opportunistic infection (Hellinger, 1992). Courses of treatment were minimal. Recent advances, especially the development of protease inhibitors and new com-binations of drugs, have made this picture less bleak. The only definitive way the syndrome can be dealt with effectively is through primary pre-vention activities, however. These encourage the reduction of sharing or using needles and of risky sexual behaviors which act as the main routes of infection (Friedman et al., 1992; Wiebel and Lampinen, 1991).

As a start to these primary prevention activities, massive education cam-paigns were begun in the 1980s. These campaigns have been largely ef-fective in delivering information about the ways in which the disease is spread. A survey of 657 addicts interviewed in the late 1980s prior to an AIDS education intervention indicated that between 71.8% and 97.6% could identify specific AIDS-related risks (Feucht, Stephens, and Gibbs, 1991). Among methadone maintenance patients there was even more consistency, with at least 80% of the 261 subjects able to identify all of the risk behaviors (Selwyn et al., 1987). The sex partners of IDUs also know a great deal about the syndrome. In interviews conducted from 1988 to 1990, between 81% and 97.8% of the 137 female sex partners interviewed knew the ways in which HIV transmission could be prevented (Corby et al., 1991). Having information about transmission does not ap-pear, at least by itself, to reduce substantially the AIDS-risk behavior of abusers, however (Lewis and Galea, 1986). Several types of interventions have been attempted to address the shortcomings of data sharing alone. These include programs to provide sterile needles, interventions into the social context (such as community organization), and interventions with nonaddicted populations (such as the sexual partners of drug abusers).

In addition to the information campaigns designed to teach about risky behaviors, education programs have been conducted to teach ad-dicts and their partners about the techniques which can be used to prevent AIDS transmission, such as rinsing needles, using condoms, and so on (Brown, 1992; Chitwood et al., 1991; McCusker et al., 1992; Siegal et al., 1991). Despite the evidence that AIDS education reduces self-reported risk behavior, there have been disquieting reports that behavior (such as sharing a needle without cleaning it if circumstances warrant this) does not necessarily change for those who are addicted (Lewis and Galea, 1986).

Drug abuse treatment, especially detoxification, is also seen as an effective way of reducing AIDS-risk behavior. Programs have been begun to encourage addicts to enroll in and complete treatment. Several studies used coupons which could be redeemed for detoxification and other forms of treatment to encourage behavior change (Bux et al., 1993; Jackson et al., 1989; Passanante et al., 1991; Sorensen et al., 1993). Results were mixed, with between 59% (Bux et al., 1993) and 84% (Jackson et al., 1989; Passanante et al., 1991) being redeemed. Further study also indicated that continuing in treatment after detoxification was essential to the maintenance of newly learned behaviors (Sorensen et al., 1993). Drug treatment has also been found to reduce the risky sexual behavior of users, including prostitutes (Bellis, 1993).

For cocaine abusers who are also opiate addicts, methadone maintenance treatment has been found to be effective in reducing HIV risk among injection heroin users. For example, one study of six clinics in three cities found that the use of cocaine during the previous thirty days declined from 46.8% at treatment entry to 27.5% among average length of stay patients (that is, those who had been in treatment for 0.50 to 4.49 years). Among long-term methadone maintenance patients (4.5 years+), the rate of cocaine use in the previous thirty days was 17.2%. These changes were statistically significant at the 0.01 level (Ball and Ross, 1991). Other studies have found similar reductions in risk behaviors following entry into methadone maintenance treatment. For example, the sharing of needles and syringes is less common among drug users in treatment than among those not in treatment (Ball et al., 1988; Longshore et al., 1993; Metzger et al., 1991).

The results of at least one study suggest, however, that such positive effects may be greater with respect to use of opiates than for cocaine use. This finding emerged from a study by Chaisson and associates (1989), in which 94% to 95% of heroin-using IDUs treated with either long- or short-term methadone stopped injecting heroin or decreased the frequency with which they had injected the drug prior to treatment entry. Yet, while 68% of cocaine users enrolled in methadone maintenance treatment for less than one year and 57% of cocaine users receiving methadone maintenance treatment for more than one year decreased cocaine injection after treatment entry, 26% began, and 6% increased cocaine injection use after entry into long-term methadone maintenance treatment. Some 12% of cocaine-using subjects also began injection use of cocaine after entering short-term methadone maintenance treatment.

Conclusions

Compulsive sexuality represents a frequent problem among cocaine abusers. Cocaine use results in strong sexual stimulation for many abusers, leading in some cases to compulsive sexuality. Sexual cues may elicit craving for cocaine and vice versa. Thus, treatment of cocaine abuse should also address the compulsive sexual behaviors associated with it. While cocaine use for both males and females results in stimulating effects on both sexual drive and behavior, cocaine also produces strong inhibiting effects (Chitwood, 1985; Macdonald et al., 1988; Weatherby et al., 1992). The relationship between cocaine and sexual behavior may also be highly contextually sensitive (see, for example, Feucht, 1993), as well as a function, for females, of economic factors related to obtaining funds for purchasing the drug (Goldstein, Ouellet, and Fendrich, 1992).

The use of cocaine, in particular crack cocaine, has been identified as contributing to the spread of HIV and other sexually transmitted diseases. This may occur through three mechanisms: increased sexual activity; sexual activity with injection drug users; and prostitution, particularly when engaged in for the purpose of obtaining funds to purchase drugs (Chiasson et al., 1991; Farley, Hadler, and Gunn, 1990; Marx et al., 1991).

Use of cocaine is common among injection drug users. This is the case even where cocaine is not their primary drug of abuse. The use of cocaine is particularly prevalent among female and African American sex partners of IDUs, placing them at increased risk of contracting HIV (Feucht et al., 1993). Such use is closely associated with other high-risk sexual activities, such as frequency of injection and sexual intercourse (Bux, Lamb, and Iguchi, 1995).

Crack smoking is associated with high rates of HIV infection and other sexually transmitted diseases. Among crack smokers, the risk of contracting diseases is increased through high-risk practices such as having sex with multiple partners, exchanging sex for drugs, and failing to use condoms (Booth, Watters, and Chitwood, 1993; Chiasson et al., 1991; Marx et al., 1991; Weatherby et al., 1992). Increased rates of crack smoking, as part of a general pattern of increased drug use, have been seen as a contributing factor in the recent rise of sexually transmitted diseases (Edlin et al., 1992; Marx et al., 1991). Of particular concern is the report that crack use is implicated in the transmission of STDs among adolescents (Fullilove et al., 1990, 1993).

The need for funds with which to purchase crack cocaine and other drugs has led to an increase in prostitution. High proportions of crack cocaine users have been found in several studies to have engaged in sex-for-money or sex-for-drugs transactions (McCoy and Miles, 1992; Weatherby et al., 1992).

A number of interventions to control the spread of AIDS were widely implemented during the late 1980s. Such interventions include education about how the disease is spread and how to protect oneself against it (see, for example, Brown, 1992; Chitwood et al., 1991), as well as drug abuse treatment (see, for example, Bux et al., 1993; Sorensen et al., 1993). In general, the results of evaluation studies have indicated that despite the acquisition of increased knowledge about how to reduce risk (see, for example, Feucht, Stephens, and Gibbs, 1991), many injection drug users still engage in a high rate of risky behaviors (Lewis and Galea, 1986).

For cocaine users who are also heroin users, methadone maintenance treatment has been found to be effective in reducing HIV risk. This risk reduction occurs through reducing both use of cocaine and sharing of drug paraphernalia (Ball et al., 1988; Longshore et al., 1993; Metzger et al., 1991). For a minority of patients, however, entry into methadone maintenance treatment has also been found to be associated with increased cocaine use (Chaisson et al., 1991), suggesting the need to develop appropriate interventions for this subgroup.

IV

Treatment

8

Major Nonpharmacological Treatment Modalities

The Goals of Treatment

The treatment of cocaine abuse has two primary goals: to initiate abstinence and to prevent relapse. These objectives may be approached by a number of means, including pharmacotherapy, psychotherapy, and other therapies. Furthermore, cocaine treatments should attempt to develop alternatives to the use of cocaine and other drugs and provide the former cocaine abuser not only with the skills needed to maintain abstinence, but also with those needed to initiate and lead a drug-free life. Treatment may take place in outpatient, partial hospitalization, or inpatient settings. Nonpharmacological treatment modalities may include psychodynamic, supportive, behavioral, and cognitive behavioral approaches, and may involve the entire range of individual, couples, group, or family therapies. Kleber (1989) makes the point that couples therapy may be needed to repair the very detrimental effects prolonged cocaine use has on relationships, and that family members must learn to recognize the early warning signs and symptoms of relapse. During and after treatment, support groups such as Alcoholics Anonymous, Narcotics Anonymous, and Cocaine Anonymous can be an important source of assistance to the recovering cocaine abuser.

It would appear that treatment for stimulant abuse should be carried out independently from treatment for more general drug and alcohol problems. There are several reasons for this. First, combined treatment may not address the problems specific to cocaine abuse, such as anhedonia and the high level of craving (Gawin and Ellinwood, 1988). Second, while patterns of psychopathology may be similar in some respects to those in abusers of other drugs (Craig, 1988), cocaine abusers appear to differ by having lower rates of borderline and antisocial features and less subjective distress (Malow et al., 1989). Treatment for cocaine abuse should, however, take into account addiction to other drugs (Condelli et al., 1991).

Any effort at rehabilitation of stimulant abusers, once the acute withdrawal period has passed and stabilization has been achieved, includes three general strategies, which have been outlined by Schuckit (1994). The first strategy is the *development and maintenance of high levels of motivation for abstinence* through education about the dangers of stimulants and the benefits of alternative, non-drug lifestyles; outreach to family members to help them assist the patient in avoiding relapse; group therapy to aid the stimulant-dependent individual in reassessing the situation and learning from other drug users how to avoid rationalization of further drug use; and the use of models to help overcome substance abuse problems. The second strategy is *helping the stimulant abuser to rebuild a drug-free life*. Here, individual counseling and self-help groups are of value in helping drug users establish a drug-free peer group; learn how to cope with the stress of daily living without abusing substances; develop options for the appropriate use of free time; and establish interpersonal relationships which focus on a healthy and enjoyable life rather than on survival and drug-related problems. The third step Schuckit describes is concerned with *relapse prevention*. Stimuli that can trigger relapse (for example, particular mood states, geographic locations, and cues associated with drug-using acquaintances) need to be identified and strategies for avoiding and coping with them practiced and established (Kirby et al., 1995). These strategies may require two to four weeks of intense treatment in an inpatient and/or outpatient setting, followed by continued involvement in counseling, self-help, and other support networks for at least several months. Schuckit estimates that the optimal likelihood of improvement following such a regimen is in the 20%–40% range for the year following treatment, regardless of the mix of therapies.

As is the case with treatment for the abuse of other drugs, successful treatment of the cocaine-addicted requires a broad understanding not only of cocaine-related issues but also of addiction in general. Gawin, Khalsa, and Ellinwood (1994) note that the knowledge needed before the clinical presentation by a drug-abusing individual can be adequately understood and interpreted and effective treatment implemented should include an understanding of recent cultural changes and older historical forces, characteristics of both acute stimulant euphoria and acute post-use euphoria, the significance of the route of administration, neurochemical effects, and medical consequences, as well as the clinical characteristics of the transition to dependence, abstinence rates and symptoms, and interactions with psychiatric disorders.

Finally, it should be noted that successful treatment of the cocaine abuser, as is the case with treatment of other addictions, is usually less a case of helping the patient to develop insight into the reasons for abusing substances than one of changing targeted drug-taking behavior(s) through carefully designed interventions which address the habits and patterns associated with such abuse. The development of insight is, of course, valuable in the treatment process. It has yet to be empirically demonstrated, however, that it is *essential* in producing behavioral change in substance abusers, despite many decades of research studies. It should also be kept in mind that while both psychotherapeutic and pharmacological interventions have been shown to have efficacy in substance abuse treatment, neither has been found to be a solution in itself to the problem of substance abuse (Platt, 1986, 1995b).

The Treatment Process

Assessment and Diagnosis

Assessment should be considered an integral part of the treatment process, a time when the patient can be oriented toward and perhaps motivated for treatment (Miller and Rollnick, 1991). Washton, Gold, and Pottash (1987) have suggested a number of techniques and elements in the evaluation process: *assessment of the reasons why the patient seeks treatment,* since failure to do so may lead to later therapeutic failure; *assessment of the potential major obstacles to the patient's success in treatment,* such as inappropriate motivation or treatment goals; *detailed assessment of past and present drug use,* including what drugs were used, how much, when, where, with whom, and how, as well as who assisted in easing the cocaine "crash"; *assessment of the patient's own view of the consequences of drug use,* including those affecting physical health, mood, mental state, occupational and social functioning, interpersonal relationships, financial status, and self-esteem; *determination of the patient's current cocaine use, abuse, or dependency; evaluation for the presence of psychiatric illness,* although it may be necessary to wait three to four weeks following the complete cessation of drug use to conduct a valid examination; and *assessment of the general lifestyle and available support network* in order to maximize recovery and relapse prevention by bolstering alternative sources of gratification and support.

Obtaining the information needed to understand the cocaine-abusing patient initially requires the development of a good working relationship between the patient and the primary treating professional. This is also the first step in developing the therapeutic alliance necessary for a successful treatment intervention. Millman (1988) noted the importance of the following components in the evaluation phase of treatment: a careful and comprehensive *drug history,* including the circumstances surrounding drug use, the psychoactive effects sought, and the route, frequency, and amount of each drug used; a complete *psychiatric history,* including the circumstances regarding the onset of psychiatric symptoms and the relationship of drug use to these symptoms; and a comprehensive *physical examination,* including laboratory toxicologies, to determine routes of administration as well as any sequelae of drug use. The evaluation process should not be limited to the initial phase of treatment, but should continue throughout the treatment process.

As has been noted, cessation of drug use is the first and primary objective of a drug treatment program. Thus, early in treatment the focus should be on practical techniques for achieving abstinence. Washton, Gold, and Pottash (1987) suggest the usefulness of a test period of about thirty days of abstinence before further treatment is attempted, both as a useful therapeutic tool and as an indicator of the patient's motivation for abstinence.

Convincing the patient in an outpatient setting that he or she is an addict is not a necessary first step in the treatment of cocaine addiction (Washton and Stone-Washton, 1993). Such attempts at encouraging acceptance of one's identity as an addict are *not* a prerequisite to a successful outcome, and are often countertherapeutic and a major cause of early dropout. Furthermore, such struggles only confirm the mistaken beliefs of misguided clinicians that patients have to "hit bottom" before becoming serious about recovery (see, for example, Miller, 1985). Nevertheless, every effort should be made to develop on the part of the patient recognition that drug use is significantly impairing certain aspects of his or her life (Millman, 1988).

Washton and Stone-Washton (1990, 1993), in discussing the treatment process with cocaine abusers, identified the formation of a good working relationship with the patient as *the* basis for positively affecting his or her behavior. In this regard they cited Zweben's (1989) dictum that allowing cocaine addicts to resist and be ambivalent about not returning to drugs fosters openness and a willingness on the part of the addict to take personal responsibility for his or her actions. Clinicians' taking an extreme anti-drug stand results in reluctance on the part of patients to share drug fantasies and a greater likelihood that they will *act out* rather than *talk out* their covert impulses to get high. Working with shared goals and establishing an empathetic, understanding, and respectful attitude can result in the clinician's ability to engage highly resistant patients in the treatment process and to explore the patient's true attachment to drugs. Thus, a patient's inability or unwillingness to accept the existence of a problem may be reflective of an early stage of change rather than of an inability or unwillingness to change (Prochaska and DiClemente, 1986, 1992). Time and respectful coaxing may be needed before a patient can move to the next stage of change.

Also, written treatment plans (with a copy to the patient), involvement of significant others, and a combination of individual therapy and a cocaine recovery group should be part of any cocaine treatment program. Such procedures have, in fact, been incorporated into the *Standards for Conducting Outcome Studies of Substance Abusers,* which is used in Germany.[1]

Finally, it bears repeating that the treatment of cocaine abusers should be directed primarily toward the presenting problem: drug abuse. Indirect approaches emphasizing psychotherapy and the acquisition of insight or understanding are likely to be ineffective in addressing cocaine abuse. The therapist may be required to take a highly directive role in treating the cocaine abuser, setting very clear limits. Such a stance may be inconsistent with the nondirective and accepting role that is aimed at allowing the patient sufficient autonomy to make his or her own personal choices and decisions (Washton, Gold, and Pottash, 1987).

Phases of Cocaine Treatment

Treatment of and recovery from cocaine abuse has been conceptualized by a number of writers, including McAuliffe and associates (1990–91), Millman (1988), and Wallace (1990b), as consisting of three phases. Though possibly artificial when viewed by clinicians, and pending confirmation by rigorous research, these conceptualizations remain useful in understanding the process of treating cocaine abuse. During the first phase, *cessation of cocaine use* (Millman, 1988), the patient is assisted in recognizing how cocaine abuse is interfering with his or her life. Drug use then ceases; termination of involvement with drug-using peers and activities occurs; drug education is provided; the individual is encouraged to enter a self-help group; regular family sessions are encouraged (if needed); and a support group is established with regular meetings.

As has been pointed out by Dackis, Gold, and Estroff (1989), this initial phase of treatment must include assessment of Axis I, Axis II, and Axis III problems. Since the presentation of problems after stabilization may differ from those at treatment entry, final assessment and determination of Axis I and Axis II problems should be delayed until two to three weeks after detoxification (Pollack, Brotman, and Rosenbaum, 1989).

The second phase, *early recovery,* lasts from two to twelve months, and involves a focus on relapse prevention and on developing new modes of living in which the patient learns to recognize and cope effectively with a number of important issues. These include learning how to recognize early signs of relapse; coping with the memory of the euphoria associated with cocaine abuse ("euphoric recall"); mastering the desire to gain control over drug use; reinforcing the negative aspects of cocaine use; learning how to avoid drug-related cues, including persons and places; learning how to prevent slips from becoming full-blown relapses; identifying and coping with internal mood states which serve as conditioned cues for drug use; and developing pleasurable and rewarding alternatives to such cues.

The third phase of treatment described by Millman (1988) is *long-term treatment.* During this phase the tasks include maintaining a commitment to abstinence; overcoming renewed denial and overconfidence; improving interpersonal skills; and, as needed, continuing involvement in self-help groups and psycho- or pharmacotherapy.

Wallace's (1990b) conception differs somewhat from the schema proposed by Millman. The first phase, *early initial abstinence/withdrawal,* covers the first two weeks following the last use of crack. This phase requires pharmacological intervention for the severe chemical disruptions produced in the brain by crack, including those attributable to dopamine depletion and receptor supersensitivity, and resulting in craving and other symptoms. The second phase, *prolonging abstinence,* refers to the first six months of recovery, when the risk of relapse is still high, and the task of avoiding a slip or relapse should be reframed in terms of the goal of extending the period of abstinence. The third phase, *pursuing lifetime recovery,* consists of a period of one to several years, perhaps a lifetime, during which the risk of relapse persists. Continuing long-term treatment may be required to assist the individual in avoiding relapse, as well as in preventing involvement in other addictive or compulsive behavior.

Both Millman's and Wallace's conceptions stress stabilization and engagement early in treatment, followed by the development of an understanding of the disease process and the identification of the risks of relapse and high-risk situations. Education in the mechanics of relapse prevention, including coping with slips to cocaine use, occurs next. Both schemas then emphasize the need to continue relapse prevention practices actively throughout one's lifetime.

McAuliffe et al. (1990–91), focusing on outpatients, have postulated three stages of recovery from cocaine addiction: the initial building of "walls" against drug triggers and supplies; the extinguishing of addiction within a protective community of recovering persons; and a gradual lowering of the walls and assisting the addict in expanding beyond the community of recovering persons in order to function more fully in conventional society. In this conceptualization heavy emphasis is placed on preventing relapse, providing intensive support at all stages of recovery, and acquiring alternative responses to the "triggers" that are likely to be encountered in the course of recovery. A special kind of alternative response is the "commitment response," which helps the recovering person meet his or her needs without drugs and binds one to an appropriate course of action while resolving ambivalence.

Treatment Settings and Modalities

As noted, treatment of cocaine abuse may be carried out in a variety of settings. These include outpatient drug-free treatment, inpatient, partial hospitalization, and therapeutic communities.

Outpatient Drug-Free Treatment

Outpatient drug-free treatment as practiced may offer any combination of a number of treatment modalities, including individual treatment sessions several times a week, individual psychotherapy, peer support groups, family therapy, couples or marital therapy, contingency contracting, urine monitoring, and education. Ideally, such treatment should also involve significant others in the patient's life. Such persons may provide valuable assistance in monitoring the patient's behavior and providing alternative activities during periods of craving for drugs (Gawin and Ellinwood, 1988). The involvement of significant others in cocaine treatment has been found to increase the likelihood of abstinence (Higgins, Budney, Bickel, and Badger, 1994).

THE WASHTON INSTITUTE MODEL

Cocaine treatment, as conceptualized by Washton and Stone-Washton (1993), emphasizes the replacement of habitual drug use with habitual attendance at the treatment program. Abstinence becomes "a singular priority." The first stage of treatment, involving a pointed focus on basic habit-breaking strategies, should begin in the first session. Achieving this goal requires five program elements: a highly structured outpatient regimen combining individual, group, and family counseling; education; urine testing; self-help; and an enhanced support network to deal with drug triggers or cues and to assist the patient in resisting readily available cocaine.

The treatment program at the Washton Institute involves three phases, each focused on a specific set of tasks and goals (Washton, 1989a). The first twelve-week phase focuses on breaking the addictive cycle through the establishment of initial abstinence, assessment of the severity of the patient's problem, and enhancement of motivation for change. During this phase patients attend four group sessions and one individual session per week. The second phase of the program, lasting four weeks, involves the same number and types of sessions per week but is focused on solidifying abstinence and learning specific relapse prevention skills. The third phase of the program involves either a twelve-week continuing care group or an open-ended, recovery-oriented psychotherapy group. The former focuses on the provision of peer support and the development of a long-range recovery plan, while the latter focuses on addressing a range of topics, including self-esteem, sexuality, and issues related to adult children of alcoholics. All members of the group are encouraged to attend self-concept meetings, and family members are involved in treatment through an initial four-week education group or through participation in a longer-term codependency group. Urine testing (at least twice per week) is continued throughout the program.

Remaining drug-free between sessions requires the use of a highly structured, moment-by-moment plan for how one's time is spent, with whom it is spent, and how to respond to offers of drugs. This plan is paired with a buddy support system, family involvement in searching for and destroying drugs in the patient's home and car, urine monitoring, and personalized planning (Washton and Stone-Washton, 1990, 1993). The emphasis throughout the program is on the patients' assumption of full responsibility for their own active role in their recovery. The program's responsibility is seen as guiding the patient "carefully through the 'minefields,' 'booby traps,' and 'steep inclines' of daily life and teach[ing] him or her how to avoid drug triggers, dealers, and users and how to manage feelings rather than chemically escape from them" (p. 17).

RAWSON'S NEUROBEHAVIORAL TREATMENT MODEL

Rawson and his associates at the California-based Matrix Center have developed a program for the outpatient treatment of cocaine abuse which they have labeled "Neurobehavioral Treatment" (Rawson et al., 1991, 1993). The neurobehavioral model "utilizes information and strategies derived from clinical research on addiction in an intensive treatment experience" (Rawson et al., 1993, p. 93). Using the techniques developed by many clinical researchers on cocaine treatment, the model attempts to address the dysfunctions present in cocaine abusers when they enter treatment.

In their six-month program, Rawson and his associates see recovery from cocaine abuse as having five distinct stages, each focusing on specific issues and problems: *withdrawal* (0–15 days post-cocaine), during which patients are depressed and disoriented, feel out of control, do not understand what is happening to them, and need explicit direction; *honeymoon* (16–45 days post-cocaine), during which cravings are reduced, mood improves, energy increases, and confidence and optimism return, but during which activity is inefficient and scattered and the risk of dropout and relapse to cocaine abuse is present; *the wall* (46–120 days post-cocaine), during which the major hurdle in the recovery process occurs and vulnerability to relapse increases, as low energy, anhedonia, difficulty concentrating, irritability, loss of sex drive, and insomnia are experienced, and patients believe that these conditions will continue indefinitely; *adjustment* (121–180 days post-cocaine), characterized by a feeling of accomplishment at having completed the wall stage, which often results in the belief that "everything can go back to normal," and during which the beginning of adjustment to a new, normal lifestyle, which began in prior stages, occurs; and *resolution* (181+ days post-cocaine), when a shift occurs from learning new skills to monitoring for signs of relapse, maintaining a balanced lifestyle, and developing new interests.

The goals of treatment are directed toward eliminating drug use and maximizing acquisition of relevant information while retaining as many patients in treatment as possible. Specific goals for the patient include cessation of drug use; remaining in treatment for twelve months; learning about issues critical to addiction and relapse; receiving direction and support from a trained therapist; receiving education for family members affected by the addiction and recovery; becoming familiar with the support available from self-help programs; and urine monitoring.

The results of an evaluation study of the neurobehavioral model conducted during 1986–1989 have been reported by Rawson et al. (1993). On the basis of this study, which was a process evaluation without statistical analysis, the authors drew the following conclusions: the primary attraction of the neurobehavioral model is the individual session (versus group sessions); the participation of family members in treatment results in higher retention rates; and the dropout rate pattern corresponds to the hypothesized stages (that is, 20% dropped out during the first two weeks during the withdrawal stage, while 10.2% dropped out during the wall stage). Subject self-selection into treatment mode complicates drawing statistical conclusions. A more formal evaluation is clearly necessary before the value of this model of treatment can be fully determined.

OUTCOME STUDIES OF OUTPATIENT TREATMENT

Relatively few studies of the effectiveness of outpatient treatment have been conducted. One of these, Kang et al. (1991), failed to demonstrate the effectiveness of psychosocial outpatient therapy in retaining patients in treatment or engendering abstinence from cocaine. Kang and associates evaluated the efficacy of random assignment to once-weekly individual supportive-expressive psychotherapy, family therapy, or group therapy led by paraprofessionals for 168 patients with cocaine or crack addictions. Approximately one-third of subjects dropped out of the study before therapy began. While significant improvement on the Addiction Severity Index (ASI) was observed for the cohort of 122 patients who were interviewed six to twelve months later as a whole, virtually all of the improvement was restricted to 23 subjects (19%) who were not using cocaine at follow-up. Furthermore, there was a strong relationship between abstinence from cocaine use and absence of addiction-related problems, especially psychiatric symptoms and family problems. The authors concluded that outpatient therapy once a week was ineffective in treating cocaine abuse disorders. The 19% abstinence rate obtained in this study most likely was reflective of spontaneous remission for those patients sufficiently motivated to seek treatment, as the number of therapy sessions attended was not related to either number of days of cocaine use or improvement as measured by the ASI. Thus, it was concluded that where improvement took place, it was almost always associated with discontinuing use of cocaine, and that either an intense level of outpatient contact or residential treatment followed by aftercare is probably needed, at least initially, while the patient is attempting to initiate and sustain abstinence.

Inpatient Treatment

The treatment of cocaine abuse is generally unlikely to require inpatient care, since the problem is usually not immediately life-threatening, nor is it associated with a medically dangerous withdrawal syndrome requiring pharmacological intervention under inpatient supervision (Gawin and Kleber, 1986a). At times, however, hospitalization may be necessary to initiate abstinence or to start treatment for those for whom outpatient care has failed. Hospitalization may also be required to address the psychiatric sequelae of cocaine abuse in addicted women during the perinatal period. During such periods of hospitalization, treatment is typically directed only at addressing acute depression or agitation, or at facilitating delivery and preventing perinatal morbidity (Galanter et al., 1992). Despite the usual lack of medical need for such care, patients applying for treatment appear to prefer inpatient treatment. Khalsa, Paredes, et al. (1993) found that fewer than 30% of patients in one treatment study were willing to accept random assignment which potentially would have excluded them from inpatient treatment.

Noting that drug addiction is a chronic disease associated with progressive deterioration (medical, psychiatric, and psychosocial), Dackis, Gold, and Estroff (1989) suggested that severely addicted patients may require hospitalization in order to break the cycle of addiction. Inpatient hospitalization also provides the opportunity for a full medical and psychiatric evaluation under controlled conditions. Roehrich and Gold (1991) recommend inpatient treatment when any of the following conditions are present: uncontrolled cocaine use by intravenous or freebase routes; serious associated medical or psychiatric conditions; previous failure in outpatient treatment; the absence of an existing abstinence support system; or addiction to another drug or drugs requiring detoxification or treatment.

Budde, Rounsaville, and Bryant (1992) largely agreed with Roehrich and Gold (1991) and suggested that inpatient treatment can be justified under several conditions, including the presence of a greater severity of cocaine use, suggesting heavier craving (and thus a diminished ability to achieve an initial period of abstinence); heavy use of other drugs, in particular alcohol; cocaine-associated impairments in social functioning and an absence of social supports necessary for achieving a drug-free state; and previous failure in treatment, indicative of the need for more intensive treatment.

Pollack, Brotman, and Rosenbaum (1989) were in substantial agreement with these other authors. They proposed the following indications for hospital care of cocaine abusers: uncontrolled or chronic use of freebase or intravenous cocaine; concomitant dependence on other substances of abuse and/or need for detoxification from alcohol, sedative-hypnotics, or opiates; serious medical or psychiatric problems, including systemic infections, cardiac events, psychosis, and suicide risk; significant impairment of psychosocial functioning and the absence of familial or social supports; refusal to participate in outpatient treatment, including court- or employer-mandated treatment; repeated failure in outpatient treatment; inability or unwillingness to stop using cocaine as an outpatient; and ready access to cocaine in large quantities.

Cocaine-abusing patients on an inpatient psychiatric service tend to differ from non-abusers along a number of dimensions. In the study by Galanter et al. (1992), cocaine abusers were found to be younger (32.9 years versus 41.6 years for non-abusers), male (78% versus 61%), African American (62% versus 31%), and homeless (52% versus 30%).[2] They were also found to have only an Axis I substance abuse diagnosis (56% versus 42%) as opposed to being dually diagnosed. And they tended to have shorter stays than other psychiatric patients (24.4 days versus 37.7 days). Surprisingly, only 6% were referred to and enrolled in an ambulatory psychiatric clinic upon discharge.

Partial Hospitalization

Partial hospitalization, in the form of either day, evening, or overnight hospitalization, has found wide applicability in the treatment of both chronically and acutely ill psychiatric patients, and its use is indicated for certain of them (Creed, Black, and Anthony, 1989). Treatment for drug addiction perhaps represents the most glaring area of underutilization in psychiatry of this modality (Guydish et al., 1993), although examples exist of the application of day treatment programs to the treatment of alcoholism from a relatively early date (Fox and Lowe, 1967). These alcohol treatment programs have been demonstrated to be less costly than (Collins, Watson, and Zrimec, 1980), and, in a randomized clinical trial, not to differ in outcome from, the more costly residential treatment for alcoholics (McLachlan and Stein, 1982). After reviewing the literature on partial hospitalization, Parker and Knoll (1990) reached the following conclusions: partial hospitalization has been used as a treatment modality for serious mental disorders for over fifty years; it has repeatedly been demonstrated to be as effective as or more effective than long-term inpatient treatment and more effective than traditional outpatient treatment; and it has substantial economic advantages over inpatient treatment. Despite these facts, partial hospitalization in general continues to be underutilized in psychiatry.

The day treatment setting is well suited to the theoretical goal of helping substance abusers become productive, drug-free individuals. Guydish et al. (1993) note several compelling reasons for application of an intensive day treatment model to drug abuse: the nonspecificity of day treatment, which allows its application to treatment populations with multiple addictions; its applicability for use with a population having dual diagnoses; and its value as an intervention midway between the residential therapeutic community and the traditional outpatient model. Day treatment may be particularly useful for patients from severely disadvantaged socioeconomic backgrounds who are treated in public hospitals. Galanter et al. (1993) described such a program for crack cocaine abusers in a general hospital setting, which involved both peer-led milieu treatment and professional services, and found that the 150 patients entering it attended an average of 44 times during the year studied, and that 39% had an acceptable treatment outcome. Platt et al. (1995), however, compared day treatment (40 hours/week) against standard outpatient treatment (3 hours/week) for cocaine abusers but did not find any differences in effectiveness. Specifically, there were no differences in retention rates or cocaine use after one month in treatment and after the complete twelve-week course of treatment. In both samples, living arrangements (structured shelter versus independent living situations) were found to be related to both retention in treatment and continued cocaine use, with those patients in a structured setting tending to remain in treatment longer and to achieve cocaine abstinence. These findings are inconsistent with others indicating that, in general, greater treatment exposure results in better outcomes (Carroll et al., 1993; Hubbard et al., 1989; Lamb, Kirby, and Platt, 1995), and that day treatment is superior to outpatient treatment in psychiatry (Parker and Knoll, 1990). Another evaluation comparing day treatment with inpatient treatment found no differential effectiveness (Alterman et al., 1994).

Residential Treatment: The Therapeutic Community

The long-term therapeutic community (TC) as a treatment modality for drug abusers is based on a model of individual change achieved through the use of the community as the change agent. The therapeutic community is intended to simulate a model family environment within which the resident optimally acquires role models, skills, and relationships not acquired during the formative years. Essential elements of this approach include firm behavioral norms; reality-oriented group and individual therapy; a system of clearly defined rewards and punishments through a communal economy of housework and other roles; a "ladder" of hierarchical responsibilities; and the potential of advancement from client to staff role (Institute of Medicine, 1990). The therapeutic community model has received substantial attention in the research literature, and the results of several nationally based multisite studies have provided evidence for the effectiveness of this modality (Hubbard et al., 1989; Institute of Medicine, 1990; Simpson and Sells, 1990). Much of the work published to date has been based on addicts, most of whom were primary opiate abusers or polydrug abusers entering therapeutic communities prior to the cocaine epidemic of the late 1980s (De Leon, 1993). Its usefulness with the cocaine-using population is thus largely untested.

Comparative Studies of Treatment Modalities

INPATIENT VERSUS OUTPATIENT TREATMENT

Several studies have compared inpatient and outpatient treatments in order to determine their differential efficacy in treating cocaine addiction. Generally, little evidence exists for the greater effectiveness of inpatient over outpatient treatment of addictive disorders.[3] Many drug abuse patients, however, perceive inpatient care as having been of greater help to them than other forms of treatment (Marsh et al., 1990). There is also some suggestion that intensive treatment may be more differentially effective for severely disturbed and less socially stable patients (Miller and Hester, 1986).

Washton and Stone-Washton (1993) reported the results of an uncontrolled treatment evaluation study of 60 drug addicts, 85% of whom were cocaine addicts, approximately evenly divided between snorters and crack smokers. Completion rates were very similar for inpatients and outpatients (77% versus 74%, respectively), as were abstinence rates following treatment (64% versus 68%). Of all abstinent patients, both inpatient and outpatient, 46% were continuously abstinent for the entire treatment and follow-up period. Slippage to the primary drug of abuse occurred at least once in 33% of all patients, while 23% slipped at least once to marijuana or alcohol but not to their primary drug. When premature dropout occurred, it was almost always associated with relapse. No relapsed patients completed treatment, whereas 87% of abstinent patients completed treatment. Cocaine smoking was associated with a lower abstinence rate (58%) than cocaine snorting (78%). While noting that the size of the subject sample and other methodological limitations prevented conclusive results, the authors suggested that these findings indicated that successful treatment of cocaine and crack addicts can take place in both inpatient and outpatient programs which are followed by intensive aftercare treatment emphasizing relapse prevention, and that for many patients, intensive outpatient treatment can be a cost-effective alternative to inpatient treatment.

In a nonrandomized, naturalistic study, Budde, Rounsaville, and Bryant (1992) examined treatment outcomes one year after treatment for a sample of predominantly male, young (under 20 years of age), and higher socioeconomic status cocaine addicts who had undergone inpatient or outpatient treatment. At admission the outpatients were more likely to have a current diagnosis of a depressive disorder, while inpatients were more likely to have a current diagnosis of alcoholism, a history of suicide attempts, and more severe ASI ratings for drugs, alcohol, family/social, and psychiatric problems. Inpatients and outpatients were compared at one year posttreatment for drug-related problems, recent drug use, treatment seeking since discharge, and current level of depression. Those patients who had received inpatient treatment, in comparison with those patients who had undergone outpatient treatment, had lower ratings of problem severity in several areas, particularly drug use, employment, psychiatric status, frequency of cocaine use, and depressive symptomatology. Alternative explanations for these findings include inpatients' having a better long-term prognosis because of higher socioeconomic status despite poorer clinical status at admission and a low rate of follow-up (64%). The authors concluded that the results supported the greater effectiveness of inpatient treatment for cocaine addiction. Nonetheless, the design weaknesses of the study were such that further confirming studies are required.

Khalsa, Paredes, and associates (1993) evaluated the effectiveness of a number of treatment interventions, either singly or in combination. Veterans Administration patients were assigned to 21-day inpatient treatment, "intermediate" outpatient treatment, or community self-help groups. The inpatient program included individual counseling, group therapy, and drug education, and was guided by a twelve-step philosophy. This intervention was often followed by other treatment modalities, but without any systematic basis for assignment to postintervention care. The outpatient program consisted of one to four visits with a physician, followed by individual counseling on an as-needed basis, and a weekly group session based on the Alcoholics Anonymous program. Thus, both programs incorporated the twelve-step philosophy. Each patient received one of six possible combinations of treatment: a single episode of 21-day inpatient care; multiple episodes of residential care lasting more than 1 month, and including admissions to both inpatient and therapeutic community programs; inpatient care of at least 21 days, followed by outpatient or self-help program involvement at least weekly for a minimum of 6 months ("high-intensity" treatment); high-intensity outpatient or self-help involvement without inpatient treatment; a single episode of inpatient treatment followed by low-intensity (less than once weekly for fewer than 6 months) outpatient or therapeutic community involvement; and low-intensity outpatient and/or self-help treatment without inpatient care.

At follow-up (a year after treatment), outcomes were evaluated according to the combination of treatments received by each patient. Overall, when the 12 month periods preceding and following treatment were compared, there was a significant reduction in cocaine use for all groups. Prior to treatment entry, patients reported smoking crack on 45% to 65% of days each month during the prior year; after treatment, the figures fell to 22% to 37% of days per month on average spent smoking crack. Similarly, cocaine use at a severe level (defined as "daily use for at least a month or a series of heavy binges or very heavy, and at least biweekly, binges") was significantly reduced. Prior to treatment entry, 65% to 75% of days per month were spent using crack at this level, while following treatment, this figure fell to 17% to 22%. At the same time, the mean percentage of time spent not using cocaine increased to 58% to 69% of days per month following treatment, compared with 5% to 20% prior to treatment entry. Following treatment, mean time spent in drug dealing also dropped, from between 18% and 22% prior to treatment to below 6% following treatment. Otherwise, little change was observed with respect to mean time spent working, engaging in stable relationships, or engaging in criminal activity (Khalsa, Paredes et al., 1993).

Treatment combinations most preferred by patients in this study, based on numbers of patients selecting each, were inpatient treatment followed by high-intensity outpatient or self-help treatment (selected by 29%) and inpatient treatment followed by low-intensity outpatient or self-help treatment (selected by 26%). The least preferred treatment combinations were low-intensity outpatient and/or self-help care (selected by 5%) and high-intensity outpatient and/or self-help treatment (3%). With respect to drug use following treatment, exposure to all treatment combinations resulted in a decrease in the proportion of time spent smoking crack. Differences between treatment combinations did not reach statistical significance on this variable. The highest rates of abstinence, however, were achieved by patients involved in inpatient treatment followed by high-intensity outpatient or self-help and high-intensity outpatient and/or self-help alone, while a significant reduction in the proportion of time spent in severe use occurred in the group receiving inpatient treatment followed by high-intensity outpatient and/or self-help. The other major outcomes were a decrease in drug deal-ing and criminal activity for all treatment combinations (with the great-est change evident in inpatient treatment followed by high-intensity outpatient and/or self-help) and a decrease in excessive alcohol con-sumption for all groups. The high-intensity outpatient and/or self-help group also showed less severe cocaine use and the highest rate of co-caine abstinence, although the multiple residential treatment group also improved, reaching the level achieved by the former group one year fol-lowing treatment.

Khalsa, Paredes et al. (1993) concluded that their findings suggested a positive outcome for any combination of treatment interventions uti-lized in the study, but with better outcomes for frequent, longer-term treatment. The importance of these findings must be somewhat tem-pered, however, by the self-selection of treatment modalities by entrants into the study, and the resultant lack of random assignment, a fact that the researchers themselves readily acknowledged.

PARTIAL VERSUS INPATIENT HOSPITALIZATION

O'Brien, McLellan, and associates (1992) described initial evaluation findings of a randomized study of day versus inpatient treatment for cocaine-abusing and cocaine-dependent men. A somewhat later report of preliminary results on 104 patients has also been published (Alterman, O'Brien, and Droba, 1993). The evaluation findings that follow are drawn from this latter source. While both programs lasted approximately a month, the day hospital program operated 6 hours Mondays through Thursdays and 3 hours on Friday (27 hours/week), while the residential inpatient program provided a total of 48 hours of treatment weekly. The major intervention in both programs was group meetings focusing on overcoming denial and helping patients cope with everyday problems and stresses. Drug abuse education, recreational therapy, and participa-tion in self-help groups were also components of both programs. Individual counseling and psychotropic medication were provided as needed. Final evaluation results (Alterman et al., 1994) indicated that, at 7 months, inpatients were significantly more likely to have completed treatment than were day patients (89.1% versus 53.6%); but while sig-nificant decreases in levels of alcohol and other drug abuse were still present in both groups, there were no significant differences between groups. Both groups had improved significantly at the 7-month follow-up in non–substance-related functioning (that is, family/social, psy-chological, and employment problem areas on the Addiction Severity Index). Furthermore, successful completion of the day treatment program followed by participation in self-help groups resulted in lower rates of alcohol and cocaine abuse during follow-up (McKay et al., 1994). Alterman, O'Brien, and Droba suggested that their data indicated that while inpatients received significantly more medical treatment, and day hospital patients received significantly more psychiatric treatment, the quantity of treatment received in the remaining five areas was equal for the two groups. Thus, if the amount of treatment received determined its effectiveness, there would be less expectation of a superior outcome for the inpatient group, unless medical treatment, the only area in which inpatients received more service, was particularly salient in treating cocaine abuse.

Chemical Dependency Treatment

Chemical dependency treatment, also known as Minnesota or Hazeltontype treatment (Cook, 1988a, b), is a term applied to the therapeutic approach used by the private treatment sector. This treatment approach is typically offered in settings such as private psychiatric hospitals and other residential milieus. In chemical dependency treatment, drug dependency is regarded as the primary disease or problem and is considered not necessarily reflective of a psychiatric disorder. This approach may be contrasted with the *psychiatric model,* in which the use of drugs is regarded as self-medication for the treatment of an underlying psychiatric disorder. Without treatment of this underlying disorder, abstinence will be difficult or impossible to attain (Millman, 1988). Chemical dependency programs may focus on the development of pleasurable and rewarding alternatives to substance abuse, since the patient is considered always to be at risk. Thus, in this model the patient is, and will always be, in the process of recovering.

While generally noting its effectiveness, Millman (1988) also observed several deficiencies in chemical dependency treatment. As one consequence of its deemphasis of the psychiatric approach, there may be a failure to recognize or appropriately treat psychopathology, particularly subtle symptomatology, as well as a failure to incorporate the latest understanding of the addiction which derives from psychiatry. Such deficits may result in patients' precipitous withdrawal from treatment, with resultant demoralization and risk for resumption of drug abuse. Chemical dependency treatment may also place undue reliance on a uniform disease model, with the result that all compulsive substance abuse disorders are treated similarly. This approach may be inappropriate in many cases, since it may fail to lead to a full understanding of the nature of the addiction. Additionally, the use of the same 28- to 30-day inpatient intervention for all substance abuse patients may not be appropriate.

Chemical dependency treatment has not been subjected to rigorous evaluation (see Platt, 1995b). It is likely, however, that this situation will change, as the demands of managed care financing will require that this relatively expensive form of substance abuse treatment provide documentation of both its effectiveness and its cost-effectiveness.

Self-Help

Twelve-step self-help programs such as Cocaine Anonymous (CA), Alcoholics Anonymous (AA), and Narcotics Anonymous (NA) may fill a void in a patient's life and contribute to reducing the risk of relapse. Such programs employ a variety of behavioral, cognitive, educational, self-control, and relapse prevention techniques to minimize craving and relapse (Millman, 1988). Thus, Washton and Stone-Washton (1993) recommend involvement in such self-help fellowships for recovering cocaine abusers. Clinician recommendations for such involvement may, however, potentially lead to "power struggles," which are to be avoided. Thus, a patient's resistance to involvement in self-help groups should be used as an opportunity to explore his or her resistance to the recovery process in general (Zweben, 1987). There is as yet relatively little evidence available regarding the efficacy of self-help interventions for cocaine abuse, although evaluation research is beginning to emerge with respect to the treatment of alcoholism (see, for example, the reviews by Bean-Bayog, 1991 and Emrick, 1987), and heroin addiction (McAuliffe, 1990; McAuliffe and Ch'ien, 1986; Nurco, Stephenson, and Hanlon, 1990–91; Nurco, Stephenson, and Naesea, 1981; Nurco et al., 1983; Zackon, McAuliffe, and Ch'ien, 1985).

Psychotherapy

Engagement

Engaging abusers of cocaine and other stimulants in treatment is a difficult task, and often remains unaccomplished. In a very early study, O'Malley, Anderson, and Lazare (1972) offered psychotherapy to 18 amphetamine users, but not one of the patients returned for even a single scheduled visit. A similar but not so complete lack of success was obtained with abusers of barbiturates and hallucinogens (Anderson, O'Malley, and Lazare, 1972).

Millman (1988) has emphasized the need for the therapist to demonstrate an "active, educational, advisory, and supportive stance" (p. 32) during the early stages of psychotherapy, when the focus is on controlling drug abuse and dealing with the patient's interpersonal and work-related difficulties. As is the case with treatment in general, the early course of psychotherapy should also focus on the development of a therapeutic relationship, and the therapist should adopt an attitude of empathy and acceptance, although these qualities must be tempered by tact, discipline, and the need to set limits. There is also a need to recognize and manage the "profound and unsettling" (Millman, 1988, p. 31) dependencies, either on the therapist or on the program, which may develop on the part of the patient. In the early stages of treatment, according to Millman, positive transference should be encouraged and negative transference should be addressed only if it becomes a threat to the therapeutic relationship. To maintain effectiveness, the therapist must also demonstrate an accurate perception of the individual patient as well as possess an adequate knowledge of abused substances and the disorder he or she is treating.

Psychotherapeutic Approaches

Psychotherapy for cocaine addiction has generally been fashioned on the twelve-step model used in Alcoholics Anonymous (O'Brien, McLellan, et al., 1992). Psychodynamically oriented psychotherapy has been applied, but without a great deal of success (Khantzian, 1985; Resnick and Resnick, 1984; Schiffer, 1988; Spotts and Shontz, 1984), as was also the case for interpersonal psychotherapy (Rounsaville, Gawin, and Kleber, 1985). More recently, behavioral (Anker and Crowley, 1982; O'Brien et al., 1988) and cognitive-behavioral (Carroll, Rounsaville, and Keller, 1991) interventions have been employed with some success, particularly in the case of contingency management (Higgins et al., 1993b; Higgins, Budney, Bickel, Foerg, et al., 1994). In general, problems associated with psychotherapy for stimulant abuse include mixed compliance and high rates of relapse after initial abstinence (Rawson et al., 1986); high rates of treatment dropout (Anker and Crowley, 1982); and failure to participate (Anderson, O'Malley, and Lazare, 1972).

PSYCHODYNAMICALLY ORIENTED PSYCHOTHERAPY

Schiffer (1988) reported the successful treatment of nine cocaine abusers with traditional long-term, in-depth psychodynamic psychotherapy in a private hospital setting. Treatment was initially begun while the patients were on an inpatient drug treatment unit, and continued after discharge. According to Schiffer, the treatment process consisted of four steps: searching for traumatic or abusive conditions in the patient's childhood which might help explain the current drug problem; establishing emotional contact; helping the patient to appreciate how the abuse had affected him; and helping the patient to master the traumatic experiences. Follow-up indicated a range of 18 to 62 months of abstinence, with only two patients having a brief relapse to cocaine, after which they maintained complete abstinence for over three years.

It should be noted that all the patients in the case studies reported by Schiffer (1988) were employed and had medical insurance. Schiffer even commented that "all nine patients were reasonably cooperative and intelligent, and each in the past had acquired some significant work skills and relationships" (p. 131). No doubt their premorbid social competence contributed to the good outcomes. Unfortunately, such backgrounds are not typically the case in most cocaine abusers today, who come from impoverished backgrounds, are unlikely to be working, and are uninsured or underinsured.

INTERPERSONAL PSYCHOTHERAPY

Introduced by Klerman and associates (1984), interpersonal psychotherapy is a brief, individual intervention which has two primary goals: the reduction of symptoms and the improvement of social functioning. The original focus of this intervention was on depressive symptomatology. This was later changed to one addressing the reduction or elimination of drug use and the development of strategies for dealing with interpersonal problems associated with the onset and continuation of drug use. The definitive characteristics of interpersonal psychotherapy, as listed by Rounsaville, Gawin, and Kleber (1985), are adherence to a medical model of psychiatric disorders; a focus on the patient's current difficulties in interpersonal functioning; brevity and an emphasis on consistency of focus; and a therapist stance similar to that used in exploratory and supportive psychotherapies.

The interpersonal problem areas used in the intervention address the kinds of problems presented by drug-abusing patients. Three subgoals of stopping drug use have been identified: *acceptance of the need to stop, and not just reduce, drug use* through rejecting the idealized, romantic view of such use, as well as accepting the costs associated with drug use; the *management of impulsiveness* through the development of appropriate cognitive structures; and *recognition of the context of drug use and of supply,* including the places, persons, affect states, and situations which trigger drug use (Rounsaville and Carroll, 1993). Strategies to improve interpersonal functioning and thus to help the patient reach these goals include uncovering the role drugs play in the patient's psychological and interpersonal life; identifying interpersonal events and mental states which result in relapse; and finding appropriate substitutes for drug use. These strategies have been applied to four interpersonal problem areas: interpersonal role disputes, role transitions, grief, and interpersonal deficits. Illustrations of interpersonal psychotherapy intervention strategies for drug abusers in each of these areas may be found in Rounsaville and Carroll (1993).

Interpersonal psychotherapy for substance abusers has been evaluated in several studies. In one, conducted with methadone-maintained heroin addicts who also had a concurrent psychiatric disorder, Rounsaville et al. (1983) compared interpersonal psychotherapy with a "low contact" condition. The interpersonal psychotherapy condition consisted of one hour of weekly psychotherapy with a psychiatrist or psychologist. The low contact condition consisted of one twenty-minute meeting monthly in which symptoms and social functioning were reviewed. Otherwise, both groups received treatment as usual in a methadone maintenance treatment setting. Dropout rates were high in both groups (62% in the interpersonal psychotherapy condition, and 46% in the low contact condition), and treatment outcomes were similar. Individual psychotherapy was seen as not adding to the benefits of a full-service methadone program, despite the fact that another study suggested the superiority of professional psychotherapy over drug counseling (Woody et al., 1984).

In one of the few evaluations of psychotherapy for cocaine abuse conducted in the form of a randomized clinical trial, Carroll, Rounsaville, and Gawin (1991) compared interpersonal psychotherapy with a cognitive-behavioral program emphasizing relapse prevention. This study randomly assigned 42 outpatient cocaine abusers to either a relapse prevention cognitive-behavioral program (Marlatt and Gordon, 1985) adapted for cocaine abusers or to interpersonal therapy, a short-term psychodynamic approach developed by Rounsaville, Gawin, and Kleber (1985). Attrition was high in both groups, but was significantly higher for patients in the interpersonal psychotherapy condition (with 62% failing to complete a twelve-week course of treatment) than in the relapse prevention condition (with 33% not completing). The two treatments did not show initial differences in outcomes. When subjects were stratified by pretreatment severity of cocaine abuse, however, severe users treated with relapse prevention methods were much more likely to become abstinent than those treated with interpersonal therapy (54% versus 9%). Among subjects with lower levels of severity, improvement or lack of improvement occurred regardless of type of treatment received. Similarly, among subjects with high levels of psychopathology, those in the relapse prevention group were significantly more likely to become abstinent than those in the interpersonal psychotherapy group (58% improvement versus 14% improvement). Furthermore, the presence of antisocial personality disorder was predictive of failure to complete treatment, as well as failure to improve in treatment. Noting the similarity of their findings to those obtained by Woody et al., (1983) for psychotherapy with opiate addicts, Carroll, Rounsaville, and Gawin (1991) concluded that some cocaine abusers can be successfully treated with a purely psychotherapeutic approach, and that patient characteristics (in particular, severity of psychiatric impairment and substance abuse symptomatology) mediate overall response to treatment as well as response to specific forms of treatment. Perhaps the most important finding of this study was that some psychotherapies can be effective in *initiating* abstinence from cocaine.

Unfortunately, the findings of the Rounsaville et al. (1983) and the Carroll, Rounsaville, and Gawin (1991) studies do not suggest as high a level of promise for these interventions with cocaine abusers as was obtained with depressed patients. Rounsaville and Carroll (1993) have, however, outlined a number of implementation issues as well as clinical differences between drug-abusing and depressed patients which may have accounted for the failure to obtain more powerful findings. Thus, the more chronic and broader problems presented by drug abuse patients as a result of the protracted nature of the illness and the need to curtail drug-taking behavior make treating them more difficult than treating depressed patients.

Behavioral Interventions

Behavioral interventions for the treatment of cocaine abuse are not new, nor have they been widely utilized. Proponents of this approach, however, have been able to demonstrate empirical evidence for their successful use. The behavioral approach conceptualizes drug taking as an operant behavior. In this model, behaviors operate in the environment, that is, they are emitted by the organism and are then maintained or modified by the consequences they elicit. Drugs of abuse serve as reinforcers which control behaviors by increasing or decreasing the probability of their occurrence. The fact that animals self-administer, without prior experience, drugs which are abused by humans, and under similar temporal patterns, allows manipulations of availability, dose, response cost, and other variables, and has led to the development of a large body of knowledge about the influence on drug use of a variety of environmental, pharmacological, and other variables (Grabowski, Higgins, and Kirby, 1993; Stitzer, Bigelow, and McCaul, 1983).[4]

One of the earliest studies to employ behavioral principles was that conducted by Chambers, Taylor, and Moffett (1972) at Philadelphia General Hospital. Once it was found that 18.5% of a sample of 173 patients in the hospital's methadone program were using cocaine, a test for this substance was included in the program's regular urine surveillance program. Positive urine test findings resulted in a confrontation between staff and patients about patient drug use. As a result of such confrontations, positive urine test results dropped from 18.5% to 10.4% after one month, to 7.9% after four months, and to 2.3% after sixteen months. Condelli et al. (1991), in analyzing the results of this study, pointed out the absence of data that would be essential to either full evaluation or replication. This included an absence of information about the following: specific programmatic details regarding the nature and implementation of the intervention, particularly the confrontation process; the consequences of drug use; how well the intervention worked when staff were not confronted with the patient's positive test results; the actual monitoring and measurement of either the implementation of the intervention or other drug use; patient dropout over the course of the study; and changes in patterns of drug use by patients. In addition, most of the knowledge in this study has been developed with respect to abuse of cocaine and other illicit substances by opiate addicts in methadone maintenance treatment (see, for example, Dolan et al., 1985; McCarthy and Borders, 1985; Stitzer et al., 1986).

An early study by Anker and Crowley (1982) demonstrated that cocaine abusers could be drawn into treatment and that contingency management could be useful in attaining abstinence. In this study, 67 daily or near-daily cocaine abusers were offered contingency contracting as an adjunct to standard clinical treatment, which was primarily a psychotherapeutic intervention consisting of brief hospitalization (if indicated); medical and psychological evaluation; weekly psychotherapy; family and couples therapy; urine monitoring; education; referral; and aftercare. A counseling component of the program was directed at developing cocaine-incompatible behaviors through increased contacts with non–drug-using friends; elimination of paraphernalia and drug stashes; termination of relationships with drug dealers; changes in phone numbers or addresses, when needed, to stop drug-related calls and visits; spousal counseling; and psychotherapy for related problem areas. A contingency contract required that the patient would participate in urinalysis monitoring and that, in the event that a specimen was cocaine-positive, the patient would receive a prearranged personalized aversive consequence.[5] Of the 32 patients who entered the contract, typically for a period of from three to six months, 31 (97%) remained abstinent during that time. In the comparison group, which consisted of the 35 patients who did not enter the contract, 29 (83%) terminated treatment within five sessions, and none was abstinent for more than four weeks.

Limitations of the study have been noted by a number of writers, including Gawin and Kleber (1987); Havassy, Wasserman, and Hall (1993); and Higgins et al. (1991). These include the following observations: patients were self-selected (they chose whether to enter the contract or the comparison group), which opens the possibility that those who entered the contract would have done well under any treatment condition; the contract was not accepted by a majority of the patients; and the use of strong aversive contingencies raised ethical concerns. Nonetheless, this study represented the first demonstration of the application of behavioral contracting, including aversive contingencies, to the prevention of relapse in cocaine abusers.

Following the initial work by Anker and Crowley (1982), Higgins et al. (1991) outlined a more detailed behavioral strategy for treating drug abuse. This strategy involved rearranging the drug user's environment and consisted of four components: the detection of drug abuse; the positive reinforcement of drug abstinence; the loss of reinforcements following continued drug use; and increased density of reinforcement derived from non-drug sources in order to compete with the reinforcing effects of drugs. As noted by Higgins et al. (1991), such a model had already been successfully applied to the treatment of alcohol (Hunt and Azrin, 1973), tobacco (Hall et al., 1987), opioid (Stitzer et al., 1984), and stimulant abuse and dependence (Anker and Crowley, 1982).

In the Higgins et al. (1991) study, the overall goal of the intervention was to use the incentives to achieve initial cocaine abstinence and to retain patients in treatment, thereby gaining time to counsel them on longer-term lifestyle changes necessary to maintain cocaine abstinence. This goal was accomplished by the inclusion of two behavioral components: the establishment of cocaine abstinence by means of a contingency management program in which incentives were provided contingent on abstinence as evidenced by urinalysis; and the positive reinforcement of appropriate social behavior through adoption of the community reinforcement approach (CRA). This approach was originally developed for the treatment of alcohol dependence by Hunt and Azrin (1973) and further defined by Azrin and his associates (see, for example, Azrin, 1976; Azrin et al., 1982). The goal of this intervention component was to increase the efficacy of non-drug sources of reinforcement by improving the patient's job status, family and social relations, and recreational activities. These goals were addressed in a nonrandomized twelve-week outpatient trial by Higgins et al. (1991) in a sample of 13 consecutively admitted cocaine-dependent outpatients. A control group consisted of 15 cocaine-dependent individuals who entered the same clinic but were instead offered a twelve-step drug counseling program for cocaine dependence. The two treatments were accepted by all 13 patients offered the behavioral treatment and by 12 of the 15 patients offered the 12-step program.

The results were very promising, in that 11 of the 13 cocaine patients in the behavioral treatment were retained in treatment for 12 weeks, compared with 5 of 12 patients in the twelve-step counseling program. Continuous abstinence from cocaine in the behavioral therapy group reached 4 weeks for 10 of the patients, 8 weeks for 6 of the patients, and 12 weeks for 3 patients. By contrast, in the twelve-step group, 3 of the patients reached 4 weeks of continuous abstinence, and none reached 8 to 12 weeks of continuous abstinence. On the basis of these findings, Higgins et al. (1991) concluded that the behavioral treatment was well accepted, was effective in retaining patients in treatment, and showed a good record in achieving abstinence. Furthermore, the use of only a few exclusion criteria increased the potential for generalizability of these results (a particularly important point given that the study was conducted in a rural setting in Vermont, where drug use is generally low). The authors did note, however, that a number of criticisms could be raised about the study. First, the study was not a randomized trial, with the result that the two groups differed on important demographic variables. Second, the incentives were costly (up to a value of $12.35 daily), preventing implementation in many community clinics. And third, the use of drugs other than cocaine continued during abstinence from cocaine. It should also be noted that the study's subject recruitment procedures (for example, the use of newspaper ads to obtain volunteers) throws its representativeness into question.

Budney et al. (1991) next applied a multiple baseline design in evaluating a behavioral intervention for cocaine abuse for two males diagnosed with cocaine dependence. The intervention consisted of contingency management and a community reinforcement approach (CRA), and the goal was to increase abstinence from cocaine and marijuana. In the initial phase, reinforcement was provided contingent on the submission of cocaine-free urine specimens. The community reinforcement approach was provided during two behavioral therapy sessions each week. During this phase, almost complete abstinence was achieved for cocaine use but not for marijuana use. During a second phase, behavior therapy was reduced to once a week, and the magnitude of reinforcement was also reduced but was still made contingent on submission of cocaine-free urine specimens. No change in cocaine abstinence or marijuana use occurred as a result of these changes. A third phase involved making the delivery of reinforcements contingent on submitting both cocaine- and marijuana-free urines. This change resulted in a sharp increase in marijuana abstinence while maintaining cocaine abstinence. At follow-up, however, marijuana use was found to have resumed. The authors concluded that this behavioral intervention, while effective in achieving abstinence from cocaine and marijuana, was effective in achieving maintenance of abstinence only in the case of cocaine. As with the previous study, one problem in this intervention was the cost of incentives, which eventually reached $12.36 daily, a cost, however, that the authors called well justified compared to the costs of either hospital treatment for cocaine abuse or the health consequences of such use. It should also be noted that the very small number of subjects ($N = 2$) reduces the strength of any conclusions that could be drawn.

Higgins et al. (1993b) conducted a randomized trial utilizing their behavioral model, and compared its effectiveness with drug counseling of the type found in standard outpatient care. Thirty-eight cocaine-dependent patients were randomly assigned to a behavioral treatment consisting of contingency-management procedures combined with counseling based on the community reinforcement approach (Sisson and Azrin, 1989). This treatment approach included urine monitoring and feedback, with incentives for cocaine-free urines; one-hour counseling sessions (twice weekly for 12 weeks, and once weekly for the next 12 weeks), including the involvement of significant others, training in recognition of antecedents and consequences of cocaine use, and skill training (drug refusal, problem solving, and assertiveness); employment counseling; recreational counseling (during which contingency-management and community reinforcement components of treatment could be integrated); and disulfirum therapy for those patients with diagnosable DSM-III-R alcohol dependence. The drug abuse counseling condition contained the following elements: urinalysis without feedback to patients; a 2.5-hour weekly group counseling session together with a 1-hour individual therapy session during weeks 1 through 12, followed by one group or individual session during weeks 13 through 24; voluntary self-help meetings (drug and AIDS education and twelve-step); and disulfirum therapy for alcohol-dependent persons only on the recommendation of their counselor.

When the results obtained from the two groups were compared, 58% of the 19 patients in the behavioral treatment group were found to have completed 24 weeks of treatment, as opposed to 11% of the drug abuse counseling group. Eight weeks of continuous cocaine abstinence was achieved by 68% of the behavioral treatment group, compared with 11% of the drug abuse counseling group. Finally, 16 weeks of continuous cocaine abstinence was achieved by 42% of the behavioral treatment group, compared with 5% of the drug abuse counseling group. Higgins and his associates considered the behavioral intervention used in this study promising for a number of reasons, including its high degree of acceptability to patients; the effectiveness of the intervention in retaining patients in treatment; the effective establishment of clinically significant periods of abstinence; the reliability of the findings, in that they replicated the findings from the earlier, nonrandomized trial (Higgins et al., 1991); the utility of the intervention with intravenous cocaine users; and the applicability of the intervention for the treatment of multiple drug abuse.

The studies conducted by Higgins and his associates is based to a significant extent on two bodies of work: the behavioral approach to the treatment of substance abuse (Griffiths, Bigelow, and Henningfield, 1980) and the community reinforcement approach, or CRA (Azrin, 1976; Azrin et al., 1982; Hunt and Azrin, 1973). Two major difficulties of community reinforcement approaches programs have been noted: their labor-intensive nature and consequent high cost, and the potentially intrusive format of such interventions. The first concern was readily addressed by Grabowski, Higgins, and Kirby (1993) in noting that the cost is no greater than that of many standard treatments presently being used in traditional treatment settings, and considerably less than inpatient treatment. They acknowledged, however, that certain aspects of the approach may be intrusive, such as when spouses or employers are informed of urinalysis results. The particular vulnerability of cocaine patients, who are in acute distress during treatment, requires clinician sensitivity to such handicaps.

Higgins and his colleagues have also examined the various components of their behavioral treatment program individually in order to assess their efficacy. For example, disulfirum therapy, which was part of the behavioral treatment program evaluated in their 1993b study, was also evaluated in a separate analysis (Higgins et al., 1993a). Outcomes for patients who had had two weeks or more on and two weeks off disulfirum therapy (at a dose of 250 mg daily) were examined. Those patients who had received disulfirum therapy showed significant decreases in both drinking and cocaine use. To evaluate the effect of incentives on treatment outcome, Higgins, Budney, Bickel, Foerg, et al. (1994) applied an incentive system to one of two groups receiving behavioral treatment based on the community reinforcement approach described earlier. Vouchers exchangeable for retail items were offered, contingent on the submission of cocaine-free urine samples during weeks 1 through 12 of treatment. During weeks 13 to 24 there was no difference in treatment of the two groups. About 75% of participants in the voucher group completed the full 24 weeks of treatment, compared to 40% of the group which did not receive vouchers. Nearly 12 continuous weeks of cocaine abstinence (11.7) was achieved for the voucher group versus 6 weeks for the no-voucher group. Additionally, the voucher group showed greater improvement on the drug use scale of the ASI, as well as on the psychiatric scale. The authors concluded that incentives delivered contingent on the submission of cocaine-free urine specimens significantly improved treatment outcome in ambulatory cocaine-dependent patients.

In a related study, Higgins, Bickel, and Hughes (1994) gave cocaine abusers a choice between cocaine (10 mg intranasal administration) versus a placebo under a double-blind condition, or between cocaine and varying amounts of money. Cocaine was exclusively chosen against a placebo, but as the amount of money was increased in the alternate choice, the monetary option was increasingly chosen. At the $2.00 per choice condition, the monetary option was exclusively chosen. This study demonstrated that cocaine use, as an operant behavior maintained by the reinforcing effects of the drug, could be altered when the magnitude of an alternative reinforcer was sufficiently large.[6]

Havassy, Wasserman, and Hall (1993) have observed that the magnitude of reinforcers may be a significant factor in the effectiveness of programs which rely on them. They noted that Magura et al. (1988), for example, had not found methadone take-home privileges contingent on decreased use of cocaine to be effective in controlling cocaine use in methadone maintenance patients. This was surprising, they observed, since similar interventions had been effective in reducing other illicit drug use in this population (Stitzer, Bigelow, and Liebson, 1980). Havassy, Wasserman, and Hall (1993) suggested that operant procedures such as contingency contracting and CRA may be more useful in initiating abstinence than in maintaining it, perhaps because of their emphasis on extrinsic rather than intrinsic motivation. Thus, the authors consider it advisable to identify intrinsic motivators early in treatment.

Not all studies of contingency management have generated evidence supportive of the contingency management approach. Magura et al. (1988) assessed the effect on the use of cocaine and other drugs of providing methadone take-home privileges contingent on stopping such use. Thirty-two "difficult-to-treat" patients in a New York City methadone program volunteered for the study. These patients were not normally eligible to receive take-home privileges at their program. The intervention provided methadone take-homes on the basis of an absence of positive urine tests for cocaine and other drugs during the prior week. The results indicated that 4 of the 19 patients who had had cocaine-positive urine tests prior to the study were successful in reducing or eliminating such use during the period of the contingency intervention. These results, however, did not reach statistical significance.

A second pair of studies (Dolan et al., 1985; Black et al., 1987) addressed the value of contingency contracting on the use of cocaine and other drugs for patients in a methadone maintenance treatment program when the contingency was withdrawal from methadone. In the first study, 21 methadone maintenance patients were selected on the basis of positive urinalysis during a sixty-day baseline period. Contingency contracting was found to reduce illicit drug use significantly, although the degree to which the use of specific drugs, such as cocaine, was reduced was not reported. The second study identified 79 patients in methadone maintenance treatment at the Dallas Veterans Administration Hospital over a six-year period for whom more than 50% of urine tests over two consecutive months were found to be positive for illicit drugs. Of 60 patients who agreed to participate in the study, 31 (52%) violated their contracts by drug use. Of these, 23 (75%) had positive urine test results for cocaine. After two months, only 23 (38% of the original 60) had urine tests positive for cocaine use. While Black et al. (1987) concluded that contingency contracting for methadone withdrawal reduced patients' use of cocaine, in retrospect several problems arise in the report of this study which preclude a straightforward interpretation. Condelli et al. (1991) have noted an absence of information about the extent to which patients in the study understood the nature of their contingency contracts; believed that the contracts would be carried out; and felt that they had other options, such as nearby methadone programs to which they could transfer should they be discharged from the VA program; as well as the fact that 19 of the 79 patients identified as frequent cocaine users did not agree to participate in the study.

Kirby, Marlowe, and Platt (1995) examined the differential effectiveness of three voucher schedules for abstinence from cocaine. In an initial, uncontrolled comparison, vouchers were awarded for cocaine-negative urines based on two different schedules of reinforcement. Greater abstinence was found among subjects who received vouchers under the following conditions: immediate reinforcement for each urine result; greater reinforcement magnitude for initiating cocaine abstinence; higher maximum possible voucher earnings; and increased intermittency of reinforcers with increasing abstinence. This schedule did not provide either a response cost or differential reinforcement for sustained cocaine abstinence. This study also replicated the voucher system used by Higgins et al. (1993b) and Silverman et al. (1994).

A later study (Kirby et al., 1995) investigated whether non-drug consumables would be useful in reinforcing abstinence from cocaine; whether such effects, if any, were obtainable during treatment; and, if these effects occurred, whether they would endure beyond the time when the contingency-management program was in effect. Using a two-group design with random assignment and a no-contingency control, the researchers assigned 95 cocaine-dependent patients to a 26-session program of cognitive-behavioral counseling and 10 sessions of interpersonal problem solving. Half of the group also received vouchers for providing cocaine-negative urines. The vouchers had a monetary value based on a schedule beginning with a $5 payment for one to two cocaine-free urines during the week, and increasing to $40 for 12 consecutive cocaine-free urines. The vouchers were exchangeable for goods and services which would promote prosocial behaviors. Results at the nine-month follow-up did not indicate any group differences in treatment attendance or cocaine use during treatment. Findings with the ASI did, however, suggest a trend toward reduced cocaine use and drug spending for the voucher group, and increased employment for the non-voucher group; this last finding suggested that the use of vouchers inhibited employment seeking, although the non-voucher group may also have had more motivation to work. It is difficult, however, to understand the inconsistency in findings between this study and those of Higgins et al. (1991, 1993b). It may well be that the differences in population characteristics and environments within which the two studies were conducted were very different. Higgins and his associates conducted their studies in rural Vermont, while Kirby et al. (1995) conducted their study in Camden, New Jersey, a city which has received national notoriety for its social and economic devastation (McLarin, 1994). Such an environment provides neither alternatives to drug use nor opportunities for community reinforcement outside those provided within the confines of the study.

Finally, it should be noted that the behavioral approach recommends equal attention to historical and concurrent circumstances surrounding drug use. In this regard, Grabowski, Higgins, and Kirby (1993) have proposed that the amount of the drug taken and the pattern of use are insufficient parameters to define the need for treatment. In addition to these elements, they suggest the need to include information concerning historical and current circumstances surrounding other aspects of behavior. Moreover, they note that an interaction exists between severity of use (as defined by pattern and dose) and the strength of other features of the behavioral repertoire. They give the example of the difficulties involved in successfully treating and maintaining as drug-free individuals who are moderate cocaine users but who have few other reinforcers, such as social supports, employment, and so on. Thus, they see a careful behavioral analysis together with the differentiation of treatment elements as necessary in cocaine treatment. Such a careful behavioral analysis is, of course, a tenet of the behavioral approach (Wolpe, 1973).

Cognitive-Behavioral Interventions

The cognitive-behavioral view of drug addiction hypothesizes that individuals with a vulnerability to drug abuse have specific beliefs, activated under particular circumstances, which increase the likelihood of continued drug use. One way such beliefs may operate is by increasing drug craving. Thus, idiosyncratic beliefs concerning the effects of drugs may be activated in "provocative" or high-risk situations, such as those in which friends are using cocaine (an external situation) or in which an internal emotionally aversive state, such as anxiety, depression, or boredom, is present. Over time, these beliefs can change or become more elaborated. Thus, initial or *anticipatory beliefs* directed toward gaining peer esteem ("my friends will think more of me if I use cocaine") or denying the likelihood of becoming addicted ("*I* won't get hooked") will lead to *relief-oriented beliefs* ("I need my cocaine; I can't function without it") following the development of dependency. Relief-oriented beliefs may in turn stimulate craving, and a *permissive belief* ("It's OK," or "I deserve it") may enter into the belief system (Beck, Wright, and Newman, 1992).

Beck et al. (1993) have also suggested a number of characteristics of the drug abuser, which may be considered predisposing to such abuse. These include a general sensitivity to unpleasant feelings or emotions (for example, a low tolerance for normal cyclical changes in mood); deficient motivation to control behavior (that is, the valuing of instant gratification over control); inadequate skills for controlling behavior and coping with problems; a pattern of automatic, nonreflective responses to impulses; an inclination toward excitement seeking and a low tolerance for boredom; low frustration tolerance, likely resulting in part from a complex set of beliefs and cognitive distortions; and a focus on present emotional states, cravings, and urges, and on the actions necessary for relieving or satisfying them, with an absence of attention to the consequences of such actions. Thus, the sequence of addiction often consists of a vicious cycle in which negative emotional states (for example, anxiety, depression) lead to self-medication (for example, drug use), which then leads to or exacerbates financial, social, and medical problems, preceding renewed negative affect. Cravings are then exacerbated by dysfunctional beliefs, inaccurate attribution of responsibility for problems, and denial. They are also strengthened by addicts' tendency to ignore, minimize, or deny problems resulting from drug abuse.

Cognitive behavioral treatment of cocaine abuse "is a structured, collaborative, directive, problem-oriented treatment based on the cognitive model of substance abuse" (Beck, Wright, and Newman, 1992, p. 186). The primary focus of such treatment is to help the patient "discover, examine, and modify dysfunctional cognitive-behavioral processes that elicit and maintain the problem" (p. 186). Such treatment includes attention to eight areas: problem conceptualization; development of a collaborative relationship; motivation for reduction of craving and drug dependency; the patient's formulation of the problem; the setting of goals; socialization of the patient into the cognitive model; the use of cognitive-behavioral interventions; and relapse prevention (Beck, Wright, and Newman, 1992). Beck and his associates are in the process of evaluating the effectiveness of treatment for cocaine abuse based on this model.

Other Interventions

Social Network Therapy

Social network therapy is intended to bolster the patient's attempts to achieve stable abstinence and prevent relapse through the involvement of his or her social network (Galanter, 1985, 1986). It is similar in concept to self-help groups such as Cocaine Anonymous, Alcoholics Anonymous, and Narcotics Anonymous which recognize the need for involving others in the process of attempting to achieve and maintain abstinence, particularly in dealing with loss of control over substance use and relapse to such use. It also resembles family therapy, which views dysfunction as a family rather than an individual problem. Galanter (1986) describes the application of the principles of social network therapy to cocaine treatment. Successful implementation requires the establishment of a therapeutic alliance; a good deal of flexibility on the part of the therapist; the availability and willingness of a member of the patient's social network to participate in the treatment process; and definition of the network and recruitment of appropriate members. The therapist's role with respect to the network should be that of a team leader rather than a family member, directing the network to assist the therapist in sustaining the patient's abstinence. In support of this role, the therapist should be committed, pragmatic in approach, and readily available, and should communicate openness in his or her style. Initial sessions, for the first month at least, should be weekly, tapering to biweekly and then monthly or less frequent sessions as progress dictates. Individual therapy, when it does begin, should be ordered so as to accommodate the goals of substance abuse therapy as well as recognize the network's existence and goals.

Aversion Therapy

Aversion therapy has been employed as a treatment for cocaine dependence. Frawley and Smith (1992) reported on such a program within the context of multimodal inpatient treatment. The program also included five sodium pentothal treatments given on alternate days, daily educational groups, information about support groups, and individual and family counseling. The aversion component of the program consisted of administration of oral emetine to induce nausea in association with the act of snorting cocaine. The substance used for inhalation was in actuality a similar appearing and smelling compound of 2% tetracaine and 1% quinine in mannitol. For freebase, white candy or a white soap, which when burned created smoke, was used. For intravenous injection, a white powder which was dissolved by the patient and taken up into a syringe was used, although no actual injection took place. Rather, the powder was extruded from the needle just above where the injection would have taken place. An artificial cocaine-like scent was also applied to the fingers to achieve the odor of street cocaine. The chemical aversion treatment consisted of timing the use of the drug substitute to just prior to the onset of nausea. Five sessions of such treatment were normally used, although when aversion treatment was applied to both cocaine (or methamphetamine) and alcohol abuse, two sessions for cocaine alone were used, followed by four additional sessions for cocaine and alcohol combined.

Alternatively, faradic aversion was employed. This consisted of the application of irritating but not painful electric stimuli in conjunction with the act of using imaging and preparing to use the cocaine or methamphetamine substitute. This treatment, which was applied separately from aversion treatment for any other drug, consisted of pairing the aversive electrical stimulus with each behavior in the chain of cocaine use (manipulating and opening the packet of white powder, pouring the powder and arranging it on the mirror, and so on), as well as imagery associated with cocaine use. As was the case for chemical aversion therapy, five sessions of faradic aversion treatment were utilized. Faradic aversion therapy was used with almost all of the freebasers and intravenous users and about half of the "snorters." Both chemical and faradic aversion treatments were used with under 10% of the sample. A follow-up reinforcement application of one session each of aversion therapy and pentothal treatment, as well as an updating of the patient's continuing care plan, took place from two to six weeks after discharge from initial treatment. Periodic call-backs then took place for two years.

Data provided by Frawley and Smith (1992) indicated that approximately half of the patients participated in follow-up treatments, and that over 40% were still participating in support groups one year later. For the total group, the abstinence rate from cocaine at one year posttreatment was 53%, and current abstinence of at least six months at follow-up was 68.6%. For the group treated with aversion therapy for cocaine alone, the one-year rate for abstinence from cocaine was 39%, with a current abstinence rate (of at least six months' duration) of 62.4%. For aversion treatment for both cocaine and alcohol, the rates were 69% at one year and a current abstinence rate of 76%. Outcomes for cocaine and marijuana were 50% at one year, 65% current; for alcohol, cocaine, and marijuana, 73% one-year total abstinence and 73% current. Similar abstinence rates were also obtained for treatments of other combinations of abused substances. Despite a number of design limitations, including the lack of a comparison group and the absence of random assignment to treatment, the authors considered these results promising and favorable compared with those of other studies, although they noted that total abstinence from all drugs was not very high, an outcome which they attributed in part to the use of alcohol after treatment being considered a treatment failure.

Neuroelectric Therapy

The application of electrical current to assist in detoxification from drugs of abuse has been evaluated in several studies. After reviewing the literature, Alling, Johnson, and Elmoghazy (1990) suggested that cranial electrostimulation (the application of small amounts of electric stimulation by means of electrodes attached to the surface of the scalp) was a promising technique for use in the nonchemical detoxification of opiate-dependent patients. One variant of this approach has been evaluated with both opiate- and cocaine-dependent patients. Neuroelectric therapy (NET) is derived from electroacupuncture, which was first reported by Wen and Cheung (1973) to stop symptoms of withdrawal from heroin, and then further developed by Patterson, who modified the technique by replacing needles with surface electrodes (Patterson, 1976, 1984; Patterson, Firth, and Gardiner, 1984). Other investigators employing variants of the original treatment developed by Patterson have not been successful (Gossop et al. 1984; Man and Chuang, 1980). A study by Gariti and his associates (1992) attempted to evaluate NET employing a double-blind, randomized, placebo-controlled study and procedures similar to those employed by Patterson's original experiments. Groups of 18 opiate-dependent and 25 cocaine-dependent addicts were studied over the course of a 12- to 14-day hospitalization. An overall completion rate of 88% was achieved, with both groups reporting a comfortable detoxification and substantial improvement over the course of treatment. The findings indicated no significant difference between the active treatment and placebo groups in the reduction of withdrawal symptoms from cocaine and heroin or in reduction of craving during detoxification, although the control groups received some amount of active current, thus possibly contaminating the design. While offering no support for the effectiveness of NET, there was some suggestion that the subjects receiving NET had cleaner urines at the one-month follow-up, although the number was too small to yield a substantive finding.

Problematic Behaviors during Treatment

Abuse of Drugs

Treatment may substantially reduce the use of cocaine and other drugs, but it may not result in abstinence from these same drugs. For example, McCoy, Rivers, and Chitwood (1993) found that substantially higher percentages of street injection drug users than injection drug users in treatment had used cocaine during a baseline period. During this period (June 1987–August 1988), 90.1% of the street sample had injected cocaine versus 40.2% for the treatment sample, 60.1% versus 32% had injected speedball, and 62.1% versus 52.1% had injected heroin. Similar findings existed for the use of crack (76.5% of the street sample versus 43.4% of the treatment group), non-injected cocaine (60.1% versus 29.7%), and alcohol (90.8% versus 79.2%).

Street methadone is a frequent drug of choice for cocaine-abusing patients in treatment since many feel that the concurrent use of methadone enhances the use of cocaine by lengthening and mellowing its effects and by providing a "floor" against the aftereffects of cocaine, resulting from the relatively long half-life of methadone combined with the relatively short half-life of cocaine. These additive effects may diminish the ability of methadone patients to abstain from cocaine use (Condelli et al., 1991).

Owing to the high probability of drug use during treatment, urine testing is essential to treatment, and is viewed as creating a safe environment for the patient, as enhancing trust between the clinician and the patient, and as providing an objective measure of progress in treatment. Such testing is seen as valuable by patients in that it helps them to counteract impulses to use cocaine and to hide such drug use. It also helps both family members and employers to relax their own vigilance and thus to be more supportive of the recovering patient (Washton and Stone-Washton, 1993).

Washton and Stone-Washton (1993) suggested that the following steps are necessary to maximize the clinical value of urine testing: supervision of sample collection in order to prevent falsification, including the use of a buddy system where staff are not available for supervision; routine collection of samples at least every three to four days in order not to exceed the sensitivity limits of standard laboratory treating methods; accurate evaluation of samples by immunoassay or radioimmunoassay methods; routine testing not only for cocaine but also for amphetamines, opiates, marijuana, benzodiazepines, and barbiturates; and regular testing throughout the entire program until the patient is solidly into recovery, when occasional testing may still be helpful.

Returns to Drug Use while in Treatment

Although potentially dangerous and never to be encouraged, "slips," or returns to drug use during treatment, may provide valuable learning experiences. In this regard Marlatt (1985) views the occurrence of slips (which he labels "lapses") as like taking the incorrect "fork in the road, with one path returning to the former problem level (relapse or total collapse), and the other continuing in the direction of positive change" (p. 33).

Such slips should be addressed as a discrepancy between a stated intention and actual behavior. Washton and Stone-Washton (1993) suggest that no absolute numbers of slips should be used as a basis for suspension from a group, since this may be tantamount to giving permission for group members to have one less than the specified number.

Treatment Problems of Special Populations

Adolescents

In general, any use of illicit drugs among adolescents is of concern; cocaine use in adolescents, however, is particularly alarming (DuPont, 1991; Kandel, Simcha-Fagan, and Davies, 1986; Kozel and Adams, 1986). Such early drug use, especially where it is intense, may lead to serious and persistent delinquency (see, for example, Kandel, Simcha-Fagan, and Davies, 1986; Watters, Reinarman, and Fagan, 1985). Early and intense cocaine use in adolescents also presents a difficult treatment problem (DuPont, 1991).

Use of cocaine and other illicit drugs generally occurs within a context of poor relationships with parents, who may or may not be using drugs themselves (although they are likely to be using hard liquor); exposure to and involvement with drug-using peers; heavy involvement with marijuana; and general deviance (Kandel, 1982). Onset of cocaine use in adolescents identified as heavy cocaine users occurs at a very early age. Smith, Schwartz, and Martin (1989), for example, reported that drug use for the group they studied had started at age 14 for almost all, with

5 of 27 respondents initiating heavy drug use by age 10. Marijuana and alcohol use were also common, at 93% each. By age 14, 21% had already tried cocaine, and more than half of these (54%) were using it weekly two months after initial use. Seventy-five percent were using 3 grams of cocaine monthly, mostly by snorting (68%). One person admitted using cocaine by intravenous injection. Morning use was present in 82%. Inability to refuse cocaine was present for 79%, with most afraid to stop using it. A quarter of the sample reported spending at least $250 weekly on cocaine during a three-month period. Funds for cocaine use were obtained through work at a steady job (21%), dealing drugs (21%), or prostitution (11%), and almost all admitted stealing (96%). Problems present before starting drug use included loneliness (31%), depression (14%), attention problems at school (52%), poor grades (28%), skipping class (43%), disciplinary actions by the school (93%), suspension or expulsion from school (71%), and attempted suicide on one (39%) or more (18%) occasions.

The developmental sequence of substance abuse leading to "hard" drug use has been the subject of a number of investigations by Kandel and her associates (see, for example, Kandel, 1975; Kandel and Faust, 1975; Kandel, Yamaguchi, and Chen, 1992; Yamaguchi and Kandel, 1984). While it has been suggested that crack use may not follow the usual progression of drug use (see, for example, Fagan, 1989; Fagan and Chin, 1991), at least two studies (Fagan and Chin, 1989; Kandel and Yamaguchi, 1993) have provided evidence for a sequential pattern of drug involvement in adolescents. This sequence involves the early use of alcohol and/or cigarettes, followed by involvement with marijuana, cocaine, and then crack. In the study by Kandel and Yamaguchi (1993), the best-fitting model, accounting for 93.5% of males in a statewide (New York State) random sample of 7,611 students in grades 7 through 12, was one in which alcohol use precedes marijuana use, marijuana and cigarette use precede cocaine and crack use, and cocaine use precedes crack use. For females, the best-fitting model, accounting for 94.2% of cases, was one in which alcohol *and* cigarette use precede marijuana use, marijuana use precedes cocaine and crack use, and cocaine use precedes crack use. Similar findings were obtained by Fagan and Chin (1989) for a New York City sample of drug arrestees, community residents, and clients in drug treatment programs. In this study, 78% had used marijuana prior to crack, and 63% had used cocaine in other forms prior to using crack.

Evidence also suggests that there may be significant underreporting of cocaine and other drug use among youths. Fendrich and Vaughn (1994) interviewed youths aged 14 to 21 about their lifetime use of cocaine (and other drugs) during 1984 and 1988 as part of the National

Longitudinal Survey of Youth. Approximately one-third of the respondents reported less lifetime use of cocaine and marijuana in 1988 than they had originally reported in 1984. Some 19% who had originally admitted to lifetime use of cocaine in 1984 completely denied such use in 1988. The authors concluded that the respondents in this study were less likely to report illicit drug use during the late 1980s as a result of the growing intolerance of drug use on the part of the public.

Craving for cocaine may be particularly problematic for youthful cocaine abusers, and may present an especially difficult treatment problem. This point is well illustrated by the fact that, despite having been in a rehabilitation program for one month, 93% of the adolescent and young adult sample studied by Smith, Schwartz, and Martin (1989) still reported experiencing cocaine craving, with the majority reporting such craving as "severe." Use of crack cocaine may be an even riskier undertaking than intranasal use of cocaine. Schwartz, Luxenberg, and Hoffmann (1991) found crack-using youth, when compared with intranasal users, to be more preoccupied with cocaine-related thoughts, to dream more about cocaine, to escalate their use more quickly, and to be less likely to refuse an offer of cocaine.

Many difficulties are encountered in recruiting youthful cocaine users into treatment. Brown et al. (1989) have described the difficulties they encountered in attempting to recruit cocaine users aged 21 and younger into a treatment program at the Addiction Research Center in Baltimore. They surmise that possible reasons may have included less severe impairment and/or dependence, as well as a greater reluctance to use available treatment resources. On the basis of their experience, the authors recommended four community resources as particularly relevant in increasing the recruitment rates of youthful cocaine users into treatment: the family, schools, the medical community, and public agencies in the areas of health, social services, and criminal justice. Such agencies have particular responsibility, given the unlikeliness of youthful cocaine abusers' themselves recognizing the dangers which derive from cocaine use. All have some capacity to observe the behavior of young people, to make intelligent referrals, and perhaps to provide services themselves, in addition to possessing sufficient weight in the community to exert an influence on the behavior and functioning of others.

Methadone Maintenance Patients

Cocaine abuse presents a significant treatment impediment to patients in methadone maintenance treatment programs. A report by the U.S. General Accounting Office (1990) indicated that of 24 methadone programs in 8 states which were studied, cocaine abuse by patients ranged from 0% to 40%, and that in over a third of the programs, more than 20% were using cocaine. Various studies have reported the extent of such abuse in programs to be 75% (Cushman, 1988; Magura et al., 1989), 71% (Kang and De Leon, 1993), 84% (Magura et al., 1991), 60% (Maier, 1989), and 50% (Stitzer and Kirby, 1991). Among applicants to methadone maintenance treatment programs, Ball and Ross (1991) reported cocaine use to be typically present in approximately 50%, although a higher figure (70%–80%) was reported by Stitzer and Kirby (1991). Yet, a study of 11 of 13 methadone programs in Baltimore found that only 15.7% (range, 5.9%–33%) of patients used cocaine (Kolar et al., 1990). Thus, there is significant variation among clinics in rates of such abuse. Rates of urines positive for cocaine in four geographically dispersed clinics were found to range from 25% to 45% (Dennis et al., 1990).

Hanbury et al. (1986) found 51% of patients in a New York City methadone program to have used cocaine at least once while in methadone maintenance treatment. A similar figure was reported by Des Jarlais et al. (1992), who found approximately one-quarter of New York City methadone maintenance patients were using crack cocaine and half were injecting cocaine. The number of methadone maintenance patients using crack in this study, however, was less than half the number of injection drug users not in treatment who were using crack (Des Jarlais, 1990). Chaisson et al. (1989) reported lower figures for San Francisco. They found 24% of patients in nine San Francisco methadone programs had started or increased the use of cocaine since entry into the programs.

As the Chaisson et al. (1989) findings suggest, entry into methadone treatment does not necessarily have an immediate effect on cocaine abuse. Hubbard et al. (1989) found, for example, that 40% of patients admitted to drug abuse treatment who had been using cocaine daily or weekly prior to admission continued to use cocaine just as frequently during their first three weeks in the program. Kolar et al. (1990), however, found that rates of cocaine use in the eleven Baltimore methadone programs they studied ranged from 5.9% to 33.0%. They observed that rates of cocaine use (and other drug use as well) based on positive urine findings are likely depressed by infrequent testing in most methadone programs, and that because of the infrequent nature of urine testing in methadone maintenance treatment programs, such testing can do little more than detect daily cocaine use.

The results of a descriptive analysis of cocaine use among methadone maintenance patients was reported by Kidorf and Stitzer (1993). They found that daily cocaine use averaged 0.23 grams daily, 3.4 days per week. Cocaine was typically used simultaneously with heroin, while a smaller group (47%) used alcohol in close temporal proximity to cocaine. Concurrent cocaine-alcohol or cocaine-heroin use was associated with higher cocaine use (mean = 1.0 gm/wk) than when cocaine was used alone (mean = 0.49 gm/wk). The authors concluded that methadone maintenance patients engaged in low-dose cocaine abuse. This was particularly the case in comparison to non–opioid-dependent patients applying to cocaine treatment programs, who have been described in other studies as using in the range of 3 to 7 grams of cocaine weekly (see, for example, Gawin, Kleber, et al., 1989; Higgins et al., 1991). Given the clear preferences of patients in this study for drugs used in combination, it was suggested that modification of such drug use combinations be attempted.

In general, there is strong evidence that abuse of opiates among patients in methadone maintenance treatment is reduced with higher doses of methadone (see Platt, 1995, pp. 59–61). The opposite relationship, however, may be true for abuse of cocaine according to a study by Grabowski et al. (1993). This study reported cocaine use as *more*, rather than less, common among patients in methadone maintenance who were receiving a dose of 80 mg of methadone daily, rather than 50 mg. Urine samples for 58% of those in the high-dose group were cocaine-positive, compared with 44% in the low-dose group. Opiate abuse was in the expected direction—lower in the 80 mg group than in the 50 mg group. The authors suggested that this finding indicated the need for caution in the choices of methadone doses for cocaine-abusing patients in methadone maintenance treatment.

Not surprisingly, the use of cocaine has been viewed by some writers as undermining the effectiveness of methadone programs (Condelli et al., 1991; Strug et al., 1985). To understand fully cocaine use in methadone maintenance treatment programs, it is necessary to know just when such use began. Is it just a continuation of behavior that occurred prior to entry into treatment, or does it reflect use begun after treatment entry? Several studies suggest that for some methadone maintenance patients, cocaine use begins before entry (Hanbury et al., 1986; Hubbard et al., 1988), although some evidence exists that such use begins after entry. The Hanbury at al. (1986) study illustrates both patterns. In this study, 33% of respondents in a survey of methadone maintenance patients indicated no use of cocaine prior to treatment entry, while 67% admitted to such use. Following treatment entry, 14% of patients with no prior history of cocaine abuse started to abuse the drug. Among those who had used cocaine prior to entry, 31% stopped. Cocaine use by methadone maintenance patients may be a route back into the lifestyle of addiction. Strug et al. (1985) noted that cocaine users may begin to use other drugs to counteract the "wired" state produced by cocaine use, as well as to relieve the negative feelings associated with the "crash" and subsequent depression. Drugs used to alleviate these feelings may include depressants such as tranquilizers, alcohol, or heroin.

Continued crack cocaine use among methadone maintenance treatment patients was found by Des Jarlais et al. (1992) to be associated with the number of noninjected drugs used, the number of intravenous drug–using sexual partners, drug injection, and the use of non-heroin opiates. Cocaine use has also been seen as part of the drug use and social lives of methadone maintenance patient. (Strug et al., 1985). Perceived as a high-status drug, it is, however, also seen as one with potentially dangerous consequences. Yet, its use is not confined to deviant methadone maintenance patients. Patients who are otherwise compliant with program rules may use it. Some patients in methadone maintenance treatment programs may even sell their take-home dose of methadone for cocaine (Culhane, 1990), and cocaine use is a common reason for treatment failure (Strug et al., 1985).

Not surprisingly, cocaine use while in methadone maintenance treatment frequently results in loss of privileges, including the loss of take-home doses of methadone. In two studies, the percentage of patients who either lost take-home privileges or were discontinued from the program ranged from 25% to 50% (Black et al., 1987; Dolan et al., 1985).

A number of interventions have been implemented to address the problem of cocaine use among methadone maintenance patients. Kolar et al. (1990) surveyed methadone programs in Baltimore in order to learn what kinds of behavioral treatments were used for the management of cocaine abuse by patients. These included increased frequency of individual and group counseling; more frequent urine testing; discontinuation of methadone take-home privileges; contingent lowering of the methadone dose; inpatient hospitalization for cocaine detoxification; and detoxification and discharge from methadone maintenance after a series of positive urine tests for cocaine. The implementation of interventions for cocaine use in methadone maintenance treatment programs is, however, far from universal. A government study indicated that of 24 methadone programs in 8 states, 5 did not address cocaine use among their patients. Only 11 of the 24 programs were found to have a goal of addressing all substance abuse during treatment, and only 8 sought to stop all drug use (U.S. General Accounting Office, 1990).

Gawin and Ellinwood (1988) have recommended that persons found to have used cocaine prior to treatment entry be referred to specialized treatment. Condelli et al. (1991) noted, however, both the absence of *ef-fective* treatment programs for cocaine use at the time of their literature review and the relative absence of treatment protocols aimed at both cocaine and opioids. Among the problems facing methadone patients who sought treatment for their cocaine use, according to Condelli et al. (1991), were the difficulties related to having to attend two different drug treatment programs, or having to forgo participation in methadone maintenance treatment; the question which program provided more benefits; and the general inaccessibility, owing to their cost and location, of cocaine treatment programs for many methadone patients.

Condelli et al. (1991) identified three behavioral interventions specifically directed at reducing cocaine use among methadone maintenance treatment patients: confronting clients and staff about positive urine tests for cocaine (Chambers, Taylor, and Moffett, 1972); withdrawing clients from methadone if they continued to use cocaine (Black et al., 1987); and rewarding clients with take-home doses of methadone for not using cocaine (Magura et al., 1988). These three behavioral interventions reduced cocaine use among methadone patients by up to 37%. These studies have not been replicated, however (Condelli et al., 1991). As a group, the three studies cited have been criticized by Condelli et al. (1991) as having limited generalizability owing to small samples, a lack of statistical power, and high or unknown attrition rates. Thus, Condelli and associates make the point that it is unclear whether the reported findings were due to the interventions or to selective program dropout. They further suggest that there is a need for additional research into what systems of rewards and costs are most effective in reducing cocaine use by patients in methadone maintenance treatment, and in determining the extent to which interventions based on a token economy or other behavioral or cognitive-behavioral models might be effective in addressing this problem.

Among the interventions noted by Condelli et al. (1991) as promising in controlling cocaine use in methadone maintenance patients are those concerned with addressing problems at various stages of recovery (Rawson, 1989); cue extinction paradigms (Woody et al., 1985); and skills training packages focusing on either the ability to manage stress and anxiety (Hawkins, Catalano, and Wells, 1986), the ability to resolve problems of everyday living (Platt and Metzger, 1987), or the management of common and personally meaningful triggers for cocaine relapse (Washton and Stone-Washton, 1990).

Dunteman, Condelli, and Fairbank (1992), studying data collected as part of the Treatment Outcome Perspective Study (TOPS), found that cocaine use by current and former methadone patients showed a decline in the year following treatment; those patients who stopped heroin use after treatment entry were more likely to stop using cocaine than their heroin-using counterparts; and the likelihood of initiating cocaine use after treatment entry was higher for those patients who continued to use heroin. The authors concluded that methadone maintenance treatment programs which increased their effectiveness in treating heroin use were more likely to reduce cocaine use among some patients. Unfortunately, the data used in this study (from a cohort entering treatment programs between 1979 and 1981) may have been outdated and thus tell us little about the current or future incidence of cocaine use among methadone maintenance patients (Barglow and Kotun, 1992). In a reply to this and other criticisms, Dunteman, Condelli, and Fairbank (1992) note that cocaine use among methadone patients was a major problem at the time the TOPS data were collected. Furthermore, a study by Magura et al. (1991) found a decrease in prior-month cocaine use among patients admitted to methadone maintenance treatment programs, from 84% to 66%, at follow-up one year later. In addition, mean days of cocaine use per month decreased from 16 to 9 over this period. While cocaine use was not associated with dropout from the program, cocaine users were more likely to be administratively discharged. Magura et al. (1991) suggested that this reduction in use of cocaine after entry into a methadone program may reflect a generally stabilizing effect of treatment on most addicts, thus reducing pressure to use any drug.

Conclusions

Treatment for cocaine abuse is directed toward two primary goals: the initiation of abstinence and the prevention of relapse. These goals may be reached by a number of means, including pharmacotherapy and psychotherapy. Although specific therapies have been developed and demonstrated to be effective for other drug problems, particularly heroin addiction (for example, comprehensive or enhanced methadone maintenance, which includes both pharmacotherapy and other therapies; McLellan et al., 1993), no such intervention has yet been developed *and* demonstrated to be effective for the treatment of cocaine abuse. Evaluation of state-of-the-art treatment for cocaine abuse does suggest the existence of promising avenues of treatment, however (for example, the behavioral approach described by Higgins et al., 1991, 1993b).

Appropriate treatment for cocaine abuse requires a carefully conducted and comprehensive assessment of the treatment-seeking patient. Such an assessment should include the reasons for seeking treatment and the level of motivation for doing so; a detailed history of past drug use, including the internal states, physical location, and interpersonal circumstances surrounding such drug use; information concerning the circumstances surrounding current drug use; assessment of the personal, familial, interpersonal, and other resources available to the patient; and evaluation for the presence of other psychopathology. It is also essential to obtain the patient's views regarding the reasons for his or her drug use, as well as the consequences of such use, as part of the evaluation process (Washton and Stone-Washton, 1993).

Effective treatment for cocaine abuse should comprise several components. These include the formation of a good working relationship with the patient; development and maintenance of motivation for change; and education of the patient with respect to learning how to recognize and avoid potential drug use situations, as well as how to cope with them, how to build a drug-free life, and how to avoid relapse (Schuckit, 1994). Ideally, it would involve intensive initial inpatient treatment with intensive follow-up or intensive outpatient/self-help treatment (Khalsa, Paredes, et al., 1993).

Treatment for cocaine abuse has been conceptualized as consisting of three phases. The initial phase is primarily concerned with cessation of cocaine abuse, and focuses on assessment, clarification of motivation for cessation of drug use, and involvement in a support network or group. The second phase focuses on relapse prevention, including the identification of cues leading to relapse, particularly mood states, learning how to cope with cocaine craving, and the development of pleasurable alternatives to cocaine use. The third phase is primarily concerned with maintaining abstinence, the acquisition of additional skills needed to maintain abstinence, and continued involvement in support groups, as well as psychotherapy and pharmacotherapy (Millman, 1988; Wallace, 1990b).

Treatment for cocaine abuse is provided in a variety of settings, including outpatient, inpatient, and partial hospitalization units, and therapeutic communities. Evidence for the effectiveness of certain nonpharmacological therapies has been demonstrated, but little or no evidence exists for the effectiveness of others. Although there are a number of widely known models of outpatient treatment, including those of the Washton Institute program and Matrix Center's Neurobehavioral Treatment, there is relatively little evaluative data available as to their effectiveness. What little is available suggests that rates of failure to complete treatment are very high (perhaps in the 75%–80% range), and that once-a-week therapy is ineffective (Kang et al., 1991). Inpatient care is not a necessary ingredient in cocaine treatment except in the case of prior treatment, where treatment is necessary for comorbid psychiatric or medical conditions, or where there is a need to intervene to facilitate childbirth or reduce the risk of perinatal morbidity (Galanter et al., 1992). Inpatient treatment is, however, generally preferred by patients over outpatient treatment (Khalsa, Paredes, et al., 1993; Marsh et al, 1990). Partial hospitalization, in particular day treatment, has been as underutilized in the treatment of cocaine abuse (Guydish et al., 1993), as it has been in other areas of psychiatry (Parker and Knoll, 1990). Evidence for the effectiveness of day treatment for cocaine abuse has yet to be provided, however (Platt et al., 1995). This is also the case for therapeutic communities, chemical dependency treatment, and self-help interventions.

With only a few exceptions, randomized clinical trials for nonpharmacological cocaine treatment (other than drug trials) are rare in the current literature. Among the examples of randomized clinical trials are studies by Carroll, Rounsaville, and Gawin (1991); Higgins et al. (1993b); Kang et al. (1991); and Wells et al. (1994).

Psychotherapy for cocaine abuse has been evaluated in a number of studies, without much evidence of its being successful. The success reported with psychodynamic insight-oriented therapy has typically been obtained in case studies (for example, Schiffer, 1988). A promising intervention, interpersonal psychotherapy (Klerman et al., 1984), which aimed at symptom reduction and the improvement of social functioning, was not found to be efficacious when evaluated in a randomized clinical trial (Carroll, Rounsaville, and Gawin, 1991).

Behavioral interventions have been the most promising, based on evidence initially developed on cocaine-abusing patients in methadone maintenance treatment. Several such studies have demonstrated the effectiveness of contingency management procedures in retaining and treating cocaine-abusing patients (Anker and Crowley, 1982; Higgins et al., 1991). In particular, the studies by Higgins and associates (Budney et al., 1991; Higgins et al., 1993b, 1994) have demonstrated the successful application of the community reinforcement approach pioneered by Azrin and his associates (Azrin, 1976; Azrin et al., 1982; Hunt and Azrin, 1973). While validation of the voucher system employed in the studies by Higgins and his associates has been obtained in other settings (Kirby,

Marlowe, and Platt, 1995; Silverman et al., 1994), the use of contingency management has not been found to be effective in all studies in which it has been employed (Kirby et al., 1995; Magura et al., 1988). This suggests the possibility that population differences may play a role in the extent to which these techniques are applicable. Sufficient evidence is not yet available to evaluate the effectiveness of cognitive-behavioral interventions, such as the one proposed by Beck et al. (1993).

The results of the several studies conducted by Higgins and his associates (1991, 1993b) indicate that behavioral treatments make an important contribution to the armamentarium of cocaine treatment interventions, particularly for initiation of abstinence. These results demonstrate the power of such interventions, particularly in light of the relative comparability of abstinence rates obtained in these studies (85% in the 1991 study and 74% in the 1993 study) to the three- to four-week abstinence rates obtained with a pharmacological intervention, desipramine (59%; Gawin, Kleber, et al., 1989).

Comparisons of modalities have generally not demonstrated the differential effectiveness of several intervention modalities (see, for example, Platt et al., 1995; Washton and Stone-Washton, 1993). Inpatient treatment followed by intensive outpatient or self-help treatment appears to be the most effective combination of treatments (Khalsa, Paredes et al., 1993). A comparison of day treatment versus inpatient treatment also failed to demonstrate the superiority of one treatment over the other (Alterman et al., 1994). The demonstration of differential effectiveness will likely require more precisely targeted interventions.

Other therapeutic modalities, for which there are some evaluation data, have also been employed in the treatment of cocaine abuse. These include social network therapy (Galanter, 1985, 1986), aversion therapy (Frawley and Smith, 1992), and Neuroelectric therapy (Alling, Johnson, and Elmoghazy, 1990; Gariti et al., 1992). For none of these, however, have promising findings been confirmed.

Special populations, including youths and cocaine-abusing methadone maintenance patients, require special programming. In particular, cocaine use is widespread among patients in methadone maintenance treatment programs. While much is known about the progression of drug abuse among adolescents (Kandel, 1975; Kandel et al., 1986; Kandel, Yamaguchi, and Chen, 1992), little research has been conducted to establish the best mode of treatment for this group. With regard to cocaine abuse among patients in methadone maintenance treatment programs, the extent of cocaine use is such that the effectiveness of these programs is undermined (Hanbury et al., 1986; U.S. Government Accounting Office, 1990).

Although there is evidence for the effectiveness of several interventions for addressing such use (for example, Black et al., 1987; Chambers, Taylor, and Moffett, 1972; Magura et al., 1988), the lack of methodological details about the interventions employed, and an absence of replication, has left the extent of their generalizability to other programs unclear (Condelli et al., 1991). Thus, there is a need for further research on the effectiveness of interventions for cocaine use in methadone maintenance treatment programs.

9

Pharmacological Interventions in Cocaine Abuse Treatment

The initial goal of treatment for cocaine abuse or addiction is complete abstinence from all mind-altering drugs (Dackis, Gold, and Estroff, 1989, Gawin 1988; Resnick and Resnick, 1985).

Pharmacological interventions, while of great value in substance abuse treatment in general, particularly in the management of acute sequelae of substance abuse, have yet to be demonstrated as having any *curative* effects in the treatment of cocaine abuse. Care must be taken in their employment, given the reliance of substance abusers on pharmacological solutions to their problems (Millman, 1988; Platt and Labate, 1976). Millman has suggested three areas in which medication may be indicated: treatment of the acute sequelae of drug abuse, including symptomatology associated with cocaine intoxication; treatment of associated pathology so disabling or severe that it reinforces the resumption of drug-taking behavior; and treatment to reduce craving or block cocaine euphoria.

Several excellent reviews have appeared which specifically address the pharmacological treatment of cocaine abuse (for example, Gawin and Ellinwood, 1988; Gawin and Kleber, 1984; Kosten, 1989, 1990, 1993). The reviews by Kosten describe work on pharmacological agents which have been utilized to achieve abstinence from cocaine and to prevent relapse to cocaine use after abstinence has been achieved.

Strategies Underlying Pharmacological Treatment

Two general rationales for selection of these pharmacological agents, one clinical and the other neurochemical, have been noted by Kosten

(1989, 1991). The *clinical rationale* is based primarily on the observation that the syndrome that follows discontinuation of cocaine binges bears a high degree of resemblance to a depressive syndrome. This has led to the suggestion that antidepressive medications may be useful in alleviating this syndrome and facilitating further abstinence from cocaine. The *neurochemical rationale* is based on cocaine's impact on dopaminergic reinforcement mechanisms in the brain. Thus, agents acting on dopaminergic transmission may be useful in treating cocaine dependence. Such effects may either substitute for cocaine, serve as blocking agents for cocaine, or reverse cocaine-induced neurochemical effects. Kosten (1989, 1990, 1993) observed that the clinical and neurochemical rationales may not be mutually exclusive, in that, for example, dopaminergic agents may have antidepressant actions as well (see, for example, Gambarana et al., 1995).

Two classification schemas of pharmacological agents useful in treating cocaine-dependent patients have appeared in the literature. Weiss and Mirin (1990) divided these pharmacological agents into four classes:

1. *Agents which block the effects of cocaine, including euphoria.* Examples of the various drugs in this class include antidepressants such as imipramine and trazodone, dopamine agonists such as bromocriptine, and other neuroleptics such as haloperidol, as well as possibly buprenorphine and lithium (the latter two suggested by animal studies).

2. *Aversive agents.* These are drugs which, when taken in combination with cocaine, produce an adverse reaction, in an analogous manner to the use of disulfiram in treating alcoholism. The only drug in this category is phenelzine, a monoamine oxidase inhibitor. Use of cocaine while taking phenelzine may, however, precipitate a severe toxic reaction.

3. *Drugs for the treatment of premorbid coexisting psychiatric disorders.* Included in this class are those drugs which can alleviate disorders that may increase the vulnerability of patients to cocaine abuse. Thus, desipramine or imipramine for the treatment of depression, lithium for the treatment of cyclothymic or bipolar disorder, and possibly methylphenidate (Ritalin) or magnesium pemoline for the selective treatment of cocaine abusers with attention deficit disorder have all been shown to be useful.

4. *Drugs that treat cocaine-induced states, including withdrawal and craving.* Desipramine, bromocriptine, amantadine, imipramine,

and flupenthixol decanoate have all been shown to have some efficacy, although the level of evidence for effectiveness for each varies greatly.

As can be seen from the specific drugs listed, there is a great deal of overlap among classes, possibly confusing the actual target of any one drug.

Another schema of treatment rationales for a number of groups of pharmacological agents has been suggested by Johnson and Vocci (1993), who proposed five categories for such agents: *blockade of cocaine and related effects*, including kindling, by the use of agents such as carbamazepine, an antiepileptic drug; *abstinence therapy*, either through the use in initiating abstinence of antidepressants (imipramine, desipramine, sertraline, and fluoxetine), antiepileptics (carbamazepine), or anorectics (mazindol), or by blocking the reinforcing qualities of cocaine with calcium channel blockers (nimodipine, nifedipine), the anti–manic depressive agent lithium, or dopamine receptor blockers (haloperidol, perphenazine, pimozide, and sulpiride); *maintenance treatment*, involving dopamine agonists which may reduce craving (amantadine, bromocriptine, methylphenidate, and L-dopa); *relapse prevention*, although there are no known agents which can be used for this purpose; and *overdose therapy*, for which, in the absence of known antagonists of the toxic effects of cocaine, supportive therapy is provided by beta-blockers to attenuate cardiovascular effects and anxiolytics to reduce the incidence of overdose and to promote feelings of well-being.

Agents Addressing Dopamine Depletion

Chronic cocaine use results in overstimulation of dopaminergic reward systems in the brain and subsequent depletion of dopamine (Dackis and Gold, 1985a, b, c). This depletion of dopamine and resultant post–synaptic receptor supersensitivity of inhibitory receptors on the dopamine neuron appears to be the basis for the withdrawal symptoms (including anhedonia and cocaine craving) seen on discontinuation of cocaine (Gawin and Ellinwood, 1988; Gawin and Kleber, 1984). In addition, cocaine use temporarily "refreshes" the dopamine system while leading to further depletion (Dackis and Gold, 1985 a, b, c).

Antidepressant agents have been employed to address cocaine abuse directly through both alleviation of underlying psychopharmacological consequences of cocaine abuse (that is, dopamine depletion) and treatment of affective and related disorders (for example, attention deficit disorder, characterological disorders) which may predispose individuals to cocaine abuse. This latter point is particularly relevant, given the significant numbers of cocaine abusers who have comorbid psychiatric disorders, particularly affective disorders (see, for example, Gawin and Kleber, 1986a; Weiss et al., 1988; Ziedonis et al., 1994).

Tricyclic Antidepressants

DESIPRAMINE (NORPRAMIN AND OTHERS)

Desipramine is a tricyclic antidepressant which has been in general use for several decades. Desipramine showed early promise and for this reason has been perhaps the most intensively studied pharmacological agent for the treatment of cocaine abuse. Desipramine and other antidepressant agents (for example, imipramine, trazodone) were shown in animal studies to reverse the decreased sensitivity to electrical stimulation in dopaminergic brain reward ("pleasure") centers similar to that induced by chronic administration of stimulants (Fibiger and Phillips, 1981; Leith and Barrett, 1976a, b). These findings led to the suggestion that desipramine and similar heterocyclic agents could ameliorate anhedonia, thus decreasing cocaine withdrawal and craving and facilitating abstinence (Gawin and Ellinwood, 1988; Gawin and Kleber, 1984; Gawin, Kleber, et al., 1989). Yet, not all studies with infrahuman organisms have yielded positive findings. Mello (1991), for example, questioned the suppressive effect of desipramine on cocaine self-administration.

What was apparently the first clinical study evaluating the role of desipramine in treating cocaine addiction was conducted by Tennant and Rawson (1983). These authors noted that studies in nonhuman primates and other animals (for example, Seiden, Fischman, and Schuster, 1975; Wagner, Seiden, and Schuster, 1979) had shown that chronic administration of stimulants such as methamphetamine significantly depleted brain norepinephrine, thus placing chronic stimulant users in a state of severe norepinephrine depletion. Reasoning that the tricyclic antidepressant desipramine was more effective in selectively blocking norepinephrine uptake than any other tricyclic antidepressant, they administered desipramine to 8 amphetamine-dependent and 14 cocaine-dependent subjects. Nineteen of 22 (86.4%) subjects reported having discontinued drug use within two to seven days, while 15 (68.2%) had urine samples negative for amphetamines and cocaine. These findings were confirmed in a number of other studies which focused either directly on cocaine use or on the alterations of mood associated with it. In an open field trial of desipramine versus placebo, desipramine was found to decrease depressive symptoms in chronic cocaine abusers (Giannini et al., 1986). Similar findings were obtained in a randomized, double-blind, active placebo-controlled, parallel group study with male cocaine abusers conducted by Wang et al. (1994). The researchers administered either desipramine (100 mg daily); bromocriptine (2.5 mg daily); trazodone (100 mg daily); a combination of 1.25 mg bromocriptine, 50 mg desipramine, and 50 mg trazodone; or a very low dose of diphenhydramine, which served as an active placebo. After two weeks, mean anxiety ratings improved relative to baseline for all groups with the exception of the placebo group, and mean depression ratings significantly decreased for the bromocriptine and trazodone groups, although mean depression ratings also decreased significantly for the placebo group. Both bromocriptine and desipramine groups differed from the placebo group in withdrawal ratings, and desipramine and trazodone differed from placebo on anxiety ratings. Thus, some beneficial effects were found for the antidepressants used in this study, although no data were presented with respect to use of cocaine.

Other studies have confirmed that desipramine is efficacious, to at least some degree, in alleviating cocaine craving and use. Gawin, Kleber, et al. (1989) found that desipramine substantially decreased cocaine use, reduced craving, and resulted in patients' achieving longer continuous periods of abstinence when compared with both lithium and a placebo. O'Brien et al. (1988) demonstrated, in a placebo-controlled study in methadone patients, that desipramine in combination with methadone produced significant improvements in psychological functioning and in reduction of cocaine abuse and cocaine craving. Desipramine did not, however, show as dramatic an improvement for cocaine use as for psychological functioning. Kosten et al. (1987), in an eight-week open trial of desipramine versus placebo at an average dose of 141 mg per day (range, 75–200 mg), found desipramine to reduce cocaine craving significantly in cocaine abusers in methadone maintenance treatment. Cocaine use was substantially, though not significantly, lower (63% versus 25%) at week 8, perhaps reflecting a threat of introduction of administrative sanctions, which appeared to have dramatically reduced cocaine use in the unmedicated groups, even if only for two weeks.

Desipramine may not be as effective, however, in suppressing cocaine craving as was previously suggested, and may in fact have differential effectiveness as a function of the presence of diagnosable psychiatric conditions. Kosten, Morgan, and Schottenfeld (1990) provided evidence for the selective clinical efficacy of desipramine in certain patient groups in a sample of 75 cocaine-abusing methadone patients. In this double-blind, randomized study, patients stabilized at an average methadone dose of 45 mg daily were administered desipramine (150 mg daily), amantadine (300 mg daily), or a placebo. Cocaine abuse was determined by twice-weekly urinalyses and self-reports. In addition, self-reports of cocaine craving were obtained, as were blood levels of amantadine and desipramine. Treatment retention was judged excellent, with 100% retention at six weeks and 70% of patients completing the study. Craving in this study was minimally reduced by desipramine (to 15% below baseline) and maximally reduced by amantadine (to 30% below baseline). Cocaine use, however, was reduced by desipramine during the first week of the study by 50%, as measured by dollars spent on the drug. A similar reduction was found in the amantadine group. By contrast, this measure in the placebo group went to 140% above baseline through week 5. Use by the placebo group past this point declined, with use by week 9 being similar to that of the desipramine group. The desipramine group, but not the placebo group, then showed a further decline in use during weeks 10 and 11. The reduction in cocaine use by the amantadine group continued throughout the study, and cocaine use by this group was always below that of the placebo group. Additionally, the amantadine group showed a greater percentage of patients abstinent for two weeks or more than either the desipramine or placebo groups. Finally, when patients with antisocial personality disorder were excluded from the study, or only depressive patients were examined, desipramine was found to have had some effect on cocaine use but not on craving. Thus, the authors concluded that desipramine had no effect on craving, and showed a significant effect on cocaine use only in patients without antisocial personality disorder, while amantadine had a significant effect on both cocaine craving and consumption in cocaine-abusing methadone patients.

Therefore, desipramine may not be effective in reducing cocaine use among patients diagnosed with antisocial personality disorder. Leal, Ziedonis, and Kosten (1994), for example, found antisocial personality disorder to be associated with a poor response to desipramine (at 150 mg daily) and amantadine (at 300 mg daily) in cocaine-abusing methadone maintenance patients. Antisocial personality disorder was also associated in this study with a poor rate of treatment retention and continued cocaine use. Similar findings were obtained by Arndt et al. (1994), who found that patients with antisocial personality disorder made few gains with or without desipramine (initial dose of 50 mg, increased to a target dose of 250–300 mg daily), while patients without antisocial personality disorder made gains with desipramine, but not with a placebo, with respect to psychiatric symptomatology, legal status, and family problems.

The intravenous users evaluated in early studies may not, however, have presented with the same picture of psychological devastation as is presently seen among chronic crack smokers. Khalsa, Jatlow, and Gawin (1994) examined the usefulness of desipramine with chronic crack smokers in a double-blind comparison of desipramine, flupenthixol decanoate, and a placebo. Minimal psychotherapy was provided in this study so as to isolate more effectively the efficacy of the pharmacological interventions. Both medications were found to be significantly superior to a placebo in engaging the crack users in treatment and in reducing cocaine use, loss of control over cocaine urges, craving for cocaine, depression scores on the Beck Depression Inventory, and SCL-90 scores. There are now a number of reports of both open trials and controlled studies which have demonstrated, to varying degrees, the effectiveness of desipramine in addressing the dysphoria and accompanying anhedonia seen in cocaine addicts during withdrawal from the drug.

Desipramine was also compared against lithium carbonate in a number of studies. In a small, open outpatient trial, Gawin and Kleber (1984) demonstrated that desipramine markedly decreased cocaine abuse and craving. In this study, the use of desipramine (at a dosage level of 3.1–3.7 mg/kg) resulted in marked decreases in craving after two to three weeks of treatment. Furthermore, the presence or absence of an affective disorder did not have an impact on outcome. Lithium was effective in reducing cocaine craving only in subjects with cyclothymic disorders. Similar findings have been obtained by other investigators (for example, Kosten et al., 1987; Rosecan, 1983).

In a later study, Gawin, Kleber, et al. (1989) compared desipramine with lithium and a placebo in a double-blind, random-assignment, six-week study involving a sample of 72 patients who met DSM-III-R criteria for cocaine abuse, but not for other substance abuse. These investigators found 60% of desipramine-treated patients were cocaine-abstinent for three to four weeks during the first six weeks of treatment. In the placebo and lithium groups, by contrast, only 20% and 25% of patients, respectively, demonstrated abstinence from cocaine. Furthermore, patients in the desipramine group attained continuous periods of abstinence more frequently than did subjects in the lithium or placebo groups. Fifty-nine percent of the desipramine-treated subjects were abstinent three to four consecutive weeks or more, compared to subjects in the placebo (17%) and lithium groups (25%). Overall, mean weekly cocaine use in the desipramine group decreased during the first week of treatment from 3.5 grams to 0.5 grams, and a statistically significant difference existed between the desipramine and placebo groups for the remainder of the treatment period. While cocaine craving was significantly reduced for the desipramine group (when compared with the placebo group), this difference did not reach statistical significance until weeks 4 and 5. Thus, desipramine initially reduced cocaine use, followed by a reduction in cocaine craving in about three weeks. This finding was interpreted as suggesting that the action of desipramine in reducing cocaine abuse was not that of a simple anti-craving agent which resulted in a decrease in cocaine use. The importance of this study lies in its demonstration of the usefulness of desipramine as an effective pharmacological agent *in the first stage* of treatment of actively cocaine-addicted outpatients.

STUDIES OF DESIPRAMINE'S MECHANISM OF ACTION

The possible mechanism of action of desipramine was examined by Kosten, Gawin, et al. (1992). These investigators administered intravenous cocaine challenges (at dosages of 0.125 to 0.5 mg/kg at a fixed desipramine dosage of 150 mg daily) to patients who had been stabilized on desipramine for ten days or more. The desipramine condition failed to attenuate the "high," the "rush," or the euphoria associated with cocaine use at any of the dosages used, although the cocaine craving associated with actual cocaine administration was attenuated. Craving was higher at baseline than during the desipramine condition and returned to baseline after cessation of desipramine administration. The authors concluded that desipramine appeared to reduce the duration of cocaine craving and may also have reduced the priming effects of a single administration of cocaine. The latter finding is of potential importance in relapse to cocaine use.

Desipramine may not affect the reinforcing qualities of cocaine, though it may interfere with its other stimulus properties. Fischman et al. (1990) reached this conclusion after examining responses to self-administration of cocaine in desipramine-maintained patients. They found a reduction in euphoria under the desipramine condition, although there was no effect on cocaine self-administration. The authors noted that their results differed from those obtained by Gawin and Kleber (1984) and Gawin, Kleber, et al. (1989), who had found a decrease in cocaine use under the desipramine condition when compared to "standard" cocaine treatment. By contrast, in the Fischman et al. (1990) study, none of the subjects was seeking treatment, cocaine was readily available, stimulus cues for self-administration were present throughout, and there were no differential contingencies associated with cocaine self-administration. The study did not, however, contain a placebo control for the desipramine condition. Additionally, desipramine levels, which averaged 134 ng/ml, may have been insufficient to achieve a therapeutic level, whereas mean levels in the Gawin, Kleber, et al. (1989) study were somewhat (but not very much) higher, at 149 ng/ml.

By contrast, Khalsa, Gawin, et al. (1993) reported that lower desipramine concentrations early in treatment, but not high levels, were related to later treatment outcome. This finding led them to suggest the existence of a dose-response relationship between desipramine and treatment outcome in cocaine abusers, with the existence of a ceiling effect. If this is indeed the case, it may explain some of the apparently contradictory findings obtained with the use of desipramine.

NEGATIVE FINDINGS WITH DESIPRAMINE

Not all studies employing desipramine have resulted in positive findings. Although the efficacy of both desipramine and amantadine in reducing cocaine abuse among depressed patients in methadone maintenance treatment was demonstrated in a twelve-week randomized, double-blind study against placebo (Ziedonis and Kosten, 1991), there was a failure to demonstrate the efficacy of desipramine and amantadine in treating cocaine abuse in non-depressed methadone-maintained patients. In a randomized placebo-controlled clinical trial conducted by Kosten, Morgan, et al. (1992), doses of 150 mg per day of desipramine and 300 mg per day of amantadine were provided. Treatment retention was judged excellent, with 75% of patients completing the full twelve-week trial. Self-reported cocaine use was significantly lower than baseline in the two medication-treated groups at week 4 (decreases of 43% for the amantadine-treated group and 67% for the desipramine-treated group), but this difference was lost at week 8. At twelve weeks only 27% of the desipramine-treated group, 15% of the amantadine-treated group, and 13% of the placebo-treated group were cocaine-abstinent. The findings of these two studies suggest that both desipramine and amantadine are efficacious only in the case of depressed cocaine abusers, and perhaps only in achieving initial abstinence.

In another study with negative findings, Fischman et al. (1990) administered desipramine to cocaine abusers for three weeks at doses (8,

16, or 32 mg) sufficient to maintain a serum concentration at a therapeutic level for the clinical management of depression. No effect was found with respect to continued cocaine administration, although heart rate and blood pressure levels were found to increase beyond the effect expected for either drug. Changes also occurred in the subjective ratings of cocaine's effects. Administration of desipramine resulted in decreases in ratings of the cocaine experience along dimensions such as "positive mood" and "vigor" while increasing those for unpleasant affects such as "anxiety" and "anger." This shift in subjective effects suggests the possibility of an increase in undesirable behaviors resulting from the interaction of desipramine and cocaine.

A failure to find an effect of desipramine on cocaine use and craving when desipramine was compared with a placebo was also reported by Arndt et al. (1990). These investigators conducted a double-blind, placebo-controlled study of desipramine in 79 male cocaine-abusing methadone-maintained patients. The twelve-week medication phase of this study aimed at a range of 150 to 300 ng/ml blood levels of desipramine. At the end of the twelve-week medication phase, improvement was observed in both the placebo and desipramine groups. The desipramine group showed increases in the categories of money earned, drug use, days of reported cocaine use, days of crime, illegal income, psychiatric status, and cocaine craving. The placebo group also showed improvement, with less drug use, fewer days of opiate use, and fewer days of cocaine use. The only significant differences between the desipramine and placebo groups were with respect to employment and psychiatric problems (with the latter showing a decrease in the active medication group versus an increase in the placebo group). Rates of cocaine-positive urines were 78% for the desipramine group and 74% for the placebo group. Similarly, the two groups did not differ with respect to the presence of other drugs of abuse (52% for the desipramine group and 53% for the placebo group). At one-, three-, and six-month follow-up, the desipramine group urines were 80%, 78%, and 80% cocaine-positive, compared with 79%, 46%, and 38% for the control group. Thus, not only was desipramine ineffective in this study, but its use may have resulted in poorer long-term outcome. Similarly, a study by Triffleman et al. (1993) failed to find desipramine efficacious in treating crack-abusing male Veterans Administration patients. In this study, desipramine or a placebo was administered on day 5 of a two-week inpatient stay with dose advanced until a level of 200 mg day was reached. Medication was continued for a total of eight weeks. While initial retention in treatment was related to desipramine levels at week 2, this difference failed to reach significance, and no overall differences emerged between the desipramine and placebo groups with respect to craving or depression scores, or on measures of subjective withdrawal symptoms.

Hall and her associates (1993, 1994) also reported negative findings for desipramine in a study which evaluated desipramine at 200 mg per day against placebo for crack cocaine abuse. This study employed a 2 × 2 design which also examined enhanced continuity of care in brief inpatient treatment followed by outpatient treatment. Under the enhanced condition, participants began attendance at outpatient groups while in inpatient treatment, thus guaranteeing therapist continuity, whereas under the standard treatment, there was no continuity of therapists. The enhanced treatment consisted of the same counselor in both inpatient and outpatient treatment. Standard treatment consisted of different counselors during inpatient and outpatient treatment. Desipramine was initiated during inpatient treatment and continued on entrance into outpatient treatment. The results indicated that the desipramine-enhanced treatment produced better outcomes at three weeks, and that the differences between the treatment groups increased when subjects with antisocial personality disorder were removed. These differences did not last for eight weeks, however. While enhanced continuity of care resulted in decreased use of cocaine, and desipramine itself increased the number of days in treatment if therapeutic levels were reached, desipramine did not affect drug use.

Adverse effects resulting from the use of desipramine have also been reported. Weiss (1988), for example, reported that three patients who had stopped heavy cocaine abuse for one to six months relapsed to cocaine use shortly after beginning treatment with desipramine. Weiss attributed these treatment failures to the development of *early tricyclic jitteriness syndrome,* which may have stimulated conditioned craving for cocaine owing to the similarity of this syndrome to the subjective effects of cocaine intoxication.[1] Weiss concluded that there may be a subgroup of individuals for whom desipramine worsens, rather than relieves, cocaine craving. Thus, unless major depression is present, use of tricyclics for longer than six to ten weeks may not be of therapeutic value, or may even result in negative effects.

Tricyclic antidepressants may also increase the toxic effects of cocaine. Desipramine when administered in combination with cocaine may have the potential for toxic cardiovascular effects, in that their combined administration resulted in a significant increase in heart rate and blood pressure (Fischman et al., 1990). Another study, however, failed to obtain such an adverse cardiovascular interaction between desipramine and acute intravenous cocaine. In this study, cocaine abusers treated chronically with desipramine showed an increased baseline heart rate of 10 to 15 beats per minute compared with a placebo group, but a substantially blunted heart rate response to intravenous cocaine (Pickett et al., 1990). Desipramine has also been found to provide protection against the lethal, but not the convulsant, effects of high doses of cocaine (Jackson, Ball, and Nutt, 1990).

Thus, despite initial promise for desipramine, it would seem appropriate to heed Weddington's (1990) warning that reports of the *statistically* significant efficacy of the drug, where present, do not necessarily translate into *clinical* efficacy, and that the latter has not been demonstrated. Given the *possibility* of cardiovascular side effects resulting from the use of desipramine (for example, postural hypotension, slowing of cardiac conduction), caution was urged in the use of this drug with cocaine addicts who do not demonstrate symptomatology of major depression or another disorder for which the use of desipramine is approved.

Nontricyclic Antidepressants

MAPROTILINE (LUDIOMIL)

Maprotiline is a tetracyclic, noradrenergic antidepressant which likely acts by blocking reuptake of norepinephrine at nerve endings, thus potentiating central adrenergic and noradrenergic synapses. Maprotiline, which possesses low anticholinergic activity, has also been evaluated for the treatment of severe cocaine abuse. In a seven-week open trial, 11 cocaine abusers in a private inpatient facility were administered maprotiline at a dose level of up to 150 to 200 mg daily (mean dose, 152 mg daily; Brotman et al., 1988). Nine patients completed the trial. Of this number, all but one achieved abstinence and remained cocaine-free at a mean follow-up of ten weeks. The authors concluded that maprotiline was well tolerated and appeared to increase treatment compliance and promote abstinence by decreasing cocaine craving and associated anxiety and depression.

PHENELZINE (NARDIL)

Phenelzine sulfate belongs to the class of drugs called monoamine oxidase (MAO) inhibitors. Phenelzine increases the presence of three neurotransmitters (dopamine, serotonin, and norepinephrine) which have been implicated in cocaine abuse. Since phenelzine increases these very neurotransmitters, Golwyn (1988) suggested its use in treating cocaine

withdrawal symptoms and craving. MAO inhibitors are typically recommended for use with patients characterized as "atypical," "nonen-
dogenous," or "neurotic," and its use is indicated for patients who have
failed to respond to more commonly used antidepressants.

Serious reactions, particularly hypertensive crises, may occur if MAO
inhibitors are used concurrently with sympathomimetic drugs such as
amphetamines, cocaine, methylphenidate, dopamine, epinephrine, and
norepinephrine, or with high-protein foods which have undergone protein breakdown by aging (*Physician's Desk Reference*, 1994). Such interactions are likely to be substantial for MAO-A inhibitors, but probably
less so for MAO-B inhibitors (Yu, 1994). In addition, MAO-A inhibitors
may be dangerous when taken in combination with some red wines and
cheese. This potentially dangerous interaction of phenelzine and sympathomimetic drugs, including cocaine, during the first fourteen days of
treatment was seen by Golwyn (1988) as another reason for its potential usefulness in treatment (Golwyn's clinical experience with
phenelzine-cocaine interactions had indicated that these side effects were
perhaps not as dangerous as thought). In an open-trial, uncontrolled
study, cocaine-abusing patients ($N = 26$) who had been in a 28-day residential program with prior pharmacological treatment of tyrosine (1,000
mg daily) and tryptophan (1,000 mg daily) were orally administered
phenelzine (15 mg. three times a day (t.i.d.), to a maximum of 90 mg
daily). Additionally, disulfiram was administered to patients with an alcohol addiction diagnosis. At six months all patients had cocaine-negative urines. Three patients who had feared "slipping" while on phenelzine
and who thus chose imipramine or desipramine reverted to cocaine
abuse. Golwyn concluded that phenelzine was a highly effective treatment for cocaine abuse, but that it should be considered as a "last resort" because of the potential risks associated with its use.

A report exists describing the use of phenelzine and tranylcypromine
sulfate (also a MAO inhibitor antidepressant) with a cocaine-abusing patient who had failed to respond to other medical and psychological interventions. No hypertensive crisis occurred when this patient used cocaine, and the deterrent effects were reported as appearing to be helpful
in breaking a pattern of cocaine abuse (Brewer, 1993). Nunes, Quitkin,
and Klein (1989) suggested that since a significant subgroup of cocaine
abusers in their study met criteria for atypical depression, the use of
monoamine oxidase inhibitors (MAOI) was indicated. Such use, however, is usually contraindicated, given the high likelihood of relapse to
cocaine use and the possibility of a potentially toxic interaction of cocaine and MAOIs.

Other Antidepressant Agents

BUPROPION (WELLBUTRIN)

Bupropion hydrochloride is an antidepressant whose mechanism of action is presently unknown, but which appears to be fundamentally different from either tricyclic or MAO inhibitors. Bupropion has mild dopaminergic activity and does not appear to act on the serotonin and norepinephrine systems. Noting that, as an effective antidepressant, it had few anticholinergic side effects, that it decreased dopamine turnover, and was well tolerated, Margolin et al. (1990) evaluated its effectiveness in the treatment of cocaine abuse. In a small open trial lasting eight weeks, 6 cocaine-abusing methadone patients were administered bupropion in doses of 100 mg three times daily while also participating in twice-weekly psychotherapy sessions. No clinical interactions were observed between bupropion and methadone or bupropion, methadone, and cocaine. Relatively few side effects, with the exception of dry mouth and jitteriness, were noted. At the end of eight weeks, cocaine use was reduced from a level of 4.5 subjects per week to 1 subject per week, and increased positive and decreased negative affect was noted, as were fewer episodes of cocaine craving consequent to dysphoric states. The authors concluded that bupropion held promise in the treatment of cocaine abuse.

These findings were not confirmed in a small double-blind inpatient study which compared bupropion (100 mg, t.i.d.) with a placebo (Hollister et al., 1992). In this study, dropout was high: at the end of twenty-one days, retention was only 8 of 22 subjects in the bupropion group, and 6 of 24 in the control group. Side effects were also evident, in particular dizziness, dry mouth, restlessness, and lethargy, which likely contributed to the high dropout rate. Data collected on the remaining subjects suggested that a high rate of spontaneous improvement also occurred in the placebo group.

FLUOXETINE (PROZAC)

Fluoxetine hydrochloride is a serotonin-uptake blocker which has shown promise in treating depression (Gram, 1994; Taylor et al., 1994), obsessive-compulsive disorder (Tollefson, Birkett et al., 1994; Tollefson, Rampey, et al., 1994), and eating disorders (Walsh, 1991; Wood, 1993), as well as being of potential value in treating alcohol craving (Gorelick and Paredes, 1992; Naranjo et al., 1994). It is chemically unrelated to tricyclic, tetracyclic, and other antidepressant agents.

A number of studies have suggested that fluoxetine may be of value in treating cocaine abuse and craving. Batki and his associates (1990) evaluated this agent for its efficacy in treating cocaine abuse in a group of methadone maintenance patients who were also receiving weekly group therapy. In an open trial lasting nine weeks, fluoxetine was administered each morning in doses ranging from 20 to 60 mgs, with a final average dose of 45 mg per day. Self-reports, urinalysis results, and plasma cocaine levels all showed a significant decrease in cocaine use over the course of the trial. Craving and monies spent on cocaine also decreased significantly, and subjects still using cocaine at week 9 reported a decrease in the "highs" obtained from cocaine. Patients receiving fluoxetine at 40 mg daily, when compared to a group receiving a placebo, stayed in treatment longer (11 weeks versus 3 weeks) and remained abstinent longer (Washburn et al., 1994). Fluoxetine at a dose level of 40 mg per day appeared to be equally effective in increasing retention of primary cocaine-dependent (crack-using) outpatients, as well as in reducing cocaine abuse and craving in secondary cocaine-dependent (methadone maintenance treatment) patients (Batki et al., 1994). These results, and the fact that fluoxetine was well tolerated by these patients (who in general had significant medical problems), suggested to Batki et al. (1994) that fluoxetine showed promise in the treatment of cocaine-abusing methadone maintenance patients.

Another study similarly obtained positive findings with fluoxetine. Pollack and Rosenbaum (1991) administered fluoxetine to 11 cocaine-abusing heroin addicts. The initial dose level was 20 mg, which was increased to 40 mg after two weeks. Three patients dropped out of the study within a few days because of lack of acute therapeutic effects. Of the remaining 8 who had received fluoxetine for at least one week, 5 were successfully treated for cocaine abuse. A preliminary report of a double-blind trial of fluoxetine by Batki, Manfredi, Jacob, Delucchi, et al. (1993) also reported promising results with respect to decreased cocaine craving and use. Covi et al. (1994) employed a double-blind, random-assignment design with fluoxetine at 20, 40, and 60 mg daily in a twelve-week study treating cocaine-dependent outpatients. Over time there was decreased cocaine use and craving, although patients in the 60 mg group showed a higher percentage of cocaine-positive urines. In a second analysis, those subjects who had achieved a fluoxetine blood level of over 100 ng/ml were compared with the placebo group and a "missing values group." All groups were found to have improved, that is, they showed lower craving scores. Finally, when stratified by initial urine positivity and assignment to treatment group, those initially scored negative for cocaine reported less overall use. Those initially scored positive decreased craving relatively more than those initially negative.

Batki, Manfredi, Jacob, and Jones (1993) conducted an open prospective study of fluoxetine (mean dose = 45 mg/day for nine weeks) in 16 cocaine-abusing methadone maintenance patients. Although none of the patients reached abstinence, cocaine use was reduced, as was craving and the quality of the high obtained. Benzoylecgonine and cocaine concentrations decreased significantly from intake to week 9 of treatment. Fluoxetine was well tolerated, with few side effects, and did not appear to affect methadone concentrations in urine.

TRAZODONE (DESYREL)

Trazodone hydrochloride (Desyrel) is a triazolopyridine antidepressant derivative unrelated to tricyclic, tetracyclic, or other depressant agents. While its mechanism of action is not fully understood, it is known to inhibit selectively serotonin uptake by brain synaptosomes and to potentiate the behavioral changes induced by the serotonin precursor 5-hydroxytryptophan. Trazodone has much less central antidopaminergic or anticholinergic activity than tricyclic antidepressants (Taylor, Hyslop, and Riblet, 1980), and does not block norepinephrine reuptake (Davis and Glassman, 1989). Trazodone has been shown to decrease the toxicity of amphetamines (Silvestrini et al., 1968), and has been reported to have value in treating cocaine-induced panic disorder where heterocyclic antidepressants were not well tolerated (Louie, Lannon, and Ketter, 1989). A case report has suggested the value of trazodone in decreasing cocaine craving and relieving withdrawal symptoms (Small and Purcell, 1985).

LITHIUM CARBONATE (ESKALITH, LITHOBID)

Early case studies reported beneficial effects of lithium carbonate on both amphetamine (Flemenbaum, 1974) and cocaine abuse (Cronson and Flemenbaum, 1978; Gold and Byck, 1978). In several studies lithium was effective in reducing euphoria associated with stimulant use. For example, lithium was found to block mood responses to methylphenidate (Wald, Ebstein, and Belmaker 1978); to block the activating effects of methylphenidate, including increased arousal, thought disorder, excitement, and depression (Huey et al., 1981); and to attenuate the euphoriant and activating effects of amphetamines (van Kammen and Murphy, 1975). Additionally, lithium was found to inhibit the development of cocaine-induced behavioral sensitization in rats while not inhibiting the development of amygdala kindling (Post, Weiss, and Pert, 1984). Another study reported that lithium inhibited hyperactivity and stereotypic activity in rats who had been administered cocaine (Flemenbaum, 1977).

A study by Gawin, Kleber, et al. (1989), in which lithium (600 mg) was compared with desipramine (2.5 mg/kg) and a placebo in a double-blind, random-assignment study of 72 cocaine-abusing patients, found both lithium and the placebo to be substantially less effective than desipramine in inducing abstinence from cocaine (20% abstinence for the placebo group, 25% for the lithium group, and 60% for the desipramine-treated groups) or bringing about a reduction in cocaine craving three to four weeks later.

Nunes et al. (1990), following up on the initial positive findings reported by Gawin and Kleber (1984), suggested that lithium may be effective with a subgroup of cocaine abusers with cyclothymic disorders. They conducted an open trial evaluation of lithium carbonate, sufficient to maintain a blood level between 0.4 and 1.0 miliequivalents (mEq) per liter, in 10 cocaine abusers diagnosed as having bipolar spectrum disorders preexisting the onset of all substance abuse disorders. Although most patients showed some reduction in cocaine use, this decrease was not statistically significant, and only 3 of the 10 patients were cocaine-free for three consecutive weeks. Thus, Nunes et al. (1990) were unable to replicate Gawin and Kleber's early (1984) positive outcomes.

Overall, then, the evidence from recent studies has failed to support the initial enthusiasm shown for this agent. It is possible, however, that lithium carbonate may have some value in certain cases where cyclothymic disorders (for example, hypomania, cyclothymia, and hyperthymia) are present. In such cases, where cocaine is used to potentiate the high, to avoid the "crash" or depression (Gawin and Ellinwood, 1988), or as a result of the impulsivity and poor judgment associated with these disorders (Weiss et al., 1988), the use of lithium may be both appropriate and efficacious.

Agents Addressing Attention Deficit Disorders

Methylphenidate (Ritalin)

Methylphenidate (Ritalin), an amphetamine-like psychostimulant, can produce euphoria indistinguishable from that produced by amphetamines (Brown, Corriveau, and Egbert, 1978), as well as other stimulant-like effects, including increased interpersonal interaction, increased talkativeness and rapport, and increased pressure of thoughts (Huey et al., 1981). Thus, the possibility existed that methylphenidate would act with respect to cocaine in the same way methadone substitution acts with respect to heroin and/or morphine use, that is, that methylphenidate would produce consistent acute cross-tolerance to stimulants while having minimal euphorigenic effects and less abuse liability (Gawin, Riordan, and Kleber, 1985; Kleber and Gawin, 1984).

Several case studies have been reported in which methylphenidate was successfully employed to treat cocaine abuse in individuals with definite or strongly suggested attention deficit disorder (Khantzian, 1983). Following these early studies, Khantzian et al. (1984) reported on three cases of successful treatment of cocaine dependence with methylphenidate, one of which involved a diagnosis of attention deficit disorder. Improvement in signs and symptoms of abstinence, as well as craving and other related behavioral disturbances, was obtained in all three cases. On the basis of these findings, Khantzian et al. (1984) suggested that cocaine dependence was associated with preexisting or resulting psychopathology, usually mood disturbances. Furthermore, it was suggested that stimulant abusers used these drugs to overcome the states of depletion, anergia, and emptiness associated with depression. Nonetheless, in an open trial study of methylphenidate at various dosages in a sample of five cocaine abusers without attention deficit disorder, Gawin, Riordan, and Kleber (1985) found no clinical improvement or decrease in cocaine use. The very small number of subjects, however, calls into question the strength of these findings in either direction.

Magnesium Pemoline

Weiss, Pope, and Mirin (1985) reported the successful use of magnesium pemoline at doses of either 75 mg daily (1 mg/kg daily) or 225 mg taken four times daily (approximately 4 mg/kg) in two cocaine-abusing patients who appeared to be self-medicating symptoms of residual attention deficit disorder. Desire for cocaine was significantly reduced in both patients, with neither patient abusing the medication. Again, the very small number of subjects calls into question the validity of the findings.

Agents Addressing Cocaine Withdrawal and Craving

Amantadine Hydrochloride

Amantadine hydrochloride, which enhances dopamine transmission, had been thought to be potentially useful in maintenance therapy because of its ability to reduce cocaine craving. Amantadine is believed to act by releasing dopamine and norepinephrine from neuronal storage sites and slowing their reuptake by the neuron, thus making increased dopamine and norepinephrine available to receptor sites (Tennant and Sagherian, 1987). Preclinical evidence for the efficacy of amantadine suggested that it held promise in cocaine treatment. Amantadine did not attenuate self-administration of cocaine in baboons, and baboons did not maintain self-administration with amantadine (Sannerud and Griffiths, 1988), suggesting a lack of reinforcing qualities for amantadine while not modifying the reinforcing qualities of cocaine.

Because of its rapid action, amantadine has been seen as being potentially effective in reducing craving during cocaine withdrawal. As noted by Gawin, Morgan, et al. (1989), the rapid onset efficacy of this drug in dopamine deficiency disorders such as Parkinson's disease and anhedonic/anergic syndromes which resemble cocaine withdrawal suggested its potential usefulness. Indeed, promising results were obtained in early studies. Kosten (1989) reported that amantadine was effective in reducing cocaine craving and use in methadone-maintained patients. Similar findings were obtained by Kosten, Morgan, and Schottenfield (1990).

In another study of methadone maintenance patients, amantadine (300 mg daily) was compared to desipramine (300 mg daily), and a placebo in a double-blind, randomized clinical trial. Treatment retention was judged excellent, with 100% retention at six weeks, 70% at the end of the trial, and no differential dropout. Cocaine craving was reduced to 70% of baseline for the amantadine group, but not for the desipramine or placebo groups. Dollars spent on cocaine were also reduced, dropping to 40% of baseline for both the amantadine and desipramine groups but not for the placebo group. Abstinence from cocaine was achieved by 45% of the entire amantadine group and 60% of those in this group who completed the twelve weeks of treatment. Cocaine use and craving were found to have been reduced even further, to 20% and 50% of baseline, respectively, a finding which was also present in the desipramine-treated group. Patients, regardless of the presence of an antisocial personality disorder, responded to amantadine, but not to desipramine, while patients without antisocial personality disorder responded to both amantadine and desipramine.

A third study conducted with methadone-maintained patients also found amantadine, at 200 mg daily for three weeks, followed by an increase to 200 mg twice daily for three subsequent weeks, decreased cocaine craving, self-reported cocaine use, and Beck depression scores (Handelsman et al., 1988). A fourth study (Morgan et al., 1988) found administration of amantadine (at a dose of 300 mg/day), to be somewhat effective in decreasing cocaine use and craving while not having any immediate anti-craving effect.

Amantadine was evaluated against bromocriptine for its relative efficacy in withdrawal from cocaine in a double-blind study by Tennant and Sagherian (1987). At doses of 100 to 300 mg daily for amantadine and 2.5 to 7.5 mg daily for bromocriptine for ten days, both drugs appeared to be effective in alleviating the intensity of cocaine withdrawal symptoms (cocaine craving, low energy, sleep disturbance), although neither was found to reduce cocaine use significantly later in treatment. Also, when amantadine was administered in single doses of 300 mg to cocaine abusers in treatment in a double-blind crossover study, it was found to be less effective than a placebo in reducing craving (Gawin, Morgan, et al., 1989). Additional negative findings were reported by Weddington, Brown, et al. (1991), who conducted a single-blind, placebo-controlled twelve-week trial of amantadine (at a dose of 200 mg daily for four weeks, followed by eight weeks of placebo) and desipramine (at a dose level of 200 mg daily) among cocaine-dependent outpatients. All groups, including a twelve-week placebo control, received individual counseling twice weekly. The results indicated that all groups, including the placebo control, showed a dramatic decrease in cocaine use, craving, and depression for the entire treatment period (for subjects who stayed in treatment), and no statistically significant differences emerged among groups.

Another study (Kosten, Morgan, et al., 1992) demonstrated that amantadine (at 300 mg/day) had a significant effect on both cocaine craving and consumption in cocaine-abusing methadone patients at week 4 of the trial but that this effect disappeared by week 8. At twelve weeks only 15% of the amantadine-treated group, versus 13% of the placebo-treated group, were cocaine-abstinent. Weddington et al. (1990), however, found four weeks of amantadine treatment at a dose of 200 mg to be no more effective than desipramine (twelve weeks at 200 mg daily) or a placebo with respect to decreasing cocaine use or craving. Negative findings were also reported in a study which employed a cue reactivity procedure to evaluate amantadine. In this study, amantadine was found to increase reactivity to drug-related cues while having no effect on craving. This study thus provided no support for the value of amantadine in reducing craving, although the cue reactivity paradigm was found to be useful in conducting medication trials (Robbins et al., 1992). One problem with all these studies is that dosage levels may not have been sufficiently high to produce a therapeutic effect (Weddington et al., 1990).

Bromocriptine (Parlodel)

Bromocriptine is a long-acting dopamine agonist used in the treatment of Parkinson's disease. This agent may potentiate or inhibit the actions of dopamine both pre- and postsynaptically. Bromocriptine may influence brain "reward" systems likely involving dopamine which may be implicated in cocaine self-administration (Hubner and Koob, 1990; Kumor, Sherer, and Jaffe, 1989). Furthermore, dopamine receptor blockers (for example, chlorpromazine, haloperidol, thioridazine, pimozide) have been known for some time to block the euphoria produced by another stimulant, amphetamine (Angrist, Lee, and Gerson, 1974; Gunne, Änggård, and Jönsson, 1972), although no changes, or only small alterations, in euphoria resulted when the stimulant was cocaine (Gawin, 1986b; Sherer, Kumor, and Jaffe, 1989).

Dackis and Gold (1985a), in a case study of two patients (again, too small a sample on which to base conclusions), found bromocriptine, administered blindly against a placebo in a single oral dose of 0.625 mg, to produce "striking and consistent" (p. 1151) relief from cocaine craving during the postwithdrawal period. Furthermore, administration of thioridazine, a dopamine antagonist, resulted in an acute increase in cocaine craving. These findings, together with the ability of bromocriptine to reverse two biological alterations associated with cocaine abuse (hyperprolactinemia and increased postsynaptic dopamine receptor activity), suggested that bromocriptine should be further evaluated for its effectiveness in the treatment of cocaine craving. Also, bromocriptine had been found to prevent the late behavioral depression that follows acute administration of cocaine in the rat (Campbell et al., 1989). A case study report (Gutierrez-Esteinou et al., 1988) also suggested that bromocriptine had a stimulation-antagonizing, anti-cocaine action in humans.

Bromocriptine was evaluated against amantadine for its relative efficacy in withdrawal from cocaine in a double-blind study by Tennant and Sagherian (1987). It was administered at a dose of 2.5 to 7.5 mg daily, while amantadine was administered at doses of 100 to 300 mg per day for a period of ten days. All participants in this study also received tyrosine (at 400 mg four times daily) and tryptophan (1,000 mg at bedtime). Both bromocriptine and amantadine appeared to be effective in alleviating the intensity of cocaine withdrawal symptoms (cocaine craving, low energy, and sleep disturbance). While 71.4% of patients in the amantadine condition remained in the study for the full ten days, a 57% dropout rate occurred in the bromocriptine group, owing to significant side effects (headache, vertigo, and/or syncope). Neither drug was found to reduce cocaine use significantly later in treatment. Tennant and Sagherian suggested that chronic cocaine use may have contributed to bromocriptine's side effects through dopamine receptor supersensitivity, and that a lower dose might have been more effective. Another double-blind trial of bromocriptine versus placebo conducted by Giannini, Baumgartel, and DiMarzio (1987), employing 0.625 mg four times daily for 42 days, resulted in rapid and significant relief from abstinence symptoms, providing support for the view that withdrawal symptoms (dysphoria and craving) are behavioral manifestations of dopamine receptor supersensitivity.

Jaffe, Cascella, Kumor, and Sherer (1989) reported that a single 2.5 mg oral dose of bromocriptine did not reduce baseline levels of craving for cocaine during the first 100 minutes following intravenous injection of cocaine. Jaffe et al. (1989) did not see an inconsistency between these findings and those of Dackis and Gold (1985a), since the form of craving (that is, postwithdrawal craving) addressed in the latter study may have been more a chronic or subacute type as opposed to the acute craving studied by them.

In a replication and extension of their 1985 study, Dackis and associates (1987) conducted a randomized, double-blind, placebo-controlled study of low-dose (1.25 mg administered orally) bromocriptine in a group of 13 recently abstinent cocaine-user inpatients who complained of cocaine craving. Compared to the placebo condition, a significant reduction in cocaine craving occurred under the bromocriptine condition. The authors concluded that the ability of a low dose of bromocriptine to reduce craving could be explained by the presence of dopamine receptor supersensitivity reflecting a functional dopamine inhibition which might underlie craving. In another study of bromocriptine on the subjective effects of cocaine, Kumor, Sherer, and Jaffe (1989) employed single administrations of 2.5 mg doses of bromocriptine, given 120 minutes before single 40 mg intravenous doses of cocaine. A 5.0 mg dose was also used with five subjects. Pretreatment with bromocriptine diminished cocaine-induced blood pressure changes and increased the heart rate after the administration of cocaine. It did not, however, significantly affect subjective responses to cocaine, although a trend in this direction was observed. This finding suggested that the craving and euphoric responses associated with single doses of cocaine may be separable.

Several studies have been conducted examining the efficacy of bromocriptine in comparison or in combination with other pharmacological agents in alleviating cocaine abstinence symptoms by addressing dopamine depletion. Employing a double-blind design, Giannini and Billett (1987) studied 36 male cocaine abusers who had been treated with bromocriptine, either alone—0.625 mg four times a day (q.i.d.) for 30 days, after which placebo A was substituted—or in combination with 200 mg desipramine before sleep (hs.) against placebo (placebo A q.i.d. and placebo B hs.) for 99 days. Abstinence symptomatology in both treatment groups declined over 90 days, and did so at a higher rate than for the placebo group. Outcomes under the combined bromocriptine-desipramine condition were better than for either placebo or bromocriptine alone. The authors interpreted these results as further supporting the hypothesis that both dysphoria and craving were manifestations of dopamine receptor supersensitivity, and that desipramine further alleviated withdrawal symptoms by inducing additional receptor subsensitivity.

Giannini et al. (1989) then compared both bromocriptine (2.5 mg every 6 hours) and amantadine (100 mg, also q.i.d.) against placebo (q.i.d.) in a randomized 30-day outpatient trial. Both bromocriptine and amantadine were more effective than the placebo in reducing dysphoria and craving for 15 days. The effectiveness of amantadine then declined, reaching the placebo level of effectiveness by 30 days. Bromocriptine, however, remained slightly more effective than either amantadine or placebo during days 15 through 30. These findings were attributed to the differing mechanisms of action of amantadine and bromocriptine. That is, bromocriptine reverses dopamine depletion, while amantadine actually releases dopamine into the synaptic cleft. Since amantadine's indirect agonist activity is dependent on dopamine release from already depleted stores, initial improvement may be at the cost of further reducing the amount of dopamine available later, thus worsening neurotransmitter depletion.

Wang et al. (1994), in a randomized, double-blind, active placebo study, compared bromocriptine (2.5 mg daily), desipramine (100 mg daily), and trazodone (50 mg daily) alone and in combination against an active placebo (diphenhydramine) for their effectiveness in cocaine treatment. Significant reductions in depression were observed in the bromocriptine and trazodone groups, although such a reduction was also found in the placebo group at two weeks. Overall, both the bromocriptine and trazodone groups differed from the placebo group in alleviating withdrawal symptoms, and both trazodone and desipramine were more effective than the placebo in reducing anxiety ratings.

Despite the effectiveness shown for bromocriptine in a number of studies, many patients experience significant side effects, including headaches, vertigo and dizziness, orthostatic hypotension, and syncope (Wang et al., 1992).

Noting the overreliance on self-report in evaluating improvement in patients treated with bromocriptine, Kranzler and Bauer (1990), in a double-blind study, evaluated autonomic reactions to cocaine-related cues as well as self-reports of symptoms in patients treated with either bromocriptine (1.25 mg twice daily) or a placebo. Bromocriptine was found not to reduce desire, autonomic reactivity, or subjective symptom severity when subjects were exposed to cocaine-related cues, leading the authors to suggest that the ability of bromocriptine to produce these effects is largely due to a positive expectation rather than to a specific pharmacological effect.

Doubt about the usefulness of bromocriptine in cocaine withdrawal was also raised by Teller and Devenyi (1988). The hypothesized mechanism of action of bromocriptine is the relief of dopamine depletion after chronic cocaine use (Dackis and Gold, 1985a, b) and the subsequent reversal of craving. Since this reversal of craving is accompanied by increases in prolactin levels secondary to dopamine depletion, prolactin can serve as a marker of inhibitory dopaminergic control (Dackis et al., 1984). The failure to find a change in serum prolactin levels pre- and post-administration of bromocriptine in an uncontrolled study of 25 heavy cocaine users raises a question about the effectiveness of bromocriptine in producing these effects. A randomized, double-blind, placebo-controlled study of bromocriptine (1.25 mg three times daily versus placebo for three weeks) in cocaine-abusing outpatients failed to demonstrate an effect in initiating abstinence from cocaine (Moscovitz, Brookoff, and Nelson, 1993).

Buspirone (BuSpar)

Buspirone hydrochloride is an antianxiety agent pharmacologically unrelated to the benzodiazepines, barbiturates, or other sedative/anxiolytic drugs. It acts by enhancing dopaminergic and noradrenergic firing and by suppressing a subset of serotonergic activity. In a study by Giannini, Loiselle, et al. (1993), buspirone (10 mg t.i.d.) or a placebo was administered to withdrawing cocaine abusers over a thirty-day period. From the tenth day on, buspirone was significantly, and increasingly, more effective than the placebo in reducing withdrawal symptoms. Thus, buspirone may be of value in the treatment of cocaine withdrawal symptoms.

L-dopa (Levodopa)

L-dopa, the precursor of dopamine long used as an anti-Parkinsonian agent, has been evaluated in several studies for its potential usefulness in maintenance therapy and for the reduction of craving. In an open evaluation, Rosen, Flemenbaum, and Slater (1986) administered 10 mg of carbidopa and 100 mg of L-dopa to several cocaine abusers. "Some response" was noted by the end of the first week of use. "Most" patients received an additional 25 mg of carbidopa and 100 mg of L-dopa two to three times daily during a second week of treatment, when additional improvement was noted. A study by Wolfsohn, Sanfilipo, and Angrist (1993) of 30 patients diagnosed as having primary cocaine dependence and who had recently used cocaine (within the previous twenty-four hours) received four doses of L-dihydroxy-phenylalanine/carbidopa (100 mg/25 mg) or a placebo the next day. Ratings late the afternoon of the same day and the next morning revealed no significant effects. The authors attributed this finding to "the rapid clearing of indices of abstinence" (p. 52) in the placebo-treated patients.

Cocaine Antagonists (Agents Blocking Euphoria)

Flupenthixol Decanoate

While tricyclic antidepressants can reduce craving for cocaine during withdrawal from the drug, the delay in onset of such an effect ranging from seven to fourteen days after administration is problematic in that it may result in low treatment compliance and, therefore, may increase the resumption of cocaine use early in treatment (Giannini et al., 1986; Gawin, Kleber, et al., 1989). Gawin, Allen, and Humblestone (1989) suggested, therefore, that the use of flupenthixol decanoate, which acts by blocking dopamine and has both an antidepressant action at low doses and a neuroleptic action at higher doses, if effective, would have an obvious treatment advantage. Additionally, flupenthixol decanoate requires infrequent intramuscular administration. Gawin, Kleber, et al. (1989) evaluated the efficacy of flupenthixol decanoate (single dose of 10–20 mg by intramuscular injection) in a preliminary, open-ended, open-label outpatient trial with 10 heavy crack users who had marked cocaine craving and who had not responded to conventional treatment. The results indicated that flupenthixol decanoate was well tolerated and appeared to reduce cocaine craving rapidly and facilitate the induction of abstinence, resulting in a 260% increase in the average time spent in treatment by patients in the study (based on their maximum previous stays).

In a double-blind study by Khalsa, Jatlow, and Gawin (1994) described earlier, the comparison of flupenthixol decanoate (10–20 mg every two weeks) with desipramine and a placebo suggested that both medications were superior to the placebo in engaging the crack users in treatment, reducing cocaine use, and improving control over cocaine urges, craving for cocaine, and dysphoria. In this double-blind study, crack cocaine abusers meeting DSM-III-R criteria for cocaine dependence were provided with flupenthixol at 10 to 20 mg every two weeks, desipramine (dose not given), or a placebo. Minimal psychotherapy was provided to help isolate pharmacological effects and "to better approximate the realities of [the] urban environment" (p. 438). Engagement in treatment by the third visit for both medications was superior to the placebo condition (30% versus 5%). Both flupenthixol and desipramine were significantly superior to the placebo in reducing cocaine urges, dyscontrol over cocaine urges, and craving for cocaine, and in improving Beck depression scores and Hopkins Symptom Checklist 90 scores.

It is likely that more work will be done evaluating flupenthixol decanoate for possible use as a pharmacological agent in the treatment of cocaine abuse. In this regard, Grabowski, Higgins, and Kirby (1993) noted three pharmacological properties which make flupenthixol decanoate particularly attractive for such use: it possesses at best modest reinforcing properties of its own (certainly not at a level where it could be considered the replacement therapy for cocaine, that is, the "methadone for cocaine"); it has few noncontingent punishing effects (that is, unpleasant side effects) when compared with other antidepressants; and it may attenuate cocaine reinforcement and thus allow extinction to occur. Each of these properties, while not alone sufficient to sustain treatment-oriented behavior, may increase the likelihood of positive treatment outcomes. Thus, flupenthixol decanoate, as an injectable, long-acting dopamine antagonist, holds promise as an efficacious pharmacological treatment agent for cocaine abuse.

Pimozide

Pimozide is a dopaminergic antagonist which has been shown to block the reinforcing properties of stimulants in rats (De Wit and Wise, 1977; Yokel and Wise, 1975) and nonhuman primates (Woolverton, 1986), although no studies of this agent in man have been reported. Pretreatment with pimozide before cocaine administration, like pretreatment with

Haldol (haloperidol), attenuates cocaine-induced increases in the in vivo reuptake of dopamine (Parsons, Schad, and Justice, 1993).

Agents Producing Aversive Reactions When Taken with Cocaine

Mazindol, like cocaine, is a potent catecholamine reuptake inhibitor. It inhibits both dopamine and norepinephrine uptake and can interact with a receptor on the dopamine uptake transporter protein which may mediate the self-administration of cocaine. It is used clinically as an appetite suppressant (Hauger et al., 1986; Ritz et al., 1987).

In an open trial, Berger, Gawin, and Kosten (1989) found mazindol, at 1 to 3 mg per day, to reduce substantially cocaine craving, euphoria, and intake in methadone maintenance outpatients. These results were obtained on the first day of administration and were sustained for one month. All patients completed the trial, and no adverse side effects were noted. A study by Diakogiannis, Steinberg, and Kosten (1991) failed to demonstrate a significant effect of mazindol (2 mg daily for one week) on cocaine use among cocaine abusers in methadone maintenance treatment. Although 7 of 19 patients bought less cocaine while on mazindol, craving appeared to increase during mazindol treatment periods versus placebo treatment periods. Furthermore, the quality of cocaine euphoria was not affected, and no difference between placebo and mazindol conditions was seen with respect to number of clean urines. Side effects, including jitteriness and agitation resulting from mazindol use, were reported by most patients in the study. The results of a study by Preston et al. (1993) indicated a lack of any effects by mazindol at doses of 0 mg, 1 mg, and 2 mg orally administered two hours prior to an injection of cocaine at doses of 10 mg, 12.5 mg, 25 mg, and 50 mg i.v. on the magnitude or profile of subjective responses to cocaine, including craving. This last study also noted the possibility of increased cardiovascular risk resulting from use of mazindol.

Other Pharmacological Agents

Agents Used in the Treatment of Opioid Addiction

BUPRENORPHINE (BUPRENEX)

Buprenorphine, a mixed opioid agonist/antagonist, has shown promise as a treatment agent for cocaine-abusing opioid addicts (see Platt, 1995b, pp. 126–132, for a discussion of buprenorphine as a therapeutic agent in opioid addiction). Of all pharmacologic agents presently under investigation, buprenorphine appeared, on the basis of early studies, to offer the most promise for the treatment of individuals dually addicted to cocaine and heroin. For both the detoxification and maintenance treatment of heroin addiction, buprenorphine offers the advantages of acceptance and cross-tolerance with opiates, while being effective in blockading the effects of narcotics and having a relatively brief and less intense withdrawal period (compared with methadone), as well as having a relatively low abuse potential. As a mixed opiate agonist/antagonist, buprenorphine acts as an agonist at low dosages and as an antagonist at high dosages (Mello and Mendelson, 1980). Buprenorphine has weak opioid agonist actions which may decrease opioid interactions with cocaine when both are used together, thus making this form of abuse less attractive. It also has the further advantage of increased antagonist activity at higher dose levels, thus possibly affecting cocaine abuse more strongly (Lewis, 1985).

Buprenorphine's promise for use in attenuating dual abuse of cocaine and heroin was suggested by a study in nonhuman primates (rhesus monkeys) in which suppression of cocaine self-administration took place at doses of buprenorphine (0.40 and 0.70 mg/kg daily) sufficient to suppress heroin administration (Mello et al., 1990a). In a subsequent study, this effect was present even when buprenorphine was used at a dose (0.237–0.70 mg/kg daily) which did not consistently suppress opioid-maintained response (Mello et al., 1990b). Furthermore, in the latter study, buprenorphine more effectively reduced the reinforcing properties of cocaine than did naltrexone across the range of dose studied (buprenorphine reductions in cocaine self-administration averaged 72% to 93% from baseline versus 25% to 28% from baseline for naltrexone). The authors concluded that their findings suggested that buprenorphine interfered with the reinforcing effects of cocaine, and thus might be an effective agent in the treatment of cocaine abuse as well as combined abuse of cocaine plus heroin. In a subsequent study (Mello, Kamien, et al., 1993), intermittent buprenorphine treatment (0.40 mg/kg every 48 or 72 hours) was found to be less effective than the daily administration used in earlier studies (Mello et al., 1990b; 1992). The suppressant effects of buprenorphine on cocaine self-administration in rhesus monkeys has been shown to persist for as long as 120 days, while tolerance to buprenorphine's suppression of food-maintained response develops over 30 to 70 days (Mello et al., 1992). Thus, consistent with findings of other studies (Mello, Bree, and Mendelson, 1983; Mello et al., 1981), the results of this study indicate that buprenorphine appears to reduce cocaine's reinforcing qualities selectively, possibly even making cocaine aversive during buprenorphine administration. An alternative hypothesis for buprenorphine's reduction of cocaine self-administration is that buprenorphine may increase the reinforcing qualities of cocaine, thus resulting in less cocaine being required to maintain response (Mello et al., 1992).

Initial evidence for the usefulness of buprenorphine in the treatment of cocaine abuse was also provided in humans in reports by Kosten, Kleber, and Morgan (1989a, b). These investigators conducted a one-month trial of the utility of buprenorphine versus methadone in addressing cocaine use among cocaine-abusing opiate addicts. Illicit cocaine use was examined in 41 buprenorphine-maintained patients and 61 methadone-maintained patients. Cocaine-positive urines averaged less than 3% in the buprenorphine-maintained sample, compared to approximately 25% in the methadone-maintained sample, strongly suggesting the utility of buprenorphine. When 12 cocaine-abusing, methadone-maintained patients were switched to buprenorphine maintenance, 5 stopped their cocaine use, and a sixth reduced cocaine use by 50%, while the other 6 showed no change (Kosten, Kleber, and Morgan, 1989a).

A number of studies have nonetheless failed to provide support for the anticipated value of buprenorphine. Buprenorphine has in fact been shown to interact with cocaine in a synergistic manner in nonhuman primates, enhancing rather than attenuating cocaine's reinforcing properties (Brown et al., 1991). In humans, Rosen et al. (1993) found that five days of sublingual buprenorphine (2 mg daily, versus placebo in a crossover design) significantly enhanced dually dependent (cocaine and opiates) patients' ratings of cocaine-induced pleasurable effects in response to intranasal cocaine challenges administered on days 3 and 5 of the treatment. This enhancement of subjective effects was greater on day 3 than on day 5, suggesting a different interactive effect with prolonged treatment.

Gastfriend and associates (Gastfriend et al., 1992; Teoh, Mello, et al., 1994) conducted an open outpatient trial of daily sublingual buprenorphine (at doses of 4 mg or 8 mg daily) in 25 male patients dually addicted to cocaine and heroin. Urine screens were negative for more than 50% of the time in both groups, while daily self-reports indicated decreases in both heroin and cocaine abuse (daily consumption of heroin weekly, down from 7 days to less than 1 day; cocaine from 5.3 days to less than 1). The results indicated a high rate of retention

(87%) for an average treatment duration of 20 weeks. This effect was dose-dependent, though not significantly so, occurring at the 4 mg but not at the 8 mg dose level (Gastfriend et al., 1993).

Positive findings regarding the value of buprenorphine in patients dually dependent on cocaine and opioids was provided also by Schottenfeld et al. (1993). In a study of 15 dually dependent (cocaine and opioids) patients given an ascending and tapering schedule of buprenorphine dosing (4 mg, 8 mg, 12 mg, 16 mg daily, sublingually) with 21 days of maintenance at each dose level, the researchers found expected dose-dependent reductions in opioid use. Opioid use was absent in 64.7% of patients at 16 mg, while 27.3% were abstinent at the 4 mg ascending dose. Cocaine use was significantly reduced during buprenorphine tapering (12 mg, 8 mg, 4 mg), compared with use of ascending doses up to 8 mg. Intermediate reductions in opiate use were present at doses of 12 mg and 16 mg of buprenorphine during the ascending phase of treatment. Cocaine craving, however, was not affected by buprenorphine at any dose level. The authors concluded that while buprenorphine significantly and substantially affected opioid use, there was a less robust (particularly when compared with buprenorphine's effects on cocaine), though still significant, impact on cocaine use, with higher doses and longer time on buprenorphine most strongly attenuating cocaine use. These data also suggest the potential value of buprenorphine in treating combined cocaine and heroin abuse but are less robust than the findings obtained by Gastfriend et al. (1992) and Teoh, Mello, et al. (1994).

More recently, Schottenfeld et al. (1994) compared sublingual buprenorphine, at 4 mg and 12 mg, against methadone at 20 mg or 65 mg in a 26-week randomized, double-blind clinical trial in 120 opioid- and cocaine-dependent patients. Cocaine use was lowest in the high-dose buprenorphine group (27%), with no significant differences found among the other conditions. The high-dose methadone group, however, had a significantly higher proportion of combined cocaine-free and opiate-free urines (32.7%) than the low-dose methadone (18.5%) or high- and low-dose buprenorphine groups (20.9% and 9.1%, respectively). The rate of opiate-free urines was highest in the high-dose methadone group (59.6%), followed by the high-dose buprenorphine (42.6%), the low-dose methadone (31.6%), and the low-dose buprenorphine group (27%). Retention was found to be highest in the high-dose methadone and high-dose buprenorphine groups, with 62% and 58%, respectively, completing the 26-week trial. Low-dose methadone and buprenorphine groups were less effective in maintaining retention, with 48% and 31%, respectively. Thus, this study found that higher doses of both buprenor-phine and methadone were more effective in addressing both cocaine and opiate abuse in methadone maintenance patients, and that high-dose methadone (65 mg) was superior to high-dose buprenorphine (12 mg).

Other recent reports have failed to provide further support for the early promise of buprenorphine for treatment of combined cocaine and opiate abuse. One report found that in a randomized, double-dummy study (all subjects received both oral and sublingual dosage forms) strat-ified by age, gender, and opiate usage, buprenorphine (8 mg), low-dose methadone (20 mg), and high-dose methadone (60 mg) were equally *ineffective* in reducing cocaine urine toxicology results, with only 43% of urines cocaine-negative during the study period. Opiate-negative urines averaged 63% in the buprenorphine group, 51% in the high-dose methadone group, and 36% in the low-dose methadone group (Johnson, Fudala, and Jaffe, 1991). Treatment retention was also poor, with only 40% of the buprenorphine group, 20% of the low-dose methadone, and 37% of the high-dose methadone group remaining in treatment for the full six months of the study (Fudala, Johnson, and Jaffe, 1991). Adverse effects were high (37%–100%) and equally distributed among the three medication groups (Johnson, Fudala, and Jaffe, 1991). Thus, both buprenorphine and high-dose methadone were equally effective in sup-pressing illicit opiate use, and both were significantly more effective than low-dose methadone, but cocaine abuse was not significantly reduced under any of the three conditions.

In another randomized trial, Kosten, Schottenfeld, et al. (1992) simi-larly found buprenorphine, at daily doses of 2 mg and 6 mg, when com-pared with methadone at 35 mg and 65 mg in a 24-week trial in 127 opioid-dependent patients, not to differ in terms of urine toxicology re-sults for cocaine at week 1, when both the buprenorphine and methadone groups had rates of 47%. At week 6, however, cocaine abuse was reduced by 71% in the 6 mg buprenorphine group versus 28% in the 2 mg buprenorphine group. Opioid abuse was also significantly lower in the methadone group than in the buprenorphine group (43% versus 68%), while there was no effect on cocaine abuse between the methadone and buprenorphine groups. Thus, buprenorphine did not appear to produce better outcomes with respect to cocaine abuse, al-though buprenorphine at 6 mg appeared to have a more beneficial ef-fect than buprenorphine at 2 mg. A study by Strain et al. (1994) also failed to find an effect of oral methadone (50 mg) or sublingual buprenorphine (8 mg) on opiate or cocaine abuse in dually addicted patients, but did find that when stepped-up doses of buprenorphine (11.2 mg) or methadone (67 mg) were used, cocaine abuse and combined cocaine and opiate abuse, but not opiate abuse alone, decreased. These results thus failed to provide evidence for a differential efficacy of buprenorphine versus methadone in the treatment of cocaine abuse.

From a safety perspective, buprenorphine maintenance has been shown not to have any major adverse side effects other than headache, sedation, nasal discharge, abdominal discomfort, and anxiety during induction and maintenance (Johnson, Jaffe, and Fudala, 1992; Mello and Mendelson, 1985). When present, these side effects have been shown to subside within 12 to 14 days. Likewise, no toxic interactions with single-dose administrations of intravenous cocaine or morphine were observed at daily doses of 4 mg or 8 mg of sublingual buprenorphine (Teoh et al., 1993). Both initiation of buprenorphine and maintenance have been found not to produce changes in blood pressure, pulse and respiratory rate, or temperature at sublingual doses of 1 to 8 mg daily (Jasinski, Pevnick, and Griffith, 1978; Teoh et al., 1993), although significant respiratory depression was produced at dose levels of 8 or 16 mg daily (Bickel et al., 1988).

Buprenorphine at doses of 0.3 to 3.0 mg/kg protects against the lethal effects of cocaine in mice. Such protective effects are also produced in mice by the opioid agonists morphine and methadone, but not by the opioid antagonist naltrexone, which at low does (0.3–1.0 mg/kg) blocked the protective effects of buprenorphine (Witkin et al., 1991). This study thus demonstrated a safety factor in situations where cocaine abuse may continue during buprenorphine treatment. In another study, pretreatment with buprenorphine (0.30 mg/kg) thirty minutes before cocaine administration was shown to attenuate the lethal effects of acute cocaine overdose (Shukla et al., 1991). Since the opiate antagonists naloxone and naltrexone were not effective in attenuating cocaine-induced mortality, the authors suggested the possible use of buprenorphine in place of naloxone in the emergency medical management of cocaine toxicity.

Buprenorphine is considered to have at least a moderate abuse potential, and thus potential for diversion to the black market (Hammerseley, Lavelle, and Forsyth, 1990; Stimmel, 1991). As a result, it has been suggested that take-home sublingual buprenorphine should be protected by the incorporation of a pure opiate antagonist—either naloxone or naltrexone (Lewis and Walter, 1992). In a study by Mello, Lukas, et al. (1993) of rhesus monkeys, buprenorphine (0.4 mg/kg daily) was found to reduce cocaine self-administration significantly, by an average of 53% compared to a saline baseline without affecting food self-administration.

With administration of naltrexone at various doses (0.05–0.40 mg/kg daily) twenty minutes before buprenorphine, there was a significant dose-related attenuation of buprenorphine's reduction of cocaine self-administration. It was concluded that naltrexone antagonized the partial μ-agonist component of buprenorphine, a potentially important element in cocaine self-administration, and concluded that the addition of an opioid antagonist to a buprenorphine preparation in order to reduce illegal diversion might compromise its effectiveness in treating combined cocaine and opioid dependence.

Several studies have addressed the effects of buprenorphine on the ability of subjects to discriminate cocaine. A study in rats found that administration of buprenorphine resulted in only small alterations in cocaine's discriminative stimulus effects, although the nature of these alterations was dose-dependent, that is, with enhanced response at low doses and reduced response at high doses (Dykstra et al., 1992). These findings were interpreted as inconsistent with buprenorphine's acting as a cocaine antagonist. Buprenorphine maintenance (4 or 8 mg/day, sublingually) was found by Teoh, Mello, et al. (1994) to have no effect on the ability of dually addicted (cocaine and opioids) inpatient males to identify intravenous cocaine injections, while still affecting the recognition of morphine. Furthermore, blockading of identification of morphine did not reliably predict cocaine or opiate use during the first four weeks of the outpatient trial. Given that there was a significant reduction (79%) in cocaine use in 9 of 16 subjects, it may well be that there is a dissociation between cocaine self-administration and the recognition of its subjective effects (Teoh, Mello, et al., 1994).

Pretreatment with buprenorphine, as well as the opioid antagonist naltrexone and the opioid agonist etonitazene (but not cocaine), has also been found to suppress the priming effects of cocaine, thus having little potential for the reinstatement of cocaine-induced response (Comer et al., 1993). Furthermore, in this study, pretreatment with buprenorphine or etonitazene, but not naltrexone, was found to have no priming effect itself on cocaine self-administration. This last finding may be a function of buprenorphine's opioid agonist actions. Thus, Comer and associates concluded that buprenorphine may be a useful adjunct pharmacological intervention in preventing relapse to cocaine abuse.

NALTREXONE

Naltrexone is a long-acting μ-opioid antagonist which suppresses heroin self-administration (Greenstein et al., 1984; Kleber et al., 1985; Santos,

1986). Several studies with rats have shown that naltrexone blocked cocaine-induced place preference or attenuated cocaine self-administration (see, for example, Bilsky et al., 1992; Ramsey and van Ree, 1991; Suzuki et al., 1992). This suggested that opioid systems may play a role in cocaine reinforcement. If this were true, an opioid antagonist such as naltrexone might have clinical utility in the treatment of cocaine abuse. Naltrexone (at doses of 100–150 mg three times daily) also was shown to decrease cocaine-positive urines more effectively than methadone (Kosten, Kleber, and Morgan, 1989b). Yet, in studies with rats, naltrexone had been found not to suppress (Ettenberg et al., 1982), and to even increase (Carroll et al., 1986), cocaine self-administration.

A study in rhesus monkeys by Mello et al. (1991) found that both low-dose (0.32 mg/kg daily) and high-dose (3.20 mg/kg daily) naltrexone effectively suppressed cocaine-maintained response (average suppression, 25%–28% below baseline) for days 1 through 10 of treatment, after which response under both drug conditions did not differ from the placebo condition. The levels of suppression of cocaine self-administration induced by buprenorphine were, by contrast, 72% to 93%. Furthermore, in several studies naltrexone was found to antagonize the partial μ-opioid receptor agonist effects of buprenorphine (Mello, Lukas, et al., 1993; Witkin et al., 1991). This led to the conclusion by Mello, Lukas, et al. (1993) that the addition of naltrexone to a buprenorphine preparation in order to reduce illegal diversion may compromise the effectiveness of buprenorphine in treating combined cocaine and opioid dependence, including buprenorphine's protective effects against the lethal effects of cocaine.

Agents to Reduce Cocaine Toxicity (Calcium Channel Blockers)

Nifedipine, a calcium channel blocker, was thought to reduce the acute effects of cocaine and to attenuate cocaine-induced euphoria, as well as to reduce cardiac toxicity from cocaine. Kosten (1993) had even suggested that it might hold promise for use with patients who experience cocaine-related toxicity. Muntaner et al. (1988) intravenously administered nifedipine (10 mg or placebo) to cocaine abusers 20 to 25 minutes before 20 mg to 40 mg of cocaine or placebo. A preliminary report indicated that pretreatment with nifedipine (10 mg) reduced blood pressure as well as decreased cocaine-related changes in heart rate shortly after injection. Cocaine-related subjective responses (elevations on general drug effects and feeling good) were also reduced under one of four dose conditions (10 mg nifedipine, 40 mg cocaine). In their later report,

Muntaner et al. (1991) concluded that pretreatment with nifedipine attenuated some subjective effects of cocaine and reduced blood pressure, but did not antagonize the cocaine-induced blood pressure effects. In a study with dogs, Hale et al. (1991) found that nifedipine ameliorated the toxic effects of cocaine on the myocardium if administered before, but not after, cocaine. The results of several other studies have, however, contraindicated a role for nifedipine in cocaine treatment. Derlet and Albertson (1989b), in a study with rats, found that pretreatment with nifedipine (at 2 mg/kg) did not provide a protective effect against cocaine toxicity. In fact, nifedipine (as well as the calcium channel blockers diltiazem and verapamil) potentiated seizures and death. Similar findings were obtained in a more recent study for both nifedipine and another calcium channel blocker, nimodipine (Derlet, Tseng, and Albertson, 1994).

Antiseizure Medications

Carbamazepine, an anticonvulsant, may reverse cocaine-induced kindling, as well as the dopamine-receptor supersensitivity resulting from chronic cocaine use. Animal studies have suggested that carbamazepine may be very effective in suppressing the development of *cocaine-induced* amygdala-kindled seizures, but that it has little effect on fully developed seizures (Weiss, Post, Szele, et al., 1989). At the same time, carbamazepine does not appear to block the development of behavioral sensitization, including cocaine-induced motor activity (Post, Weiss, and Pert, 1984). While carbamazepine may be effective in blocking cocaine-induced seizures when administered chronically, it may not be effective when administered intermittently, and may even worsen seizures (Weiss, Post, Szele, et al., 1989). The seizure-related effect of carbamazine appears to be related to inhibition of mechanisms related to cocaine's local anesthetic actions, but not of cocaine's stimulant effects (Weiss et al., 1990).

Carbamazepine has been evaluated in a number of open clinical trials (Halikas et al., 1989; Halikas and Kuhn, 1990; Halikas et al., 1992; Kuhn, Halikas, and Kemp, 1990), as well as in a case report (Sherer, Kumor, and Mapou, 1990). In a nonrandomized trial of carbamazepine, Halikas et al. (1989) examined the effects of carbamazepine in 21 long-term cocaine users who had taken carbamazepine for three days or more. Of the 13 patients who took carbamazepine for longer than three days, clear success was obtained with 6 patients, for whom abstinence ranged from one to eight months where carbamazepine was used regularly in a dose of 200 to 400 mg daily. The 7 other patients who had also taken carbamazepine for three days or more had at least partial success. Cocaine use in the successfully abstinent group dropped from 78.5 of 100 days to 0.55 of 100. Cocaine use in the intermittently successful group dropped from 73.4 of 100 days to 28.4 of 100 while in treatment. By contrast, cocaine use in the 8 cocaine abusers who had refused treatment fell only from 78.5 days to 60.9 days per 100. Self-reports of the 13 full and partial successes showed that craving "was significantly reduced even . . . in high-risk situations which often stimulate craving" (Halikas et al., 1989, p. 623). These studies suggested beneficial effects of carbamazepine in reducing acute withdrawal, reducing or eliminating cocaine craving, and blocking the euphoric effects of cocaine.

Since motivation and coercion may have played a role in the earlier studies, Halikas and associates (1991) attempted to control for these variables by studying paid, chronic crack-cocaine users who were unmotivated for treatment. In the first double-blind, placebo-controlled crossover study of carbamazepine, conducted with 32 subjects, these researchers found carbamazepine to lower significantly the mean number of positive urine specimens, when compared with a placebo. Higher serum concentrations (above 4 micrograms per ml) were associated with better outcomes. Thus, this study linked outcomes with therapeutic dose levels of carbamazepine and suggested a beneficial effect of the compound.

Carbamazepine, like desipramine, decreases norepinephrine turnover. As with cocaine, overdose can cause seizures and tachycardia (Sullivan, Rumack, and Peterson, 1981), although none appear to have been thus far reported in the studies which have been conducted. A single dose of smoked cocaine has been found to increase both heart rate and diastolic blood pressure in patients receiving a therapeutic dosage of carbamazepine (400 mg daily; Hatsukami et al., 1991). One animal study suggested a paradoxical effect of carbamazepine. Cocaine administered to rats receiving chronic administration of carbamazepine showed reduced kindling seizures following cocaine administration; the opposite effects resulted from intermittent administration of carbamazepine, however. Similarly, the administration of carbamazepine to rats chronically self-administering cocaine did reduce cocaine intake, but resulted in seizures and lethality (Carroll et al., 1990). Thus, Pentel and Thompson (1993) concluded that "high doses of carbamazepine may increase the toxicity of high doses of cocaine in rats but the occurrence of this interaction may depend on the manner and timing of carbamazepine administration" (p. 167).

A side effect reported by subjects in the study of cocaine abusers by Halikas et al. (1989) was the appearance of early opioid withdrawal symptoms (for example, insomnia and global apprehensiveness), or "methadone effect wearing off" about 18 to 24 hours after a dose of carbamazepine. The authors suggested that the enzyme induction effect of carbamazepine may have accounted for this effect. Minor side effects, including transient drowsiness, slowness and sluggishness, transient itching, or skin disturbances, were also reported in this study, although the results of another study found no statistically or clinically significant side effects resulting from carbamazepine administration (Halikas, Nugent, Pearson, et al., 1993).

Other Agents

Amino Acids (L-Tryptophan, L-Tyrosine)

Cocaine produces a depletion of neurotransmitters (mainly dopamine, norepinephrine, and serotonin) in the brain, by first causing their discharge and then blocking their reuptake. In addition, deficits in neurotransmitters have been linked to the drug hunger (craving) and withdrawal symptoms seen in cocaine abuse (Gold et al., 1983). Since amino acids are the precursors for such neurotransmitters, the suggestion has been made that increasing the supply of amino acids may increase the supply of neurotransmitters, thus contributing to the restoration of normal functioning (Chadwick, Gregory, and Wendling, 1990).

L-tyrosine and L-tryptophan are amino acids which have been implicated in the treatment of cocaine abuse. While their roles in treatment are unclear, it is known that dopamine and norepinephrine are depleted by chronic cocaine use, and their precursors tyrosine and tryptophan may increase the presence of these two neurotransmitters in the central nervous system (Tennant and Sagherian, 1987). Providing support for a possible role for tyrosine in cocaine abuse, Truelson et al. (1986) found chronic cocaine use to result in a long-term loss of tyrosine hydroxylase in rats. Tennant (1985) found plasma levels of tyrosine to be somewhat depressed when central nervous system norepinephrine was also depressed. Wallace (1987) suggested that the use of L-tryptophan and L-tyrosine could result in improved outcomes in detoxification from cocaine. In an open, non-blind trial, Gold et al. (1983) administered tyrosine (0.1 gm/kg) to 6 cocaine addicts and found that it had consistent antiwithdrawal effects. Chadwick, Gregory, and Wendling (1990), however, conducted a double-blind, double crossover, placebo-controlled study of L-tryptophan (1 gm/day) or L-tyrosine (1 gm/day) for 14 days each in 29 cocaine-abusing inpatients and found no significant effects on drug craving and withdrawal symptomatology. While participants in the study by Tennant and Sagherian (1987) received tyrosine (at 400 mg four times daily) and tryptophan (1,000 mg at bedtime) in addition to either amantadine hydrochloride or bromocriptine mesylate, their role in the study remained unclear.

Diazepam (Valium)

Diazepam has been widely used in the treatment of withdrawal states (including those characterized by severe agitation and catecholamine excess) associated with other drugs of abuse. Among these are sedative-hypnotics (see Sellers, Naranjo, and Harrison, 1983) and ethanol (Thompson, 1978). Cocaine-induced tachycardia and hypertension have been found to be blunted by diazepam, suggesting a central mediation of cocaine's peripheral sympathetic effects (Schrank, 1993). Diazepam has been found to have protective effects against cocaine intoxication, whether administered before or after cocaine exposure. Employing a rat model, Derlet and Albertson (1989b) demonstrated substantial sedative effects of diazepam after exposure to high doses of cocaine. Diazepam did not, however, totally suppress cocaine-induced cortical EEG seizure activity. Similarly, while diazepam (1–10 mg/kg) was found to be dose-dependently protective against cocaine lethality at low does of cocaine, it was not effective in protecting against cocaine convulsions in mice at higher doses (Witkin and Tortella, 1991). Similar findings to those for diazepam (1–10 mg/kg) were obtained for phenobarbital (30–100 mg/kg). In this study, the noncompetitive NMDA antagonists MK-801 (dizocilpine) and phencyclidine produced dose-dependent protection against cocaine convulsions.

Lisuride

Lisuride, a nonaddictive ergot derivative whose actions are similar to those of bromocriptine, including dopaminergic agonist effects, has been demonstrated to reduce signs of psychostimulant withdrawal in animals (Pulvirenti and Koob, 1993; Pulvirenti et al., 1991). Such findings have yet to be demonstrated in humans. A controlled, double-blind, parallel design test of lisuride, in doses up to 4.0 mg daily, was conducted in hospitalized stimulant (cocaine or amphetamine) abusers during acute withdrawal (Gillin et al., 1994). While REM latency was prolonged and reduced REM time observed, lisuride-treated patients did no better than placebo-treated patients in terms of reduction of other withdrawal signs. Since both groups displayed low self-ratings of craving, Gillin et al. (1994) concluded that further studies in groups displaying more severe withdrawal symptoms were needed to test fully the efficacy of lisuride.

Nutrition and Herbal Medicine

Many of the therapeutic agents just described are neurotransmitter releasers or uptake blockers. With regard to releasing agents, Blum et al. (1988) noted that they may be effective only if there are neurotransmitters to release, and that they will not remediate a state of dopamine depletion. The authors evaluated the usefulness in freebase and intravenous cocaine users of the neuronutrient Tropamine. This agent provides a greater supply of L-tyrosine, a preparation containing precursor amino acids needed for dopamine synthesis, as well as providing vitamins and minerals known to be depleted in cocaine abusers.[2] In an open-trial study, Tropamine was evaluated against the neuronutrient SAAVE (which provides a greater supply of D-phenylalanine), an enkephalinase inhibitor, and a no-supplement control in a group of 54 patients. In a 30-day inpatient program, significant reductions in treatment dropout (4.2% for Tropamine versus 28.6% for SAAVE and 37.5% for controls), as well as in agitation, drug craving, and acting out, were obtained with Tropamine, when compared with the groups receiving SAAVE or no supplement. Blum et al. (1988) concluded that Tropamine accelerated recovery during cocaine withdrawal through facilitating retention in treatment and reducing drug hunger.

Management of Conditions Associated with Cocaine Abuse

Toxicity, Euphoria, Withdrawal, and Overdose

The toxic effects of cocaine appear to result, in large part, from the direct stimulatory effects of cocaine on the central nervous, cardiovascular, and respiratory systems, although inhibition of catecholamine reuptake (the proposed primary mechanism for cocaine's actions) may amplify such effects. Ultimately, overstimulation and subsequent catecholamine depletion may result in depression of these systems (Goldfrank and Hoffman, 1993). Toxicity may also result from the cumulative effects of continued cocaine use. For example, the development of a toxic psychosis in an individual who has repeated the administration of cocaine every fifteen minutes may be the result of the accumulation of cocaine on the nasal mucosa, and the persistence of cocaine in the plasma for from four to six hours (Van Dyke et al., 1976).

Acute Cocaine Toxicity (Overdose)

Medical management of cocaine toxicity is dependent on clinical signs and symptoms, and generally involves supportive therapy. Treatment of hyperthermia, close monitoring of cardiac and neurologic status, and symptomatic relief should be instituted. Cocaine-induced seizures may require administration of a short-acting barbiturate such as pentobarbital sodium (Nembutal); phenothiazines such as chlorpromazine (Promapar, Thorazine) or haloperidol (Haldol and others) should be avoided in managing acute reactions because of possible lowering of the seizure threshold by neuroleptic drugs.[3] In extreme cases of overdose, hospitalization and respiratory assistance (including life support) may be necessary. Cocaine psychosis, if it persists for three to five days after discontinuation of use, or if the patient becomes increasingly difficult to manage, and where psychotic symptoms do not appear to be anxiety-related, may require reevaluation of the diagnosis and use of a neuroleptic medication such as haloperidol (Gold, 1992; Millman, 1988).

Cocaine overdose is a life-threatening emergency, and requires rapid intervention. Interventions found useful in managing this severe adrenergic crisis–like condition include the administration of barbiturates (secobarbital or amobarbitol) or diazepam (Valium) in order to prevent seizures, as well as to address the severe agitation and overstimulation typically present (Estroff and Gold, 1986; Gay, 1982). Propranolol (Inderal) is administered either orally or intravenously to control tachycardia, tachypnea, and hypertension. Lidocaine is used in the event that ventricular arrhythmias are present (Gay, 1982; Roehrich and Gold, 1991). Cocaine overdose frequently occurs in combination with use of other drugs of abuse, including heroin and alcohol, and this fact should also be taken into account.

The treatment of cocaine toxicity generally addresses the following specific symptomatologies: *acute behavioral toxicity,* including psychosis, agitation, and delirium; *long-term toxicity,* including neurotoxicity, kindling (that is, seizures and psychosis), and stroke damage; *convulsions,* although some are resistant to standard anticonvulsant therapy; and *lethality,* through effects on the cardiovascular, respiratory, and thermoregulatory systems (Witkin and Katz, 1993). Acute cocaine toxicity may result in outcomes including a progression from ischemia to stroke, with consequent neurological damage. Although there is currently no specific pharmacological treatment to prevent this outcome, Meldrum and Garthwaite (1990) have suggested the use of excitatory amino acid antagonists, such as ketamine, in order to minimize neurological impairment.

The need for a number of pharmacological agents for the treatment of cocaine toxicity has been noted by Witkin and Katz (1993). These include agents to protect against neurological damage, kindled seizures and psychosis resulting from repeated high doses of cocaine, and medication-resistant convulsions, as well as agents to increase the chances of survival after exposure to life-threatening cocaine toxicity. Commenting on the current status of knowledge concerning the management of both acute and chronic cocaine toxicity, these authors noted that such toxicity is not fully understood, and that treatment strategies, although generally effective, have yet to be perfected.

Acute behavioral toxicity appears to be best controlled by heavy sedation induced with benzodiazepines and barbiturates. Haloperidol and chlorpromazine are less effective in controlling such toxicities (Witkin and Katz, 1993). Haloperidol, though a dopamine-receptor blocking agent, does not prevent the development of seizures resulting from cocaine kindling (Karler et al., 1989). It is, however, effective in preventing lethal consequences of amphetamine overdose (Witkin and Katz, 1993).[4] More rapid means of drug delivery are needed (Witkin and Katz, 1993).

In general, the management of acute psychiatric complications of cocaine intoxication requires supportive care and involves the reduction of external stimuli. At the same time, minimization of risks to other patients and staff is required. Successful management of the neuropsychiatric manifestations of cocaine toxicity can also positively affect emergent cardiovascular complications, at least in the emergency or initial care situation (Goldfrank and Hoffman, 1993).

Cocaine Euphoria

Stimulants may potentially "block" (that is, replace) the euphoria resulting from cocaine use, much as the synthetic narcotic methadone blocks heroin euphoria by occupying opiate receptors. Thus, Estroff and Gold (1986) have suggested that the amphetamines, methylphenidate (Ritalin), and pemoline (Cylert) could all theoretically serve this purpose, although, as they also note, strong objections exist to the substitution of one addicting agent for another. Among other agents which have been suggested as being of possible value in overcoming the cocaine high are tricyclic antidepressants.

Haloperidol has been evaluated for its effectiveness in altering cocaine-induced euphoria. In a report by Gawin (1986a), four cocaine users with histories of stimulant-induced paranoid psychoses were treated with haloperidol or chlorpromazine (both dopamine blockers) for cocaine-induced paranoia. Use of these agents during the presence of pre-paranoid anxiety did not eliminate the euphoria induced by cocaine, although the development of paranoia appeared to be eliminated. In a randomized, double-blind trial (Sherer, Kumor, and Jaffe, 1989), pre-treatment with an 8 mg dose of haloperidol before intravenous administration of cocaine (40 mg) was found to attenuate cocaine-induced increases in systolic and diastolic blood pressure, but not heart rate, thus suggesting some degree of dopaminergic, as well as adrenergic, blockade. Although some euphoric subjective effects of cocaine were reduced by pretreatment with haloperidol (unlike in the cases described by Gawin, 1986a), no effects were found relative to the "rush" associated with cocaine use. Sherer, Kumor, and Jaffe (1989) concluded that haloperidol appeared to have little clinical effect on cocaine self-administration. This finding is reinforced by other findings that showed that about 21.7% of patients receiving depot neuroleptics (haloperidol, fluphenazine) at levels expected to achieve dopamine blockade were concurrently abusing cocaine (Stone et al., 1993).

These data find parallels in the drug discrimination literature, where pretreatment with neuroleptics such as chlorpromazine, pimozide, and haloperidol only modestly decreased the detection of the cocaine stimulus in animal studies (see, for example, Järbe, 1978, 1984). Yet, relatively selective dopamine (D1) antagonists were highly effective in blocking the stimulus effects of cocaine, as well as other cocaine-induced behavioral effects such as stereotypy or the effects on food intake (Woolverton, 1991).

Cocaine Withdrawal

DSM-IV criteria for a diagnosis of cocaine withdrawal are as follows: cessation or reduction of heavy use after a prolonged period of use; dysphoric mood and two or more of a number of physiological changes, including fatigue, vivid and unpleasant dreams, sleep disturbance (insomnia or hypersomnia), increased appetite, and psychomotor retardation or agitation; the presence of clinically significant distress resulting from the preceding symptoms, or impairment in social, occupational, and other important areas of functioning; and the ruling out of a general medical condition or another mental disorder which might account for the observed symptoms.

As noted previously, cocaine is believed to act by facilitating the actions of endogenous catecholamine neurotransmitters. This is accomplished by the blocking of physiologic inactivation by high-affinity uptake of these neurotransmitters, particularly of dopamine (Grabowski and Dworkin, 1985). Agents which mimic or increase the central nervous system activity of catecholamines include (other) stimulants, antidepressants, and bromocriptine. Withdrawal from cocaine is generally not dangerous from a medical viewpoint, and detoxification requires only abstinence. Symptoms of withdrawal, particularly dysphoria, may, however, be so disturbing to the patient that cocaine use is resumed to avoid these symptoms. Thus, any intervention that relieves withdrawal symptoms is of enormous assistance, and significantly improves prognosis (Gold, 1992).

The management of cocaine withdrawal generally involves addressing the acute symptoms of cocaine toxicity. No specific antidote for cocaine poisoning is known (Estroff and Gold, 1986). Several agents have been suggested as potentially effective in cocaine withdrawal, particularly as they affect craving. Among these agents are the dopamine agonist bromocriptine (currently marketed as the anti-Parkinsonian drug Parlodel), the amino acid tyrosine, the tricyclic antidepressants desipramine (Norpramin, Pertofrane), imipramine (Tofranil), and nortriptyline (Aventyl, Pamelor), as well as serotonin uptake blockers such as fluoxetine (Prozac). Cocaine addicts may self-manage withdrawal from cocaine by using sedating drugs such as heroin, alcohol, sedative/hypnotics (including benzodiazepines and, to a lesser extent, barbiturates), or stimulants such as methylphenidate (Ritalin). These drugs are often used by addicts in an attempt to manage the dysphoria present between cocaine highs and during withdrawal (Estroff and Gold, 1986).

Agitation and Seizures

According to Goldfrank and Hoffman (1993), to manage the agitation and seizures resulting from cocaine intoxication, the exaggerated central nervous system activity must be addressed. This management includes the rapid control of motor activity while protecting the patient's airways and achieving adequate ventilation and oxygenation. Thus, restraints may be needed in order to ensure the successful installation of an intravenous line. Restraining blankets, if used, should be constructed of strong netting or mesh to allow for dissipation of body heat, thus avoiding increases in the patient's temperature. Seizures should be controlled initially by the use of diazepam or other benzodiazepines. The control of seizures may also be achieved through the use of phenobarbital or phenytoin, although Goldfrank and Hoffman (1991) note that no studies exist comparing the efficacy of the two compounds. The sedative effect obtained with the use of phenobarbital may be desired, however. In the event that these agents do not provide rapid control of seizures, the introduction of nondepolarizing muscular blockade with the use of pancuronium bromide, or the introduction of general anesthesia, may be necessary. The use of succinylcholine, a depolarizing-type skeletal muscle relaxant, is contraindicated because of the risk of hyperkalemia with severe cocaine-induced rhabdomyolysis, as well as the risk of prolonging the clinical effects of both cocaine and/or succinylcholine.

The management of hyperthermia is essential to avoid cerebral, hepatic, and muscular cellular damage (Callaway and Clark, 1994). Hyperthermia can be controlled by rapid body cooling. This can be achieved with an ice and water bath, the use of mist and a fan, or the topical application to the skin of 70% alcohol. Specific pharmacological agents such as verapamil, esmolol, labetalol, or propranolol may be needed to control tachyarrhythmias. Use of these agents following prior sedation limits the risks associated with seizures. By contrast, the use of lidocaine for the treatment of ventricular arrhythmias may exacerbate cardiac conduction abnormalities as well as increase the risk of seizures and death.[5]

Finally, Goldfrank and Hoffman (1991) suggest the use of sodium nitroprusside for the management of hypertension which remains unresponsive to sedation, as well as phentolamine, which may both serve as a vasodilator and improve coronary perfusion.

Combined Psychotherapy and Pharmacotherapy

Evidence from the treatment of opiate addicts strongly suggests the advantages of combining psychotherapy and pharmacotherapy in producing good outcomes (see, for example, McLellan et al., 1993). It would not be unreasonable to expect that such an approach would apply to cocaine abuse as well, although there is much less of a research base presently available. Several studies have, however, begun to provide data concerning the additive effects of psychotherapy and pharmacotherapy. Ziedonis and Kosten (1991), for example, found that relapse prevention could be somewhat effective for non-depressed, cocaine-abusing methadone patients, while depressed patients responded poorly to relapse prevention alone. Comparing abstinence rates achieved under varying combinations of psycho- and pharmacotherapy, Carroll (1993) observed that the combination of the two forms of intervention exerted effects more rapidly than did psychotherapy alone. Interpersonal psychotherapy plus desipramine resulted in a 58% abstinence rate. Psychotherapy alone, whether relapse prevention or interpersonal psychotherapy, resulted in similar abstinence rates at six weeks posttreatment (33% and 29%, respectively). At twelve weeks the abstinence rate for relapse prevention alone improved to 57%, suggesting, according to Carroll, that additional time for this skills training approach was needed for coping skills to be practiced and implemented. Interpersonal psychotherapy plus placebo resulted in a lower abstinence rate (17%) than interpersonal psychotherapy alone (29%). Carroll concluded that non-pharmacological treatments may increase treatment retention; pharmacotherapy may act more rapidly than psychotherapy for cocaine abusers; and the combination of desipramine and psychotherapy only partially addresses the limitations (e.g., high attrition rates, only moderate success rates) of psychotherapy alone.

Carroll (1993) suggested two models of psychotherapy as treatment for cocaine abuse: a model viewing psychotherapy as a necessary though nonspecific adjunct to pharmacotherapy, as suggested by Gawin, Kleber, et al. (1989), and a model in which psychotherapy itself may be an effective and at times sufficient treatment (Carroll, Rounsaville, and Gawin, 1991). Drawing on evidence from studies of treatment for opiate addiction, Carroll (1993) suggested that the methadone model may not be appropriate for the treatment of cocaine addiction, since pharmacological agents equivalent to methadone are not available for the treatment of cocaine addiction, and studies such as those by Rawson et al. (1986), as well as her own, suggest that pharmacological intervention is not essential for the treatment of cocaine addiction. Research in the area of depression may be more appropriate as a model for psychotherapy for cocaine abuse, in that response to any of the available treatments is incomplete; relapse after symptom remission is frequent; and psychotherapy and pharmacotherapy may address different and distinct symptom areas. There is, however, no current treatment available as the "standard" for cocaine abuse as antidepressant therapy is for depression. Thus, Carroll (1993) suggested that the current state of treatments for cocaine abuse may be similar to that of treatments for depression, and the latter may serve as a guide for evaluating the efficacy of psychotherapy and pharmacotherapy for cocaine abuse.

Carroll (1993) also discussed the advantages and disadvantages of the several models of psychotherapy as treatment for cocaine abuse. The first is *the model of psychotherapy alone as treatment*. This model, for which there is some evidence of efficacy (see, for example, Carroll, Rounsaville, and Gawin, 1991; Rawson et al., 1986), leads to several research questions. For example: Which subgroups of cocaine abusers will respond to purely psychotherapeutic interventions? What is the comparative effectiveness of psychotherapy when compared with pharmacotherapy? When in the course of treatment may one intervention be more effective than another? Will intervention at one point result in a more enduring outcome compared with intervention at another point? Are there specific effects associated with each form of treatment? And are different forms of psychotherapy equally effective with all cocaine users?

The second model, that of *psychotherapy as support to pharmacotherapy*, is one in which psychotherapy serves as a baseline against which the efficacy of drug-based interventions can be compared, without which compliance with treatment and retention would be difficult to obtain. In this model, in which psychotherapy is viewed, in effect, as an inert ingredient, the question often is, "What is the relative effectiveness of active medication or placebo in the context of minimal supportive clinical management?" (Carroll, 1993, p. 126). Thus, any contributions to outcome attributable to psychotherapy may be underestimated.

The third model, that of *psychotherapy as a complementary treatment*, typically involves the evaluation of psychotherapy or pharmacotherapy alone against a combination of the two. In this model the unique contributions of each are considered, as well as their interactions with each other. The model allows evaluation of psychotherapy administered "at full strength . . . [thus allowing] maximal effects to emerge and be evaluated" (Carroll, 1993, p. 127). According to Carroll, this model is the one most likely to identify and address the potential benefits of psychotherapy-pharmacotherapy interactions and complexities. Her discussion is highly recommended for its contribution toward developing an appreciation of the theoretical issues underlying research involving pharmacotherapy.

In the absence of data from studies directly comparing psychotherapy and pharmacotherapy, Carroll (1993) compared results from her study of psychotherapy outcomes (Carroll, Rounsaville, and Gawin,

1991) with those from a previously published controlled clinical trial of psychopharmacotherapies for cocaine abuse (Gawin, Kleber et al., 1989), both conducted at Yale.

Utilizing data from the two studies on the basis of an argument that the subjects in the Gawin, Kleber, et al. (1989) trial could be considered historical controls for the 1991 study, Carroll (1993) contrasted rates of treatment retention and initiation of abstinence in the two studies. This comparison yielded the following findings: treatment retention was higher with interpersonal psychotherapy alone in the psychotherapy study (52%) than with interpersonal therapy plus placebo in the pharmacotherapy study (42%); retention through six weeks for relapse prevention alone in the psychotherapy study (71%) was comparable to that for the interpersonal psychotherapy plus desipramine condition in the pharmacotherapy study (75%); abstinence rates for subjects receiving interpersonal psychotherapy plus desipramine (58%) were greater than the abstinence rates in the two psychotherapy alone conditions (relapse prevention, 33%; interpersonal psychotherapy, 29%); the abstinence rate for relapse prevention required an additional six weeks to reach a level (57%) similar to that for the pharmacotherapy-psychotherapy condition at six weeks; and the abstinence rate at six weeks for interpersonal psychotherapy plus placebo in the pharmacotherapy study (17%) was below that for interpersonal psychotherapy alone (29%) in the psychotherapy study. Carroll concluded that the results of the comparison suggested that nonpharmacologic treatments can have an important role in fostering treatment retention; pharmacotherapy may be more rapid-acting than psychotherapy for cocaine abusers; and limitations of psychotherapy in the treatment of cocaine abuse, such as high attrition and moderate rates of treatment success, are only partly addressed by combining psychotherapy with a pharmacotherapy such as desipramine.

In a randomized clinical trial evaluating psychotherapy and pharmacotherapy, alone and in combination, Carroll et al. (1994) assigned cocaine abusers to one of four conditions: relapse prevention plus desipramine (at an initial dose of 50 mg, increased to 200 mg daily by the end of week 1, to a maximum dose of 300 mg/day); clinical management plus desipramine (at the same dose levels); relapse prevention plus placebo; and clinical management plus placebo. Psychotherapeutic interventions were manual-guided, delivered by experienced therapists, and monitored to ensure integrity of delivery. While all groups showed significant improvement, significant main effects were not found for either medication or psychotherapy with respect to treatment retention, reduction in cocaine use, or other outcomes at twelve weeks. A differential response to the interventions occurred depending on baseline level of severity. High-severity patients had better outcomes when treated with relapse prevention rather than with clinical management, while among low-severity patients, treatment with desipramine resulted in an increased rate of abstinence initiation. Other findings were that desipramine was more effective than a placebo in reducing cocaine use over six but not twelve weeks; and that depressed patients had greater reductions in cocaine use than did non-depressed patients. Depressed patients also responded better to relapse prevention than to clinical management. The authors concluded that these results underscored the heterogeneity present among cocaine abusers and the need to develop specialized treatments for clinically distinct subgroups.

NIDA Medications Development Program

The Anti-Drug Abuse Act of 1988 included, for the first time, funds for the development of new and approved medications with which to fight drug abuse. The act also provided for the establishment of the Medications Development Division (MDD) at NIDA. Among the division's goals are to conduct studies to identify, develop, and obtain approval for new medications to be used in the treatment of drug abuse and other diseases of the brain, as well as behavioral disorders; to develop innovative biological and pharmacological treatment approaches for the addictions, to be accomplished through establishing and administering a national program of basic and pharmaceutical research; and to establish close working relationships between U.S. pharmaceutical and chemical companies and medications development programs in this and other countries (Sorer, 1993).

The Cocaine Treatment Discovery Program, established under NIDA's Medications Development Division, recognizes that cocaine abuse has proved refractory to most standard methods of treatment. Thus, the program aims at identifying new pharmacological entities of potential use in the treatment of cocaine abuse (Sorer, 1993). There is increasing recognition, however, that medications such as those expected to be developed under the auspices of NIDA's Medications Development Division will be not magic bullets but rather "part of a comprehensive treatment program addressing the psychological, social, and behavioral aspects of addiction" (Sorer, 1993, p. 2).

Conclusions

Several important points regarding pharmacological approaches to cocaine-dependent individuals must be kept in mind in evaluating the many agents which have been proposed for treatment of cocaine abuse. As outlined by Schuckit (1994) and Meyer (1992), these include the fact that all interventions, particularly medications, have attendant costs and dangers, thus requiring a balanced approach to their use; that substance abuse problems fluctuate in intensity over time and have a measurable rate of remission, requiring that treatments prove they work better than the passage of time alone; and that evaluating the efficacy of pharmacological interventions requires double-blind control, including comparison with placebo or standard therapy, a large sample, and an extensive follow-up period. Few of the currently examined pharmacological agents for the treatment of cocaine abuse have met these standards.

Pharmacological agents with antidepressant effects have been extensively investigated for their usefulness in treating cocaine abuse. Interest in these agents has arisen because of their potential value in alleviating the physiological consequences of cocaine abuse and in treating disorders which may increase vulnerability to cocaine abuse (for example, affective disorders, attention deficit disorder). Initial findings (see, for example, Gawin, Kleber, et al., 1989; Giannini et al., 1986; Kosten et al., 1987; Kosten, Morgan, and Schottenfeld, 1990; Tennant and Rawson, 1983) suggesting the efficacy of tricyclic agents such as desipramine in treating cocaine abuse have not been substantiated in more recent studies (for example, Arndt, et al., 1990; Hall et al., 1993, 1994; Kosten, Morgan, et al., 1992; Triffleman et al., 1993; Ziedonis and Kosten, 1991). Desipramine may have selective effects, being most effective during the early stages of treatment (Gawin, Kleber, et al., 1989) by diminishing craving (Kosten, Morgan, et al., 1992) and by increasing the length of time the patient is retained in treatment (Hall et al., 1994).

Antidepressants other than the tricyclics have had mixed success in addressing cocaine abuse. Fluoxetine is among those agents which have shown some limited success (Batki et al., 1990, 1993; Washburn et al., 1994). Monoamine oxidase inhibitors such as phenelzine may have some value in treating cocaine abuse (see, for example, Brewer, 1993; Golwyn, 1988), but their employment is limited by the risk of potential interactions with cocaine, which may trigger a hypertensive crisis. Other agents for which little promise appears to exist are bupropion (Margolin et al., 1990), lithium carbonate (Gawin and Kleber, 1984;

Nunes et al., 1990), and trazodone (Louie, Lannon, and Ketter, 1989; Rowbotham et al., 1984).

The evidence for a relationship between attention deficit disorder and cocaine abuse suggests that pharmacological interventions for the former disorder may have some value in treatment of the latter (Eyre, Rounsaville, and Kleber, 1982; Horton et al., 1987; Rounsaville, Anton, et al., 1991; and see Chapter 5). Despite the success noted in early papers, mostly case studies (Khantzian, 1983; Khantzian et al., 1984), an open trial study did not show clinically meaningful improvement (Gawin, Riordan, and Kleber, 1985).

Craving has been a particular target for evaluating medication in the treatment of cocaine abuse. Although tricyclic antidepressants can reduce cocaine craving, there is a significant delay in onset of such effects—up to two weeks (Gawin, Kleber, et al., 1989; Giannini et al., 1986), resulting in the likelihood of low compliance with treatment regimens. Several agents have shown promise in reducing craving. Flupenthixol decanoate, which acts by blocking dopamine binding at receptors, has appeared in several studies both to reduce cocaine craving rapidly and to facilitate initiation of abstinence (Gawin, Allen, and Humblestone, 1989; Khalsa, Jatlow, and Gawin, 1994). Flupenthixol decanoate may well be the first pharmacological treatment to have demonstrated effectiveness in the treatment of cocaine abuse.

Pharmacological agents which produce aversive reactions when taken in conjunction with cocaine do not appear to have efficacy. Mazindol, which inhibits both dopamine and norepinephrine uptake, was found in a open trial study to reduce cocaine craving, euphoria, and intake (Berger, Gawin, and Kosten, 1989), although further studies did not confirm this finding (Diakogiannis, Steinberg, and Kosten, 1991; Preston et al., 1993).

The dopamine agonists amantadine and bromocriptine have shown evidence of effectiveness in addressing the withdrawal and craving associated with termination of cocaine abuse. Amantadine, an indirect dopamine agonist, appears in animal studies to share a common pharmacological mechanism (delay of dopamine uptake), while not sharing cocaine's reinforcing qualities (Sannerud and Griffiths, 1988), and also to have rapid onset of action in dopamine deficit disorders such as Parkinson's disease (Gawin, Morgan, et al., 1989). Several randomized clinical trials of amantadine demonstrated reductions in cocaine craving (Gawin, Morgan, et al., 1989; Handelsman et al., 1988; Kosten, Morgan, and Schottenfeld, 1990), although later studies did not confirm the earlier promise of effects on craving, at least not beyond the early withdrawal period (Gawin, Morgan, et al., 1989; Weddington, Brown, et al., 1991). Bromocriptine is another anti-Parkinsonian dopamine agonist which held early promise in treating cocaine abuse (Dackis and Gold, 1985b). Initial positive findings regarding its value in cocaine withdrawal (Dackis et al., 1984; Gutierrez-Esteinou et al., 1988) were not borne out (Jaffe et al., 1989; Teller and Devenyi, 1988; Tennant and Sagherian, 1987). The side effects associated with the use of bromocriptine have also been unacceptable to many patients (Wang et al., 1992).

Buprenorphine, a mixed agonist/antagonist used as a therapeutic agent in opiate abuse, has shown particular promise in treating mixed cocaine-opioid abuse. Buprenorphine may decrease cocaine-opioid interactions because of its weak opioid agonist actions, and it has antagonist actions at higher doses. Both animal and human studies suggest that buprenorphine may suppress cocaine and opiate self-administration by interfering with the reinforcing properties of cocaine (Mello et al., 1990a, 1990b; Mello, Lukas, et al., 1993), although the possibility exists that it may enhance cocaine's reinforcing qualities (Brown et al., 1991; Johnson et al., 1990; Kosten, 1993). Buprenorphine has been found to suppress the priming effects of cocaine (Comer et al., 1993). Buprenorphine may be particularly valuable in treating cocaine abuse in methadone-maintained patients (Gastfriend et al., 1992; Kosten, Kleber, and Morgan, 1989a; Schottenfeld et al., 1993; Teoh, Mello, et al., 1994), although not all the results have been promising in this regard (see Fudala, Johnson, and Jaffe, 1991; Johnson, Fudala, and Jaffe, 1991; Kosten, Schottenfeld, et al., 1992; Schottenfeld et al., 1994; Strain et al., 1994). While side effects of buprenorphine are relatively weak, this agent may have significant potential for abuse.

Carbamazepine has been evaluated, with some success, with respect to its ability to reduce cocaine toxicity. Carbamazepine has been suggested to reduce acute withdrawal effects, craving, and euphoric effects associated with cocaine administration (Halikas et al., 1989, 1990, 1991), and further research with this agent seems well justified.

Amino acids have been investigated for their value in reversing neurotransmitter depletion produced by cocaine, which has been linked to cocaine craving and withdrawal symptoms. The roles of amino acids such as L-tyrosine and L-tryptophan have been investigated in several studies (Chadwick, Gregory, and Wendling, 1990; Golwyn, 1988), but their effectiveness is still unclear.

Many pharmacological agents evaluated for the treatment of cocaine abuse, even if otherwise efficacious, may have significant side effects which limit their potential clinical usefulness. Desipramine and other tricyclic antidepressants may trigger the appearance of the tricyclic jitteriness syndrome, which itself may stimulate conditioned craving (Weiss, 1988). Tricyclics may also have toxic cardiovascular effects (Fischman et al., 1990). Mazindol's side effects also include jitteriness and agitation. The risks of using monoamine oxidase inhibitors likely far outweigh the benefits, although it has been suggested that this may not be the case (Margolin et al., 1990). Bromocriptine's side effects include headache, vertigo and dizziness, orthostatic hypotension, and syncope, while carbamazepine may elicit opioid withdrawal symptoms (Halikas et al., 1989).

It is clear that external cues (for example, drug paraphernalia) and internal cues (for example, mood states such as depression) play an important role in relapse to cocaine abuse (see Chapter 3). Thus, pharmacological interventions must have demonstrated efficacy in situations in which relapse-triggering cues are present. Several studies have demonstrated the relatively rapid decline in craving in inpatient treatment settings. Thus, there is a need for careful testing of prospective pharmacological interventions for cocaine abuse in settings other than inpatient ones (Margolin, Kosten, and Avants, 1992).

A survey of pharmacotherapies used by physicians belonging to the American Academy of Addiction Medicine for the treatment of cocaine abuse found that the four most commonly prescribed (and preferred) medications (of the 10 most frequently used) employed in detoxification were, in descending order, amantadine, bromocriptine, L-tryptophan, and desipramine (Halikas, Nugent, Crosby, et al., 1993). In detoxification, these four medications accounted for 75.5% of patients with whom medication was used. Bromocriptine was judged to be the most effective and L-tryptophan the least effective for use in detoxification. In abstinence maintenance treatment, the four most commonly used medications were, in descending order, desipramine, amantadine, L-tryptophan, and bromocriptine. These four medications accounted for 72.3% of patients treated. Desipramine was judged to be the most effective and L-tryptophan the least. In terms of preference, bromocriptine (at a dose range of 1.25–7.5 mg twice or three times daily) was clearly the preferred medication for cocaine detoxification. Desipramine (at a dose range of 75–200 mg once or twice daily) was the preferred medication for cocaine abstinence maintenance. As the study noted: "Physician's perceptions of medication effectiveness may not necessarily correspond to that medication's true effectiveness" (p. 137).

The most effective treatment programs for cocaine abuse involve a combination of psychotherapeutic and pharmacotherapeutic elements (Carroll,

1993; Gawin, Kleber, et al., 1989). This should not be surprising, given the evidence available from the evaluation of treatments for opiate addiction (see, for example, Platt, 1995b, chap. 3), where the provision of medication or psychotherapy alone rarely has resulted in as good an outcome as when the two interventions have both been used. As has been pointed out by Carroll (1993), however, an even closer parallel exists in research on the efficacy of treatments for depression (see, for example, Childress et al., 1991; McLellan et al., 1993; Woody et al., 1983). That is, the utility of combined interventions is perhaps most valuable in the initial phases of treatment, when attrition rates are highest.

10

Improving Treatment Outcome and Preventing Relapse

Evaluation of Treatment

Until recently, treatment outcome studies in the drug abuse field have usually not considered broader measures of functioning and have not generally made use of standard outcome measures which would facilitate comparison of cocaine abusers seen in different settings. Instead, they have typically focused on relatively short-term outcomes, usually only a few months after presentation for treatment (Carroll et al., 1993). Outcomes which have been measured in treatment evaluation have included treatment exposure and involvement, retention in treatment, dropout, reduction in drug use–related behaviors, and abstinence. Furthermore, findings from research underscore the complexity of the relationship between treatment and outcome which illustrates the difficulties involved in using some of the measures, such as retention in treatment, as an outcome. For example, in the Carroll et al. (1993) study, variables which powerfully predicted poorer outcome also predicted greater involvement with treatment. Thus, the total number of treatment days was not related to factors of substance abuse, psychiatric and psychosocial problems, or alcoholism, while greater treatment involvement was related to variables predicting poorer outcomes, such as ASI psychological severity, a number of Research Diagnostic Criteria non–substance abuse psychiatric variables, and number of previous substance abuse treatments.

Further complicating evaluation outcomes are the differing definitions which can be applied to the same term. For example, retention in treatment has variously been described as attending up to some point between the first and fourth week (Agosti et al., 1991), having attended 8 of the 17 sessions (Gainey, et al., 1993), or having completed 9 or more sessions over 12 weeks of treatment (Carroll, Rounsaville, and Gawin, 1991).

Predictors of Outcome

A number of predictors of outcome for opiate abusers have proven robust. Carroll et al., (1993) briefly summarized them: stable premorbid functioning (Rounsaville, Tierney, et al., 1982); a lesser degree of psychiatric impairment (McLellan et al., 1983; Rounsaville et al., 1986); and retention in treatment versus early dropout (Bale et al., 1980; Kosten et al., 1986; McLellan et al., 1982). The literature with respect to cocaine abusers, however, is much sparser on this issue.

Both psychopathology and severity of dependence have been found to predict outcome in cocaine abusers. In a sample of 94 cocaine abusers who had been seeking treatment at baseline, Carroll et al. (1993) found improvement at a one-year follow-up in a substantial proportion of the sample, particularly in those areas which had been most problematic at baseline. In this study, three variables emerged as consistent predictors of outcome across a number of domains: severity of drug use, severity of psychological symptoms, and presence of concurrent alcoholism. While all treatment domains (substance abuse, psychiatric and psychosocial problems, and alcohol use) were moderately related to one another, all were correlated with substance abuse, suggesting the centrality of this dimension. Abstinence was found to be associated with improvement in many areas, but it was not universally related to all areas. Specifically, improvement was shown on the employment, drug use, family/social, and psychological scales of the ASI, while no improvement was found with respect to the ASI medical, legal, and alcohol scales. With respect to cocaine use, at follow-up approximately one-third of the sample reported no use during the previous twelve months. Additionally, there were significant decreases in the mean frequencies of cocaine, alcohol, and cannabis use when 30-day periods preceding the baseline and follow-up interviews were compared. Number of days worked each month increased, and there were reductions in the number of days of family conflict and involvement in illegal activities. Rates of psychiatric disorders were stable, with only the rate of current anxiety disorders showing an increase. The percentages of subjects who met Research Diagnostic Criteria for drug abuse and alcoholism also dropped significantly, from 100% to 54% for drug abuse, and from 27% to 14% for alcoholism.

In another study, Carroll, Rounsaville, and Bryant (1993) found cocaine abusers who were also alcoholics at baseline to be likely to remain alcoholics following treatment, but not to differ from non-alcoholic cocaine abusers on other measures of outcome. This finding, although inconsistent with those of previous studies (for example, Rounsaville et al., 1987; Schuckit, 1985), does suggest that outcomes may *not* be worse for alcoholic cocaine abusers, although alcoholics may be in greater need of services during treatment.

The likelihood of a good treatment outcome has been found to be a function of route of cocaine use prior to treatment. Intranasal use appears to be a better predictor of good treatment outcome than crack smoking (Hall, Havassy, and Wasserman, 1991; Washton and Stone-Washton, 1990). This may be a function of the rapidity and height of peak blood levels attained via the smoking route (Miller, Gold, and Millman, 1989). Alternatively, it may reflect the fact that intravenous users generally had more severe patterns of addiction (more cocaine used on each occasion, more money spent on drugs each week, more cocaine use per week, more negative consequences of addiction), and fewer personal resources (that is, lower educational levels, less-skilled employment, less likely to be married) than did intranasal users (Budney et al., 1993).

While ethnicity appears to be related to relapse, with African Americans at greater risk of relapse than whites, this finding may be a function of differential route of administration. As noted earlier, Hall, Havassy, and Wasserman (1991) found that African Americans tended to smoke crack (82%), while whites tended to use cocaine intranasally (63%). Relapse to cocaine use is more closely associated with crack smoking than with intravenous cocaine use (Hall, Havassy, and Wasserman, 1991; Washton and Stone-Washton, 1990).

Retention in Treatment

Typically, the rate of failure to complete is high in cocaine treatment. Agosti et al. (1991) reported a 55% dropout rate by four weeks after treatment entry for a placebo-controlled trial of imipramine. Completers were found to be more likely to be white, female, or depressed. This figure is similar to that reported by other investigators. Gawin and Kleber (1984) reported a dropout rate of 54% before entry into an open-field trial of desipramine or lithium carbonate, following which the dropout rate fell to 6%. Another study, however, found a dropout rate of 44% between entry into and completion of four weeks of treatment in a double-blind clinical trial of desipramine, lithium, and placebo treatment for cocaine abuse (Gawin, Kleber, et al. 1989). Gainey et al. (1993) found that 56.4% of clients attending two clinics offering psychosocial treatments (cognitive-behavioral and twelve-step treatments) attended fewer than eight of the seventeen sessions offered. Dropout from outpatient therapy, in one study, was 42% between research interview sessions and therapy. For persons who attended at least one session, 30% dropped out before the third session, and 28% dropped out between the third and fifth sessions. Only 42% of those who attended one session were retained for six or more sessions (Kleinman et al. 1992).

Poor retention is likely to have an adverse impact on treatment outcome since length of exposure to drug abuse treatment is one of the strongest predictors of favorable outcomes (De Leon, 1986, 1991; Hubbard et al. 1989. McLellan et al., 1986; Simpson, 1979, 1981). As indicated earlier, retention of cocaine abusers in treatment is generally poor, regardless of the targeted drug problem. The same can be said regardless of whether the intervention is pharmacological (Agosti et al., 1991; Gawin, Kleber, et al., 1989; Tennant and Sagherian, 1987), psychosocial (Carroll, Rounsaville, and Gawin, 1991; Gainey et al., 1993; Kang et al., 1991; Kleinman et al., 1990; Rounsaville et al., 1983), or a combination of the two (Agosti et al., 1991; Gawin, Kleber, et al., 1989; Means et al., 1989).

Retention in treatment does not appear to be a function of primary drug of abuse, since this variable does not consistently predict either long- or short-term retention. In one study (De Leon, 1993), rates of retention in treatment at 30, 90, 180, and 360 days among admissions to a therapeutic community were examined as a function of primary drug of abuse. Retention rates for primary cocaine abusers did not appear to be different from those for any other primary drug abuse group, with the exception of primary cocaine and alcohol users having higher retention rates at 30 days.

Among the variables which have been related to retention in substance abuse treatment are demographic characteristics, including age, years of education, residential stability, and socioeconomic status (Baekeland and Lundwall, 1975; Gainey et al., 1993; Means et al., 1989); motivation (Miller, 1985; Miller and Rollnick, 1991); length of abstinence from cocaine (Means et al., 1989); involvement in a functional relationship (Means et al., 1989) as opposed to disruptive or problematic social ties, social isolation, and residential instability (Gainey et al., 1993); involvement of family and significant others in treatment (Higgins, Budney, Bickel, and Badger, 1994; Siddall and Conway, 1988);

employment stability and involvement in prosocial institutions (Gainey et al., 1993; Hawkins and Catalano, 1985; Lamb, Kirby, and Platt, 1996); extent of cocaine use and cocaine-related problems (Carroll, Rounsaville, and Gawin, 1991; Gainey et al., 1993); and plasma concentration of cocaine on admission to treatment (Tennant, Tarver, and Seecof, 1986). Each will be discussed in further detail in this chapter.

Variables predicting treatment completion at two psychosocial clinics studied by Gainey et al. (1993) included:

1. *Demographic variables,* among which age was the only predictor, with older clients being more likely to complete treatment. Gender, education, occupational status, and income were not related to treatment completion.

2. *Social isolation,* as reflected in living alone, which was strongly related to treatment completion. (Living alone is not a preferred measure of social isolation, but it has been found to predict outpatient cocaine treatment attendance; Means et al., 1989.) Length of residence, marital status, and family and social problems were not related.

3. *Drug involvement,* as reflected in the use of multiple substances, length of cocaine use, and involvement in illegal activities, all of which were negatively related to treatment retention. Cocaine use patterns and the number of cocaine-related problems were not related.

4. *Motivation,* in which both behavioral indicators (number of days of inpatient treatment in the preceding month) and external motivators (involvement with the criminal justice system) were found to be related to treatment retention.

The authors then developed a model of retention in which living alone, use of multiple substances prior to treatment, length of time since initiation of cocaine use, and the presence of external (legal) motivation for treatment remained significant predictors of treatment retention.

Lamb et al. (1994) identified the following patient and demographic variables related to treatment retention: low levels of anxiety, significant depression, previous involvement with Narcotics Anonymous, no current legal involvement, and living in the city where the clinic was located. For patients with prior involvement with Narcotics Anonymous, lack of current legal involvement and legal residence were particularly strong predictors of retention. Variables which did not predict retention in treatment included graduation from high school, income, marital status, living arrangements, gender, age, frequency of cocaine use, previous Alcoholics Anonymous involvement, and number of past treatment attempts. Lamb, Kirby, and Platt (1996) attributed the fact that this study did not find the number of past treatment attempts and patient age to be predictive of retention (whereas others have) to its focus on short-term retention (orientation to first counseling session), while others have examined longer retention periods.

Carroll et al. (1993) found treatment *retention,* as measured in number of days, to be related to four variables: psychiatric severity as measured by the ASI, with poorer baseline psychological functioning being related to treatment retention; number of non–substance abuse psychiatric disorders, as measured by Research Diagnostic Criteria; number of previous substance abuse treatments; and race, with whites reporting more treatment days.

On the basis of a factor analysis, the following predictors of treatment *outcome* were identified by Carroll et al. (1993): severity of substance abuse; psychiatric functioning; psychosocial functioning; and alcohol use. The ASI drug severity score was a predictor for all four factors, while alcohol use (either RDC or ASI scored) predicted substance use, psychiatric functioning, and alcohol use. Chronicity of cocaine use predicted psychiatric functioning and alcohol use, while the presence of a current Research Diagnostic Criteria psychiatric disorder or severity of current psychiatric functioning predicted psychiatric and psychosocial functioning as well as alcohol use. Abstinence after treatment was predicted by race, with whites more likely to report abstinence; gender, with more females abstaining; ASI drug subscale severity scores; ASI psychiatric severity subscale score; the presence of a lifetime Research Diagnostic Criteria attention deficit disorder; and lifetime Research Diagnostic Criteria diagnosis of alcoholism. Abstinence was not, however, related to improved outcome in all areas. In particular, abstinence was not found to be strongly related to reductions in rates of psychiatric disorders other than drug use, suggesting that outcome among cocaine abusers should not be considered unidimensional.

In the Agosti et al. (1991) study, dropouts were more likely to be male, African American or Hispanic, and without a history of primary depression. Gawin, Kleber et al. (1989) found African Americans and Hispanics more likely to drop out of treatment. Agosti et al. (1991) suggested that this disproportionate dropout from treatment by minorities may, in part, have been reflective of a greater likelihood of cocaine smoking and a more addictive route of use than snorting, which was more common among whites. The greater likelihood of completing treatment

on the part of patients with a history of primary depression was interpreted as reflecting a greater motivation for treatment on the part of
this group. In the Kleinman et al. (1992) study, a large number of parameters (including sociodemographic, treatment, psychiatric symptomatology, criminal history, and drug use variables) were analyzed with
respect to their relationship to retention. None was found to predict
short-term retention, while being white (versus African American) was
associated with greater long-term retention. Kleinman et al. (1992) concluded that patient variables may be less important in predicting retention than therapist and program variables.

Finally, Tennant, Tarver, and Seecof (1986) found that cocaine abusers
in whom toxicological analyses indicated the presence of detectable
plasma concentrations of cocaine on admission to treatment were significantly less likely to be retained in treatment (4.6 days) than were cocaine abusers without cocaine metabolites (13 days). Additionally, those
without cocaine in plasma on admission were less likely to produce
cocaine-positive toxicologies during treatment (78.6% versus 22.2%).
The authors suggested that these findings indicated either higher levels
of dependence or lower levels of motivation in admissions with cocaine
in their plasma.

Dropout has been a problem plaguing intervention studies. Carroll,
Rounsaville, and Gawin (1991), for example, reported a 62% dropout
from the interpersonal psychotherapy condition in their study versus a
33% dropout in the relapse prevention condition. Eighty percent of
dropouts in these programs, which were twelve weeks in length, dropped
out by week 6. In the study by Carroll et al. (1993), the follow-up rate
achieved at one-year posttreatment was 63%. By contrast, in the study
by Rounsaville et al. (1986), the follow-up rate at 2.5 years was 76% for
opiate addicts, the difference likely being the result of the latter having
been engaged in methadone maintenance treatment.

Dropout may occur as early as after the initial contact with the treatment clinic or agency. While a number of studies have addressed client
variables (that is, marital status, socioeconomic status, and previous
treatment history) associated with early dropout, with few exceptions
(Means et al., 1989; Stark, Campbell, and Brinkerhoff, 1990), most of
these reports have been for general psychiatric patient populations
which, while inclusive of substance-abusing patients, have not focused
on this population. While most of the variables studied have been patient characteristics which are not subject to change, one series of studies has addressed a variable which is under the control of treatment
agents: delay between initial contact with the clinic and intake.

Consistent with earlier findings that decreased delays between initial contact and scheduled appointment increased attendance (see, for example, Benjamin-Bauman, Reiss, and Bailey, 1984; Stark, Campbell, and Brinkerhoff, 1990), several more recent studies have addressed this issue in cocaine abusers. Festinger et al. (1995) found that shorter times between initial telephone contact and scheduled intake resulted in higher attendance rates at orientation sessions. Attendance at same-day sessions increased attendance from 57% to 83% over appointments scheduled for the next day. A randomized assignment to accelerated intake (that is, the same day or next morning) versus standard intake (scheduled for 1–3 days later) similarly resulted in a significantly higher rate of attendance at the intake session (59% versus 33%; Festinger et al., 1995).

Duration of Treatment

Time in drug abuse treatment has repeatedly been shown to be an important element related to outcome (Hubbard et al., 1989; Simpson, 1979, 1981; Simpson, Savage, and Lloyd, 1979). Most of these findings, however, have emerged from the opiate treatment literature. Specifically with respect to cocaine treatment, there is relatively little empirical data, and at least two of the few available studies have not found this relationship to exist for cocaine abusers (Carroll et al., 1993; Hubbard et al., 1988). A study by Lamb, Kirby, and Platt (1996), however, found that this relationship did hold for cocaine-abusing methadone patients.

Six months of treatment has been suggested as the minimal amount of time for a reasonable chance of continued abstinence following treatment (Washton, 1987; Washton, Gold, and Pottash, 1985). More intensive treatments, such as group therapy five times a week (intensive form) versus two days a week (minimal form), or adding psychotherapy and family therapy to either form of group therapy, are more effective in increasing retention of patients in treatment, and in encouraging higher levels of treatment participation (Hoffman, Caudill, and Koman, 1993). Furthermore, the combination of group therapy five days a week, individual psychotherapy, and family therapy is much more effective in increasing retention and participation than is any other combination of treatments. Washton and Stone-Washton (1990) similarly reported that "intensive" outpatient treatment was most effective. This program was highly structured and included behavioral counseling, cocaine-specific education, supervised urine testing, and encouragement to attend self-help groups. Rawson (1990) found outpatient treatment to be more effective than inpatient or no treatment.

Sequencing of Treatment Components

Khalsa, Anglin, and Paredes (1992) provided very useful data concerning the effects on treatment outcome of the sequencing of various treatment modalities. This study may be the only one to have reported data of this kind. Following a group of 300 cocaine-dependent males who had sought treatment at a Veterans Administration Medical Center, the researchers collected data on the various sequences of participation in treatment modalities. These included inpatient, outpatient, self-help; inpatient, self-help; inpatient, outpatient; inpatient, therapeutic community; outpatient, self-help; and inpatient only. The sequence of inpatient, outpatient, and self-help group treatment resulted in the most highly favorable outcomes, compared to the inpatient only treatment, while outcomes for the other treatment combinations generally fell between these two extremes. These findings are particularly important in terms of demonstrating treatment effectiveness for a range of combinations of different treatments and demonstrating differential effectiveness for different treatment combinations when applied to groups of cocaine abusers who were essentially similar at the point of treatment entry.

Matching Patients to Treatments

The matching of drug abuse patients to treatment has proven to be a difficult task. Ball (1994) has suggested several reasons which have accounted for this: *conceptual issues,* including the definition of how treatment differs from rehabilitation, and what operations actually take place under this term; *semantic problems,* including the problem of defining what exactly is meant by the term "treatment"; *substantive uncertainty,* including questions about appropriate psychiatric diagnoses and viable therapies, as well as how and to what populations they should be applied; *methodological issues,* including how the type, amount, and quality of treatment and rehabilitation services can be measured, as well as how treatment services provided in diverse environments can be compared; *political and financial realities,* including the inability to match patients to treatments when the full range of treatment services is not available; and *cultural issues,* including the fashioning of drug abuse treatment to match a specific culture's needs and resources, as well as its value system, with respect to drug abuse, treatment, and other issues. A general question raised by Ball (1994) during his discussion of matching relates to the need to differentiate between clinical and programmatic success. That is, what is appropriate treatment for one patient is not necessarily the same for another patient and thus requires that success be determined on an individual, not a programmatic, basis. Nevertheless, this approach does not consider treatment from a process perspective, which, if its premises are accepted, raises questions about the appropriateness of one-time matching.

Recommendations Regarding Treatment and Research

Leukefeld and Tims (1993) have developed a comprehensive and thoughtful list of recommendations concerning what direction research on the treatment of cocaine abuse and dependence should take. These recommendations fall into several broad categories. The first is *research on client populations,* including studies investigating the demography, psychopathology, natural history, and treatment-seeking behavior of cocaine-dependent clients; addressing client need, availability for treatment, and diagnostic subtypes that may indicate differential responses to treatment; focusing on client diversity, including the treatment needs of pregnant women and cultural minorities, mentally impaired, and HIV-positive chemical abusers; addressing clients with differing sets of natural contingencies, including employed clients as well as those with different kinds of social networks; and focusing on the long-term natural history of the context and dynamics of cocaine treatment.

The second category, *treatment modalities and therapy research,* includes expanding research related to the effectiveness of cocaine treatment interventions; continuing treatment studies identifying and evaluating pharmacological agents useful in achieving abstinence from cocaine and decreasing the likelihood of relapse, further understanding of the processes and outcomes of existing treatments through follow-ups of one year and longer, and evaluating the efficacy of psychosocial treatments, including psychotherapies, behavioral treatments, and relapse prevention strategies; recognizing the need for theory-based treatments; field testing promising pharmacotherapies in clinical programs to improve understanding of compliance with medication regimens; evaluating the relative efficacy of inpatient versus outpatient treatment; conducting studies to improve retention and rigorously test inpatient versus outpatient treatments for specific client subgroups; systematically investigating interventions regarded as experimental or nontraditional, such as acupuncture; evaluating twelve-step approaches; systematically attempting to integrate research and treatment; developing and testing criteria for patient-treatment matching; increasing our understanding of the role of motivation in retention of cocaine abusers in treatment; increasing our understanding of the role of self-help in the treatment of cocaine abusers; understanding the relationship between compulsive sexual behavior and compulsive cocaine use, with the aim of strengthening relapse prevention; examining the high rates of initial dropout from treatment during the first sixty days; and increasing outreach efforts to engage those who are reluctant to enter treatment, with an aim of reducing the risk of HIV infection.

The third category of recommendation concerns *research design issues,* and involves documenting the training and experience of treatment providers in treatment outcome studies; including both behavioral and intrapsychic outcome measures; including survival rates in outcome analyses; and improving reconciliation of differences among study findings.

Finally, *implications for practice* of these recommendations are discussed. They include understanding the potentially negative aspects of cocaine treatment; starting "where the client is" in order to address high dropout rates and low motivation; improving retention in treatment through maintaining program flexibility, open attitudes, and attention to boundaries; clearly stating treatment contracts and contingencies; recognizing the differences between cocaine abusers and alcoholics; incorporating elements which lead to greater program effectiveness, including structure, intense and planned interventions, frequent attendance, flexibility, definition of treatment stages, urine testing, and targeted counseling; increasing patient motivation through frequent group meetings, educational lectures, and individual counseling; recognizing the present limited efficacy of pharmacological interventions; attending carefully to medication dosage and compliance issues as more efficacious medications become available; maintaining a balanced approach for matching patients to treatment, given the difficulties inherent in treating addicts; and maintaining knowledge of current research findings on the part of practitioners.

Other issues raised by Leukefeld and Tims (1993), and for which they make recommendations, are *diagnosis,* including awareness in treatment planning of the multiple problems associated with cocaine abuse (including route of administration, psychiatric comorbidities) and the implications of Axis II diagnoses (in particular, antisocial personality); *drug testing,* which should be an integral part of treatment; *legal issues and legal involvement,* both of which are important considerations in cocaine treatment; *HIV and AIDS,* as both a major complication of compulsive cocaine use and an important aspect of treatment; *relapse,* as a frequent and repetitive characteristic of cocaine abusers; and *training,* with respect to the development of modules for cocaine treatment, regarding the specific characteristics of cocaine abusers, as well as emphasizing the need for counselors to seek out current research findings as a means of increasing their effectiveness.

Relapse and Relapse Prevention

Relapse, or return to drug use after a period of abstinence, is a defining characteristic of substance abuse disorders. This should not be surprising to those familiar with the recent drug abuse treatment research literature, which views drug dependence as a "chronic relapsing illness with an unfavorable diagnosis" (Kleber, 1989, p. 81). This is no less true of cocaine addiction than it is of heroin or other addictions (Platt, 1995a). Relapse in the addictions may run as high as 80% for any single episode (Hunt, Barnett, and Branch, 1971; Marlatt and Gordon, 1980, 1985). While cocaine abuse may share with other addictions this high rate of relapse, addiction to cocaine differs from addiction to other drugs in that cocaine use is characterized by high-dose binges, not necessarily daily doses; and the euphoria produced by cocaine may be more compelling than that produced by other drugs (Hall, Havassy, and Wasserman, 1991). These characteristics present difficult problems which have yet to be overcome by treatment programs.

One property of cocaine which greatly increases the likelihood of relapse after abstinence is the powerful "priming" effect of a single dose of cocaine. That is, an initial dose of cocaine can act as a stimulus for another dose, increasing craving or "wanting" (Jaffe et al., 1989). This phenomenon has been demonstrated in both laboratory studies with rats (de Wit and Wise, 1977) and humans (Fischman et al., 1990), and in clinical studies with humans (Childress, Ehrman, et al., 1988a). It may well be that craving for cocaine is stronger than craving for other drugs, including heroin (Kaplan, 1992), but more empirical data are needed on this point.

Acute craving for cocaine occurs soon after cessation of cocaine use (Gawin, 1991; Gawin and Kleber, 1986). The use of cocaine itself appears to increase the desire for further use. Several studies have demonstrated such a "priming effect" of cocaine. Jaffe and associates (1989), for example, found subjects' ratings of "wanting" and "craving" significantly increased about fifteen minutes after the administration of a 40 mg intravenous dose of cocaine, but not after a similar injection of a placebo. Similar findings have been obtained by other investigators. Fischman et al. (1990), for example, found that cocaine self-administration acted as a stimulus cue for the statement "I want cocaine" before the initial administration of desipramine, as well as on desipramine maintenance, but not during the initial baseline period of desipramine administration (Kosten, Kleber, and Morgan, 1989b).

In cocaine use, frequent short intervals of abstinence may be the rule rather than an exception. A review of conceptual issues in relapse to cocaine use (Havassy, Wasserman, and Hall, 1993) noted the differences which exist in the literature with respect to defining relapse, and the particular difficulty in distinguishing relapse from episodic use. These authors decided on a definition of relapse in their work as "the first occasion of resumed use (or first lapse) . . . regardless of the amount used on that occasion or whether there were subsequent occasions of use" (p. 204). Recognizing the absence of an ideal definition, they saw the one they used as having the advantages of accounting for the potential priming effects of even a single use of cocaine during a lapse; the conceptual ambiguity associated with this definition; and the ability reliably and validly to measure this event biochemically. They noted, however, that this definition provides only limited information if it is the only outcome variable; is used in the absence of knowledge about whether a lapse inevitably predicts further use; and may not be an unequivocally negative outcome, in that it may help the individual identify the circumstances leading to cocaine use.

Gawin and Ellinwood (1988) note the centrality of relapse prevention as a crucial component of treatment for cocaine abuse. After reviewing a number of treatment studies, the authors concluded that they all provided (although not always by design) a hierarchy of four stages for the treatment of conditioned craving. These were the linking of enforced isolation from drug abuse and the strict avoidance of conditioned cues during initiation of abstinence; the partial reintroduction of mental imagery during psychotherapy within the context of developing strategies for managing temptation for stimulants; the reintroduction of the patient, under controlled conditions, to the cue-rich environment; and the use of maintenance therapies, including self-help and aftercare groups and resumption of treatment. Furthermore, these four steps often take place within the context of long-term group psychotherapy modeled after groups such as Alcoholics Anonymous.

Situations Leading to Relapse

Both psychosocial and biologic factors appear to play a role in relapse to cocaine abuse (O'Brien, Ehrman, and Ternes, 1986). Among these factors are exposure to drug-related cues which elicit cocaine-craving owing to the presence of Pavlovian conditioned responses produced by the repeated use of drugs in situations associated with such environmental cues (O'Brien, McLellan, et al., 1992). Relapse to drug use may thus be occasioned by any number of cues which may serve to "trigger" craving and relapse and, as has been noted, may be very difficult to avoid even in the case of highly motivated patients. While this is true of all drug-taking behaviors, the power of such cues appears to be particularly great in the case of cocaine use (O'Brien et al., 1990b; 1993). High-risk relapse situations include those with both internal cues (for example, negative affective states, including depression, feelings of loss) and external cues (for example, presence of the drug, presence of persons with whom the drug was used, being in a location with which drug use was associated, use of other drugs). While affective states may be less salient in the case of cocaine use than in the case of alcohol use, they are still powerful (Cannon et al., 1992).

Although drug treatment programs recognizing the power of drug-related cues warn patients to avoid people, places, and things associated with previous drug abuse, such avoidance is very difficult to maintain. O'Brien et al. (1990b) therefore applied a treatment strategy of systematically exposing patients to stimuli which they were likely to encounter on leaving the treatment program, thereby making an active attempt in their treatment protocol to reduce the strength of Pavlovian or classically conditioned cues which were apt to elicit craving that could lead to relapse. Such cues were addressed in an individualized manner to a number of categories, including pharmacological, social, occupational, medical, legal, and family areas.

Interventions have also been directed at identifying situations which place the individual at high risk for relapse to drug use, and then reducing that risk through appropriate strategies (O'Brien et al., 1990a, b; O'Brien, Childress, et al., 1992). There may, however, be considerable individual variability in response to situational factors (Hatsukami et al., 1990). Kirby et al. (1995) interviewed 265 cocaine-experienced methadone patients in order to learn about situations that occasioned cocaine use and the strategies employed to avoid such use. Respondents identified a median of seven such situations leading to cocaine use. The most frequently cited situations were the presence of the drug (reported by 86% of respondents); being offered the drug (85%); having money available (83%); feeling bored (74%); and having nothing else to do (72%). The number of situations occasioning drug use was directly related to abstinence, in that those abusers reporting fewer situations also reported longer periods of lifetime abstinence. The number of situations provided was not related to demographic variables, employment status, or treatment experience. Michalec and associates (1992) have developed a survey to identify high-risk situations for cocaine abuse, although their results indicated that the frequency of *ongoing* cocaine abuse is not determined by specific situations. These results suggest the need for general, as opposed to specific, relapse prevention training.

There is a wide range of psychological and environmental determinants of relapse. Among these, Wallace (1989) has identified the following: *psychological/personality determinants,* including painful emotional state (present in 40% of the sample), denial/narcissistic denial (28.5%), failure to enter arranged aftercare treatment (37.1%), refusal of aftercare treatment (11.4%), and drug craving (5.7%); *environmental/interpersonal determinants,* including environmental stimuli (34.3%), interpersonal stress (24.4%), escalation from use of marijuana, alcohol, and intranasal cocaine to crack cocaine (14.3%), hard time handling money (11.4%), homelessness or lack of familial support (14.3%), and therapeutic community failures (20%); and *number of determinants of relapse,* with the distribution being one determinant only (14.3%), two determinants (37.1%), three determinants (40%), and four determinants (8.6%). The most common combinations of determinants were painful emotional state and interpersonal stress (20%) and narcissistic denial and/or fails or refuses aftercare treatment (22.8%). Negative life events occurring between three and nine months after treatment entry, as well as the absence of social support under conditions of high stress, were found by McMahon et al. (1994) to predict relapse to cocaine use.

Cocaine abusers, having to cope with sometimes incessant craving for the drug, must employ avoidance strategies on their own. One study identified the most commonly employed strategies used by cocaine-experienced methadone maintenance patients as avoiding people and places where cocaine was present (reported by 81% of respondents); thinking about what they could lose (76%); and leaving the situation (66%; Kirby et al., 1995). Neither the total number nor type of strategies (that is, reactive versus proactive) employed for avoiding cocaine use was systematically related to abstinence from cocaine, although four of the specific strategies (thinking about what could be lost, leaving the situation, moving to a new area, and using a different drug) were related to abstinence from cocaine. The authors of the study concluded that these findings suggested the need for individually tailoring treatment for cocaine abuse as opposed to providing general relapse prevention interventions. These findings confirm studies examining other addictions. Providing individually tailored relapse interventions is an approach which has been successful in improving rates of abstinence from smoking (Stevens and Hollis, 1989). Furthermore, alcohol intake, a behavior which itself may serve as a cue triggering cocaine use, is reduced when disulfiram is prescribed for alcohol-abusing cocaine abusers in conjunction with behavioral intervention (Higgins et al., 1993a).

Examining characteristics related to relapse in cocaine use among both freebase and/or crack smokers and intravenous users, Hall, Havassy, and Wasserman (1991) identified several variables which predicted a lower risk of relapse in the first twelve weeks of follow-up: endorsement of a goal of absolute abstinence; the presence of positive mood, or a feeling of well-being; more frequent use of coping strategies, although this was more true for whites than for African Americans, perhaps reflecting the strategies measured in the study; and greater expected likelihood of success. Life stress (that is, life events, difficulties, and physical problems) did not predict likelihood of relapse.

Psychosocial variables later identified by Havassy, Wasserman, and Hall (1993) as potentially important in successful cocaine abstinence included *having something to lose,* or negative contingencies to continued cocaine use, although these may not always be easy to identify in cocaine users who have few or no resources or who have hit bottom; *commitment to absolute abstinence; social support,* or resources provided by other persons, including contingencies provided by others (for example, social support, actual or perceived acceptance by others, and greater social integration), and arising from or enhanced by routes such as family or social network therapy, self-help programs such as Alcoholics Anonymous, and social skills training; *the ability to cope with drug-related cues,* either through removal from the setting or, more appropriately, by extinction through cue exposure interventions paired with increased self-efficacy and diminished expectations of positive outcome; *addressing psychopathology,* which may precede or precipitate substance abuse or attenuate treatment effects; and *mood states and subjective well-being,* which may play a significant role in relapse.

Havassy, Hall, and Wasserman (1993) also noted various treatment implications of their own findings and findings of others (although they observed that these implications may not be equally applicable to all socioeconomic and ethnic groups because of sample and design limitations of their own work). These included the identification and application of positive and negative reinforcers which are effective in competing with the reinforcing effects of cocaine, preferably under careful monitoring, and accompanied by the provision of coping skills training, employment, and similar opportunities; a goal of absolute abstinence; the identification of multiple potential sources of social support, both familial and extrafamilial; the development of coping skills for dealing with both internal and external drug-related cues, preferably in the natural environment; evaluation for the presence of psychiatric disorders, with treatment if necessary; and the enhancement of a subjective sense of well-being and development of alternative routes to reaching such states.

Finally, it should be noted that time to relapse can be very short for many cocaine abusers. In a study of admissions to a specialized crack treatment unit for a second detoxification in New York City, 35 subjects, 74% of whom were males and 94% African Americans, were examined. Wallace (1989) found for this sample the following times to first relapse after detoxification: within 1 week (31.4%); 2 weeks to 1 month (24.3%); 60 to 90 days (20%); 3.5 to 4.5 months (8.6%); and 6 to 7 months (5.7%). Thus, 76% relapsed with the first 90 days, and 94.3% within 6 months. While yielding some useful information concerning the temporal aspect of relapse, this high rate of relapse should not be surprising. In general, there is also a high rate of relapse for opiate addicts following detoxification (see, for example, Lipton and Maranda, 1983; Newman, 1979; Resnick, 1983; Simpson and Marsh, 1986).

Relapse Prevention Interventions

As Wallace acknowledged, "no treatment program seeking to provide efficacious [cocaine] treatment in the 1990s should fail to include relapse prevention as a vital component" (1990b, p. 149). Recognizing the difficulties inherent in treating crack cocaine addiction, Wallace suggested that a relapse prevention program for crack addicts requires the provision of adjunctive pharmacological intervention; education regarding the determinants of relapse; and remediation of the underlying psychological and emotional problems of crack-dependent individuals.

Thus, relapse prevention is "a set of strategies encompassing multiple interventions" (p. 150).

The most widely used intervention model for preventing relapse to cocaine abuse is the general one derived from Marlatt's theory of relapse prevention (Marlatt and Gordon, 1985). This model, originally developed for problem drinking, is based on cognitive-behavioral principles and focuses on the development of self-control strategies. Applications of this model to the treatment of drinking problems, smoking, and polysubstance abuse can be found in Marlatt et al. (1988). Carroll, Rounsaville, and Keller (1991) have adapted and applied Marlatt's relapse prevention to cocaine abuse. This adaptation focuses on issues specific to cocaine abuse, emphasizing the early phases of treatment, when cocaine abuse is likely to be an ongoing problem. Thus, relapse prevention is directed toward initiation and maintenance of abstinence, in preparation for longer-term treatment.

For their relapse prevention program, Carroll, Rounsaville, and Keller (1991) recommend stratified sequential implementation. The initial focus is on strengthening the patient's resolve to achieve abstinence, followed by supporting the start of abstinence. Thereafter, and subsequent to the achievement of stable abstinence, the intervention focuses on promoting the long-term prevention of relapse. The primary methods employed include *addressing ambivalence* through the fostering of a therapeutic alliance, enumeration of the consequences of continued cocaine use, and clarification of the patient's stated and unstated treatment goals; *reducing the availability of cocaine* by curtailing exposure to conditioned cues (for example, cocaine paraphernalia, drug-using individuals, locations where cocaine use has taken place), informing cocaine-using associates that the patient is no longer using the drug, and turning over cash to significant others; *the identification of high-risk situations and of coping strategies* such as the availability of money, use of other drugs, continued contact with drug-using peers, or the availability of unstructured time, as well as effective strategies for coping with such situations; *coping with craving elicited by conditioned cues* such as exposure to white powder and/or cocaine paraphernalia by the employment of exposure and extinction procedures; *the management of seemingly irrelevant but nonetheless high-risk decisions, rationalizations, and minimalizations of risk* which bring the patient closer to cocaine use by initiating a chain of behaviors resulting in cocaine use, but which, on their face, seem unrelated to such use; *lifestyle modification,* leading to the development of rewarding alternatives to cocaine use; and *the appropriate handling of abstinence violation effects,* or a slip to drug use being followed by negative self-attribution, feelings of guilt and failure, and return to bingeing, and which includes putting such slips into perspective and viewing them as opportunities for learning appropriate coping strategies.

Carroll, Rounsaville, and Keller's (1991) model emphasizes the need to address other problems which the cocaine abuser brings to treatment, in addition to applying relapse prevention methods. For instance, the presence of psychopathology requires intervention, during which relapse prevention can serve a valuable role in symptom control while preparing the patient for long-term treatment. These authors emphasize their view that relapse prevention is not necessarily an exclusive intervention but one in which techniques can be integrated into other psychotherapeutic approaches, such as supportive-expressive, behavioral, and twelve-step models. Relapse prevention may be particularly well suited for integration into other approaches, given its orientation toward abstinence; its flexibility in use at different points and phases of treatment; its applicability to cocaine abusers, who are a heterogeneous group; its accessibility and acceptability (because of its commonsense approach) to cocaine-abusing patients, many of whom have little experience with talking therapies, and also because of the ability to provide drug use control techniques early in treatment; and the provision to the patient of a broad repertoire of generalizable skills which will help to maintain abstinence through generalization to other behaviors and situations.

Carroll, Rounsaville, and Gawin (1991) conducted a clinical trial of relapse prevention and interpersonal psychotherapy. Their findings indicated that subjects in the relapse prevention condition were more likely than subjects in the interpersonal psychotherapy condition to attain three weeks or more of abstinence (57% versus 33%). Furthermore, subjects in the relapse prevention condition were more likely to be categorized as recovered at the point of treatment termination (43% versus 19%) and to complete treatment (67% versus 38%). These differences did not reach statistical significance, however, until subjects were stratified by severity of substance abuse. At that point high severity subjects in the relapse prevention condition were significantly more likely to achieve abstinence (54% versus 9%), while among low-severity patients, no difference between conditions was present. The authors concluded that these findings suggested that high-severity cocaine abusers may require greater structure and direction focused on learning and rehearsal of specific strategies to interrupt and control cocaine use, and also that the large increment in abstinence between weeks 6 and 12 suggested that treatment outcome is enhanced when rehearsal of coping strategies takes place.

The effectiveness of a cognitive-behavioral relapse prevention treatment was compared with that of a twelve-step recovery support group in an outpatient setting by Wells et al. (1994). Both interventions used group treatment formats. Patients in both treatment conditions reduced cocaine and marijuana use at six months posttreatment, although there were no differential effects on such drug use as a function of treatment condition. Furthermore, the two programs did not differ in their ability to retain patients or in their ability to increase role-playing skill levels. Other findings indicated that at six months, patients in the cognitive-behavioral condition showed better maintenance of reductions in drug and alcohol use than did patients in the twelve-step condition, and that attendance at treatment sessions was positively related to reductions in cocaine and alcohol use at six months posttreatment. Thus, the researchers concluded that approaches that can retain patients in treatment may hold greater promise for successful treatment of the addictions, and that weekly treatment may not be sufficient to hold patients in treatment.

Another approach to relapse prevention addresses conditioned reactions to environmental and internal stimuli or cues which trigger relapse to drug use. Strongly influenced by the conditioned withdrawal conception of relapse originally proposed by Wikler (1965), this model attempts to identify conditioned associations which play a role in relapse to drug use as well as the stimuli which elicit them and to develop effective extinction procedures for them (Childress, Ehrman et al., 1988b; O'Brien, Childress, and McLellan, 1991). Ideally, such programs should be part of a comprehensive cocaine treatment program.

Current research findings suggest a number of essential elements for an effective treatment program addressing conditioned responses in cocaine abuse. These include *active (versus passive) extinction procedures*. A study conducted by O'Brien et al. (1993) found that extinction through the use of passive cue exposure procedures resulted in decreased cocaine use as reflected in a higher proportion of cocaine-free urines in outpatients. While the results were encouraging, full extinction of the conditioned responses did not occur, and it was suggested that an active extinction procedure was called for to enhance the effect of the passive extinction procedure. A second element is *increased generalization from the laboratory*. One approach to increase generalization from the laboratory to the real world environment involves the use of even more realistic stimuli (including actual use of cocaine) together with realistic stimulus contexts, such as in vivo repeated exposures near "copping" corners or shooting galleries. Such methods have their risks, however.

Other less dangerous possible in vivo procedures suggested by O'Brien et al. (1993) include use of the patient's own home, or neighborhood videotapes obtained from a moving car; *training in alternative behaviors* as competing responses, including thought blocking and relaxation responses as adjuncts to more conventional treatments (counseling, therapy, relapse prevention); *giving individualized cocaine reminders* for those patients who do not respond strongly to standard test stimuli; *increasing the number of extinction sessions* in an attempt to extinguish persistent physiological arousal elicited by cocaine cues; and *using cue reactivity methodology to screen medications*.

Conclusions

Outcome studies of cocaine treatment, like outcome studies of drug abuse treatment in general, have suffered from a number of deficiencies. These have included an emphasis on short-term outcomes (usually only a few months after presentation for treatment), the absence of standard outcome measures, and a lack of consistency in defining outcome measures. Addressing these last two points could greatly facilitate comparisons of cocaine abusers seen in different settings. Additionally, there has been a general absence of consideration of broader measures of functioning in outcome studies (Carroll et al., 1993).

There are a number of predictors of positive treatment outcome which have proven robust. These include stable premorbid functioning, less psychiatric impairment, less severity of drug use, absence of concurrent alcoholism, and retention in treatment (Carroll et al., 1993). Other variables related to treatment outcome for cocaine abuse include route of administration, with intranasal use more closely associated with positive outcome than crack smoking (Hall, Havassy, and Wasserman, 1991; Washton and Stone-Washton 1990), and ethnicity, with African Americans being at higher risk of relapse (Hall, Havassy, and Wasserman, 1991).

Rates of retention in cocaine treatment are low, with rates of treatment completion also being relatively low (Agosti et al., 1991; Carroll, Rounsaville, and Gawin, 1991; Gawin and Kleber, 1984; Gainey et al., 1993; Kleinman et al., 1992). The relationship of length of time in treatment to outcome, a finding that has been well established in the treatment of other addictions, including those to alcohol and opiates (De Leon, 1986; Hubbard et al., 1989; McLellan, Woody, and O'Brien, 1979), appears to hold for cocaine as well (see, for example, Wells et al., 1994). Low rates of retention hold true for pharmacological, psychosocial, and combined interventions (see, for example, Agosti et al., 1991; Carroll, Rounsaville, and Gawin, 1991; Gawin, Kleber, and Byck, 1989; Kleinman et al., 1990; Means et al., 1989). Variables related to retention in cocaine treatment include pattern and extent of involvement with drugs, demography (gender, ethnicity, place of residence), presence and severity of psychopathology, psychosocial functioning/social competency, prior treatment history, social isolation, motivation (both internal and external), legal involvement, abstinence, and employment status (Agosti et al., 1991; Carroll et al., 1993; Gainey et al., 1993; Kleinman et al., 1992; Tennant, Tarver, and Seecof, 1986).

Duration of treatment, an important predictor of outcome in opiate treatment, has not been definitively demonstrated to play the same role in the case of cocaine treatment. Relatively little evidence exists on this issue with respect to cocaine abusers, and what does exist is inconsistent. One study has documented this relationship for cocaine abusers (Lamb, Kirby, and Platt, 1995), while two others have not (Carroll et al., 1993; Hubbard et al., 1989). Six months has been suggested as the minimal duration of treatment for cocaine abuse in order to ensure a reasonable chance of achieving and maintaining abstinence (Washton, 1987; Washton, Gold, and Pottash, 1985), although there is little empirical evidence available on this point.

The sequencing of treatment elements may play an important role in outcome. The results of the study of cocaine treatment by Khalsa, Anglin, and Paredes (1992) suggest that the sequence of inpatient, outpatient, and self-help group treatment resulted in the best outcome, while inpatient-only treatment resulted in the worst outcome. Further knowledge of the relative effectiveness of different treatments, together with a reliable system for matching patients with treatment, is likely to have a significant impact on treatment outcomes.

Recent recommendations for the future direction of treatment research, if followed, are likely to result in improved treatment for cocaine abuse and addiction. Such recommendations stress the need to learn more about patient populations, including the natural history of cocaine addiction and the role of variables relating to patient diversity in response to treatment; the need to understand better the differential effectiveness of different treatment interventions in retaining patients in treatment and improving outcome, particularly when considered in conjunction with patient motivation; the need to apply improved research design and measurement, as well as to reconcile apparent differences among research findings; and the need to implement in treatment programs practices known to be related to improved retention and outcomes.

The application of relapse prevention paradigms and strategies to the treatment of abuse is relatively recent. Although only a few studies evaluating its application have appeared (for example, Carroll, Rounsaville, and Keller, 1991; Wells et al., 1994), relapse prevention appears to be a promising intervention for the treatment of cocaine abuse, and it is likely to be the subject of further investigation (Carroll, Rounsaville, and Keller, 1991; Gawin and Ellinwood, 1988; Havassy, Wasserman, and Hall, 1993). Among the areas being investigated with respect to relapse prevention are the roles of cues, affective states, and other psychological and environmental determinants in eliciting cocaine craving and relapse (see, for example, Cannon et al., 1992; Kirby et al., 1995; O'Brien et al., 1990a, b, 1993; O'Brien, Childress, et al., 1992; Wallace, 1989). Variables which have been related to relapse have been numerous and varied (Hall, Havassy, and Wasserman, 1991; Wallace, 1989), suggesting the need for individually tailored relapse prevention interventions (Kirby et al., 1995).

11

Conclusions and Recommendations

Cocaine and/or crack abuse has become epidemic in the United States, with about 2 million individuals reporting current use in 1991, ten times more than those who abuse heroin (U.S. Bureau of the Census, 1994). This epidemic has been particularly evident among the young. For those aged 12 to 25, 1.4% admitted to current use (U.S. Bureau of the Census, 1994). Cocaine abusers are likely to have psychiatric impairments (Jonas, 1992; Weiss et al., 1988) and to be poor (Dunlap and Johnson, 1992). The sexual behavior accompanying crack use has been cited as one of the most important vectors for heterosexual AIDS transmission in the United States (Chaisson et al., 1989; Lindsay et al., 1992; Platt, 1995b; Siegal et al., 1993). In 1990, at least $18 billion was spent on cocaine by users (Bureau of Justice Statistics, 1992). Billions more are expended by government to stop drug importation and sales and to treat addicts, with additional billions lost to the economy through lost productivity and increased crime.

While the magnitude of the problem is generally understood, the solutions to it are less well known. From the review of the pharmacological and psychosocial approaches to cocaine treatment in Chapters 8 and 9, several broad conclusions can be drawn.

Treatment: What Works?

First, for most, if not all, of the pharmacological interventions cited, early open trials of the drugs have shown promise in providing a treatment for addicts or acting as an antagonist to cocaine itself. Later double-blind studies have not, however, been nearly as promising. Aside from the obvious explanation of not as yet having found the "right" drug, these disappointments may be due to differences in beliefs about the drug between those enrolled in open trials and those who know they might receive a placebo. Those enrolled in open trials or in early stages of controlled trials may also be more highly motivated to stop drug use.

Second, the value of some preliminarily effective psychosocial or combined pharmacologic and psychosocial interventions have yet to be thoroughly evaluated. Early work in the use of contingency management techniques, either alone or in combination with other interventions, has shown great promise in cocaine treatment for at least a substantial (25%–33%) minority of those with whom it has been tried (Anker and Crowley, 1982; Higgins et al., 1991, 1993b). Long-term outcomes have not been assessed, however. The one study which did try to assess the effect of contingency management on the long-term outcomes of treatment for cocaine addiction found no differences between the treatment and control groups at nine months after treatment (Kirby et al., 1995). The observed variation in outcome may be due to a variety of factors, including the differing population characteristics and environments used in the studies. These differences remain to be effectively analyzed.

Third, many variables which can affect treatment outcome have yet to be addressed. For example, the wide variety of treatment approaches which have been tried, ranging from outpatient through day hospital to inpatient treatment, have not yet been compared as to their effectiveness, including retention rates and outcomes for completers versus noncompleters.

Fourth, the "failure" of some treatment interventions may be a product of faulty patient matching. Appropriate treatment for cocaine abuse requires a carefully conducted and comprehensive assessment of the treatment-seeking patient. Issues such as motivation for treatment, drug history, the circumstances (both physical and personal) surrounding drug use, the physical and psychosocial resources available to the patient, and the patient's other psychiatric involvement must all be understood before treatment needs can be met. The specific elements needed for an appropriate assessment await further identification, however.

Fifth, in the absence of a "single best treatment approach" for all cocaine abusers, it would appear to be wise to follow the advice given by Weiss and Mirin (1990), who suggest that clinicians should adopt a flexible multimodal approach to treatment. Such an approach should include a careful psychiatric evaluation to rule out comorbid psychopathology; measures to help the patient identify and understand environmental and internal cues which may trigger drug urges; assistance for the patient in understanding the necessity for abstaining from all drugs, including alcohol; encouragement for the patient to attend and participate in self-help groups; and careful consideration of the use of adjunct pharmacotherapy.

Special Treatment Issues

Situational or "Recreational" Cocaine Abuse

It has been suggested that there are individuals for whom cocaine use is limited to very specific, self-defined "recreational" situations (see O'Malley, Johnston, and Bachman, 1985; Siegel, 1984). As a rule, however, the belief that cocaine can be used recreationally or "in moderation" is a sad case of self-deception. While "controlled" use of cocaine does exist, few individuals know their own "addiction liability," or the likelihood that they will progress from experimentation to addiction. Few also know the medical liabilities they may have which will result in life-threatening consequences of even a single episode of cocaine use. Moreover, the likelihood of an individual's being objective about his or her own use is very small. Gold (1992) found that even among callers to the National Helpline who reported "moderate" or "recreational" use of cocaine, severe problems resulting from this use were found. In fact, the only way in which "recreational users" and "everyday" users differed from each other was in their length of use. "Everyday" users had been using drugs for more than five years, while only one-quarter of recreational users had been using drugs for this long.

Women

Women cocaine users have been found to be less happy and to have higher levels of anxiety or depressive symptomatology than their male counterparts in several studies. Kandel, Murphy, and Karus (1985), for example, found that both male and female users of illicit drugs felt less happy about life than those who had never used drugs. The least unhappy, however, were women cocaine users who had used no other drugs. Griffin et al. (1989) found women to have a lower level of social adjustment, and to be more likely to be using cocaine in response to a variety of symptoms of distress. Women were also more likely to have an Axis I disorder, particularly major depression, while men were more likely to have an Axis II disorder. Cocaine use by women relieved guilt feelings, while similar use by men increased such feelings and may possibly have hastened the course of addiction. These results were consistent with those from the Epidemiologic Catchment Area (ECA) study (Helzer and Pryzbeck, 1988) which found a generally stronger relationship between alcoholism and other diagnoses, including substance abuse, among women than among men: a second diagnosis was found for 65% of women versus only 44% of men.

Despite (or perhaps because of) this acknowledgment of a higher level of psychopathology, women are not retained in treatment as well as men (Moise, Reed, and Connell, 1981). This lack of retention further exacerbates the tendency of researchers to study men only, even though women can be treated as successfully as men (De Leon and Jainchill, 1991; Kosten, Gawin, Kosten, and Rounsaville, 1993). The studies which have been conducted suggest that additional attention should be paid to pharmacotherapy which addresses the underlying depression that is particularly prevalent among female drug abusers (Kosten et al., 1993).

What data are available suggest that there are similar outcomes for addicted males and females (Simpson and Sells, 1982). Length of stay has been related to better outcomes for both men and women with respect to criminal activity and drug use, although women tend to stay longer in treatment. Gains in psychological functioning, however, appear to be higher for women than for men (De Leon, 1984; De Leon and Jainchill, 1981–82). Dropout rates for women are higher earlier in treatment (Moise, Reed, and Connell, 1981), undoubtedly reflecting their greater child care responsibilities.

Research Issues

Methodological Issues in Cocaine Research

In each of the several areas discussed, it is obvious that additional, well-designed research must be conducted. Gorelick (1992) has observed that almost all data on abnormalities associated with human cocaine use are derived from cocaine abusers seeking treatment, from those volunteering for research studies, or from case-control studies comparing cocaine users with control subjects matched on demographic characteristics. Confounding variables arising from such "naturalistic" studies may preclude drawing appropriate conclusions on the pathophysiology of cocaine abuse. Among these confounding factors are the unknown purity of the cocaine used; uncertainty about the quantity and duration of cocaine exposure, owing to the failings of self-report as well as to the negative effects on memory of the drug itself; complicating effects of other substances used in addition to cocaine; abnormalities associated with the route of administration of the drug and with the drug lifestyle; and selection bias, as reflected in the likelihood of patients with medical abnormalities to be overrepresented in studies of cocaine abusers in treatment. Gorelick concluded that the remedy for these problems includes the use of more sophisticated research designs, including prospective, longitudinal follow-up of large representative samples of cocaine abusers; case-control comparisons of well-characterized cocaine users with appropriately matched groups; and experimental administration of cocaine under safe, controlled conditions. (While studies involving the experimental administration of cocaine to well-characterized subjects provide the most control, and thus the most unambiguous findings, they are costly, however, and do not completely replicate the dose, frequency, and duration of cocaine exposure among actual abusers.)

Noting that our knowledge about the psychotherapy and pharmacotherapy of cocaine are at a primitive stage (particularly when compared with our knowledge about the treatment of other disorders such as depression), Gawin, Khalsa, and Ellinwood (1994) have delineated a number of methodological considerations for future research. These fall into five categories.

1. *Severity issues.* Treatment studies, to date, have not stratified samples according to any generally accepted index of severity of drug abuse, and thus have not allowed for comparison across samples.

2. *Self-selection artifacts.* There has been an absence of systematic assessments of treatment engagement, leading to little knowledge about those populations that find involvement in particular treatments aversive or inadequate. There has also been an absence of understanding about those for whom a particular treatment is especially attractive.

3. *Recovery issues.* There is an absence of consensus about the length of time needed for abstinence before recovery is effected or treatment is no longer needed.

4. *Heterogeneity of study samples.* How does the heterogeneity of samples affect outcome? Variables to be considered include so-

ciodemographics, psychiatric symptomatology, psychosocial resources, patterns and duration of cocaine and other drug use, degree of impairment, treatment history and perspectives, and
so on.

5. *Course and neuroadaptation issues.* There is an absence of information concerning improvement, stability, and deterioration in
   treatment. A more systematic assessment of the clinical course of
   cocaine addiction is required.

In 1984 Kleber and Gawin (1984b) observed that "single focus approaches are generally ineffective in drug abuse treatment . . . [I]t currently appears no more likely that any unimodal approach to cocaine
abuse treatment will arise than it has for opiate abusers. Integration of
various approaches based on the needs of the patients seems indicated
instead . . . Before any such schema is used in clinical practice, however,
detailed comprehensive research will be needed" (p. 122). It appears that
such advice has yet to be thoroughly heeded.

Generalizability of Findings with Opiate Addicts to Cocaine Abusers

It is still not clear whether, and to what extent, the many findings which
have been developed on other drug-abusing populations, primarily opiate abusers, can be applied to cocaine. Carroll et al. (1993) have outlined a number of such issues: the multidimensionality of outcomes for
opiate users, with only modest relationships among dimensions (Kosten
et al., 1987; McLellan et al., 1981); the likelihood of substantial improvement, in some cases, without treatment (Robins, Helzer, and Davis,
1975); and the cyclic nature of opiate addiction, with cycles often being quite lengthy (Vaillant, 1973).

New Research Methods

Attention must also be paid to promising new research methods which
will help further refine our understanding of drug use behavior. Among
these methods is interesting work being conducted in behavioral economics, which attempts to understand human behavior through the
concept of product consumption (Hursh and Bauman, 1987). Among
the methods used is cost-benefit analysis, which is now beginning to be
applied to our understanding of illicit drug use (Bickel, DeGrandpre, and
Higgins, 1993). Early results of several studies seem to indicate that drug
(in this case cigarette) use behavior can be explained at least partially

by the dose of the drug, the cost, and the amount of effort which must be expended to obtain the cost (Bickel, DeGrandpre, and Higgins, 1993). Available income was also found to be related to drug (or in this case cigarette brand) substitution (Bickel, DeGrandpre, and Higgins, 1993).

Societal Forces Resulting in Cocaine Use

Any discussion of cocaine use and addiction must begin to address the reasons why people turn to such a harmful substance. Theories have been postulated as to why individuals begin to use "hard" drugs and why they become psychologically dependent on them. The self-medication hypothesis and psychoanalytic theory have both been used to explain cocaine abuse and have been discussed in this volume (Chapter 3). Yet not all those who begin to use cocaine continue to do so. The subjective effects associated with cocaine use (that is, the experience of intense anxiety, including panic attacks, paranoia, apathy, and so on) or the fear of losing control because of the drug's effects may lead some experimenters not to proceed with further use of the drug. Later on, perceived risks to health, social disapproval, establishment of a relationship, and even loss of interest in drugs may be salient factors in stopping, or decreasing, cocaine use (Erickson et al. 1987). Erickson and Murray (1989), for example, found that cocaine users who perceived "great harm" from regular use of the drug were more likely to quit than to continue use (62.5% versus 36%). "Fear of addiction" (with addiction defined in terms of ever having experienced a craving or an uncontrollable urge to use cocaine) was also likely to be associated with quitting cocaine use (29.2% versus 16.3%). Since the use of cocaine to treat the underlying anxiety and depression of addicts or hidden childhood psychological trauma which abusers may have experienced does not completely explain cocaine use, and since not all cocaine experimenters continue to use the drug, other explanations must also be explored. Newcomb, Maddahian, and Bentler (1986) identified ten societal/social variables which are strongly related to later drug use. In decreasing order of influence they are peer drug use, deviant behavior, adult drug use, early alcohol use, sensation seeking, poor relationship with parents, low religiosity, poor academic achievement, psychopathology, and problems with self-esteem.

Larger societal issues are also related to cocaine use. Since the 1980s, young people in the inner city have been increasingly involved in the sale and distribution of drugs (Dunlap and Johnson, 1992; Fagan, 1992).

This change became particularly evident after the start of the crack epidemic, especially in those neighborhoods "that had experienced profound social and economic deterioration" (Fagan, 1992, p. 102). As the surplus of city-based jobs dried up, largely as a result of the outmigration of businesses to the suburbs, the number of licit employment opportunities paying more than minimum wage was drastically reduced (Dunlap and Johnson, 1992; Fagan, 1992). "The economic restructuring of . . . American cities resulted in large scale exclusion of their nonwhite residents from constricting labor markets that also were transforming from manufacturing to services . . . Cocaine and crack distribution thus represented new economic opportunities in neighborhoods where legitimate economic activity had been lost" (Fagan, 1992, p. 103). One author writes:

> In the day-to-day experience of the street-bound inner-city resident, unemployment and personal anxiety over the inability to provide one's family with a minimal standard of living translate themselves into intra-community crime, intra-community drug abuse, and intra-community violence. The objective structural desperation of a population lacking a viable economy and facing systematic barriers of racial discrimination and ideological marginalization becomes charged at the community level into self-destructive channels. (Bourgois, 1989, pp. 627–628)

The underground economy can thus be described as the ultimate equal opportunity employer (Bourgois, 1989). For those who cannot use the drug trade to lift them economically out of the community, the drug itself can provide at least temporary escape. From this one can conclude that the solution to the problem of cocaine and other drug abuse cannot be found only in the remedies usually proposed. Broader social solutions, which consider the necessity of having a way up and out, must be discussed and implemented (Platt, 1986).

Legalization

As discussed in Chapter 1, cocaine was initially viewed as a benign, even beneficial substance. It was found in cough drops, wine, tea, and even soda. By the late nineteenth century, in the face of increasing evidence of its destructive characteristics, however, progressively tighter forms of regulation were imposed. The Harrison Act of 1914 incorrectly grouped opiates and cocaine together, and removed these substances from over-the-counter use to controlled dispensing by licensed physicians and pharmacists. With the introduction of amphetamines, cocaine was prescribed less frequently. The drug was now not only illegal but also legally unavailable, and, like all drugs so characterized, became a commodity obtainable only through underground sources. The value of keeping drugs illegal has long been disputed. One scholar writes: "Drug laws themselves appear to be responsible for much of the 'drug problem.' In addition to the criminal production, sale and purchase of drugs, many drug users resort to robbery, burglary, and prostitution to pay for high-priced illegal drugs. Most of the violence associated with drugs is due not to the physiological effects of drugs but rather, to the illegal markets in which they are sold" (Nadelmann, 1991b, p. 3).

Would legalizing drugs reduce their ability to attract new users because they would no longer be "forbidden fruit"? Would legalization eliminate crime associated with the sale and purchase of drugs? Would legalization save the government large sums of money currently expended on interdiction, source country control, and domestic law enforcement? Would legalization provide a new source of income through the creation of a newly acceptable cash crop? The quick and immediate answer to all these questions is yes, and this position has been openly espoused (Nadelmann, 1989; 1991a, b; 1992). Advocates of this position sometimes embrace the idea that drugs are less harmful than would be supposed but generally propose that methods other than legal sanction be used to discourage drug use.

Yet, those who favor legalization fail to propose a concrete plan for implementation and therefore do not consider the difficulties which would be faced. Inciardi and McBride (1989) summarize the potential problems:

- What drugs would become legal, and who would decide which drugs made the list?
- How would appropriate and legal dosages be determined?
- Would there be a legal drug-taking age, and if so, what would it be?
- Would individuals be allowed to start using the drug, or would use be limited to those already involved?
- Would there be a "use limit" imposed on those permitted to obtain the drug?
- Where and how would a person get the drug?
- Where would the drugs be grown or manufactured?
- Should new substances be permitted to enter the United States?

- Should the industry be private or controlled by the government?
- If the market were a private one, how would issues such as purity, price, potency, and advertising be handled?
- Would restrictions be placed on the use of drugs for those in dangerous or public occupations?
- Would there be any restrictions on when and where the drugs could be used?
- Which part of the government would be charged with the enforcement of these statutes?
- Would legalization encourage people from other countries (particularly Mexico and Canada) to cross the border for the sole purpose of obtaining drugs?

Even if each of these questions could be satisfactorily addressed, a careful evaluation of the effect of legalization in other countries would argue against it. Courtwright (1993) espoused this side of the debate and claimed that legalization would result in the following:

- increases in the number of addicts of between 12% and 55%, as has been experienced in Thailand
- significant increases in drug use among those professions, such as physicians, where drugs are readily available but where use is currently discouraged
- increases in the use of drugs among those already involved because of the reduced cost (see Bickel, DeGrandpre, and Higgins, 1993)
- increased drug use by young people, including those who are under the legal age, owing to diversion by adults who could legally obtain the drug (as occurs for cigarettes and alcohol)
- maintenance of some level of criminal behavior owing to this diversion
- increases in drug use among those in dangerous or public safety professions, as well as among others viewed to be at risk, such as pregnant women, the mentally ill, parolees, and so on
- increased drug smuggling in the prison system
- increases in the "white collar" crime of tax evasion
- increases in interstate smuggling of drugs, owing to inequitable tax structures or differences in legal status of the drug

- maintenance of the role of organized crime in the supply of the drug in any situation where smuggling or sale to at-risk groups was involved

Courtwright (1993) concluded that the legalization debate is "an argument about a colossal gamble, whether society should risk an unknown increase in drug abuse and addiction to eliminate the harms of drug prohibition, most of which stem from illegal trafficking . . . It would be more accurate to ask whether society should risk an unknown but possible substantial increase in drug abuse and addiction in order to bring about an unknown *reduction* in illicit trafficking and other costs of drug prohibition" (p. 56).

Jarvik (1990) speaks specifically to the issue of legalization of cocaine and recommends the reduction of both demand and abuse while emphasizing the need for the application of new technologies and the use of empirically derived answers. These suggestions include

- reducing demand through "social therapy" preventive techniques, such as family planning, job programs, school-based prevention/intervention programs, and mass media campaigns
- the investigation of currently available treatment techniques, especially pharmacological approaches, which are at least less harmful than cocaine itself
- comparison of supply-reduction versus demand-reduction techniques to determine the most cost-effective
- extension of community sanctions, and electronic and chemical control techniques (though these may raise Fourth Amendment considerations)
- development of new pharmacological techniques
- more effective criminal justice responses, including intensive probation as an intermediate step

The most reasoned view of the legalization debate is perhaps that presented by Goldstein and Kalant (1990), who note that a rational drug policy must strike a balance between harm reduction on the one hand and strict legal prohibitions and enforcement on the other. They argue that since psychoactive drugs have always been present in society and are thus unlikely to be eliminated through legalization or criminalization, drug policy should focus on the reduction of harm from these drugs. This can be accomplished by reducing the number of new initiates into drug use through price and supply control and by treating present drug users, who should be seen as "victims of a life-threatening disease ... requiring compassionate treatment" (p. 1516).

Treatment Policy

Elsewhere I have provided a list of recommendations concerning public policy and treatment effectiveness issues related to the control and treatment of heroin addiction (Platt, 1995a, b). Most of these recommendations are equally applicable to the problems associated with cocaine as a drug of abuse. In this section I discuss the recommendations that are most salient with respect to cocaine addiction.

Public Policy Issues

Addiction is chronic and endemic. Addiction to drugs such as cocaine and heroin is not likely to disappear anytime soon, if ever, without massive intervention. But such massive intervention is unlikely to be acceptable to Americans because of both its cost and the infringement on personal rights and liberties likely needed to accomplish it. Yet, Americans see drug abuse as a major problem facing the country. An extensive public health campaign, involving both public education and substantial treatment expansion is absolutely necessary to prevent maintenance of the status quo, which should be unacceptable to all Americans.

Our society must muster the will to address the root causes of drug abuse. The toleration of poverty, poor (or absent) education, inadequate housing, and racism provides fertile breeding ground for drug abuse. Addressing these problems will require a close coordination of drug treatment resources with those allocated for other purposes, such as the "war on drugs," as well as the integration of drug abuse treatment with other health and welfare services at both federal and state levels.

Interdiction of drugs, while an important priority of national drug policy, should not be the primary one. The costs of treatment are far lower than the costs of interdiction, and the potential savings to society, whether calculated in human or in financial terms, are greater.

Adequate financing of drug abuse treatment is essential to any serious approach to the drug problem. In particular, the current two-tiered system, that is, private treatment for those with sufficient personal resources or insurance and publicly sponsored treatment for those without, should be unacceptable in a democracy that views itself as the wealthiest nation in the world.

The availability of geographically accessible, sufficiently staffed clinics to provide treatment on demand should be a clear goal. Such a goal is cost-efficient, in terms of both dollars and human costs, in avoiding the consequences of drug abuse. These consequences include crime and the resultant incarceration and poor health, disease, and otherwise unnecessary medical treatment.

Communities need to be involved in fighting drug abuse. Drug abuse has flourished, and continues to flourish, in environments in which there is apathy, resignation, and indifference. These characteristics are just as applicable to the "national neighborhood" as to the "local neighborhood." Drug abuse is a problem which requires active involvement and persistent attention in order to overcome it.

Finally, entry into treatment should be encouraged and facilitated. This goal should be approached in the same manner in which health maintenance organizations, hospitals, and physicians now advertise and otherwise compete to recruit patients into treatment. This is particularly the case for private drug and alcohol treatment programs. Why should this not also be the case for publicly funded programs? Incentive policies could result in dramatic increases in the number of persons attending substance abuse treatment. While all cocaine abusers may not be ready for treatment, appropriate incentives could be developed to encourage such readiness. That this is possible is evident in the work of Higgins and associates (1991, 1993b).

Issues Related to Effective Treatment Programs

Several decades of research on drug abuse treatment has taught us many of the essential elements of successful treatment programs, yet they are not always applied. While these elements are not as fully understood in the case of cocaine as in the case of heroin, some generalization is certainly possible. These elements include clinics staffed with competent and appropriately trained personnel who are conversant with the full range and relative efficacy of drug abuse treatments; adequate numbers of such personnel; availability of personnel at both on-site and off-site locations, to allow for appropriate referral and follow-up; development and implementation of an *individualized*, comprehensive treatment plan for each patient; attention to the remediation of social, vocational, familial, and other problems of individual patients; and attention to the medical and psychiatric problems of the patient.

Drug abuse patients require stabilization in order to make the fullest use of drug abuse treatment services. As soon as possible following treatment entry, patients need to receive the necessary medication, counseling, social work intervention, and other services needed for stabilization. Failure to provide stabilization will likely undermine the patient's course of treatment. Such stabilization is best provided within a highly structured and supportive environment which offers appropriate incentives to maximize retention.

Effective drug abuse treatment is both comprehensive and intensive. Evidence from the heroin treatment field clearly indicates that more comprehensive and intensive levels of treatment result in better outcomes (McLellan et al., 1993).

Maximally effective treatment involves coordination among elements of the treatment system, as well as follow-up and relapse prevention, which many programs do not provide. Coordination between the criminal justice and treatment systems, for example, would both facilitate earlier recruitment into treatment and enable the making of appropriate referrals for treatment.

Treatment programs must provide habilitation for patients if they are to prevent relapse. Such habilitation can include cognitive, social, and vocational development. The provision of skills in these areas is essential if relapse is to be avoided. Furthermore, the development of skills will likely increase program retention, leading in turn to better outcomes.

A Final Note

Of the strategies being used in the United States to control cocaine use (that is, control of the growth of the coca plant in source countries, interdiction of the drug at U.S. borders, domestic enforcement of existing laws against possession and sales of cocaine or crack, education programs to prevent new use, and treatment for those already addicted), *the most cost-effective of these is drug treatment.* A 1994 Rand Corporation study estimated the sums that would be needed annually to reduce cocaine consumption by 1% (Drug Strategies, 1995). Most expensive was source country control, which would cost $783 million per year. Next was interdiction at $366 million per year. Third was domestic enforcement of laws at $246 million per year. The cost of reducing cocaine use by 1% through treatment was only $34 million per year. Given that at least $18 billion was spent by cocaine users in 1990 (Bureau of Justice Statistics, 1992), for each dollar spent on drug treatment almost $5.30 would be saved. What stands in the way is a prevalent belief in this country that treatment is an inappropriate approach for combating drug use. As Kleber has said, "Nobody ever lost an election over voting against drug abuse treatment" (quoted in Kemper, 1993, p. 5).

In order for this money to be saved and cocaine abusers treated, several changes will have to occur, in accord with the recommendations made in previous sections. In their most concise form these are, first, that research which accurately measures the effectiveness of promising treatment approaches will have to continue. Such research must assess the long-term outcomes of shorter-term interventions, as well as address the question what works for whom. The search for the one perfect treatment which will work for all addicts will have to be abandoned, a proposition which is often avoided by those espousing a particular approach to treatment. The cocaine treatment field, with a few notable exceptions, suffers from a lack of controlled clinical trials, particularly with respect to psychosocial interventions. Given the magnitude of the cocaine problem, more such trials of both existing and new interventions are clearly needed. The most effective intervention for cocaine abuse and addiction is likely one which will incorporate both pharmacological and behavioral and/or psychosocial components. Second, funding from government and other sources will have to be made available both to finance the necessary research and to pay for whichever treatments are found to be effective. Monies for research will have to be available for enough time so that long-term effects can be assessed; funds for treatment may be needed by individual addicts throughout their lifetime. Third, the public at large will have to be educated so that they understand that more extreme methods of drug control (for example, mandatory minimum sentences) are unlikely to be effective in reducing drug use and will therefore be ineffective in restraining the sequelae of drug use, including crime and welfare costs.

Notes / References / Indexes

Notes

1. The Problem of Cocaine Abuse and Addiction

1. The term *erythroxylon* was coined in 1749 by Antoine Laurent de Jussieu because of the red color of the wood of some species of the plant. *Coca* was added to the term in 1786 by Lamarck as a phonetic translation of the Incan *khoka*, meaning "plant" (Dowdeswell, 1876; Johnston, 1853).

2. Evidence of cocaine has been found in a 3,000-year-old Egyptian mummy, although the means by which a native American plant made its way to Africa are unknown (Karch, 1993; Parsche, Balabanova, and Pirsig, 1993). Such a finding does, however, lead to interesting speculation (see, for example, Brothwell and Spigelman, 1993; Moore, 1993).

3. Catarrh was "an early catch-all phrase for all that might ail you, from runny nose to tuberculosis" (Gay et al., 1973, p. 415).

4. Interestingly, caffeine has recently been found to potentiate the effect of cocaine in animals (Musto, 1992).

5. There is some dispute over the amount, with Gold (1992) reporting that in 1900 an 8-ounce serving of Coca-Cola contained 60 mg of cocaine—quite a substantial dose.

6. There appear to be several areas of dispute about this event, however. Early literature, produced approximately 25 years after the fact, asserts that the isolation of the alkaloid occurred in 1859 (Freud, 1884, reprinted 1984; Koller, 1884), while later scholarly work claims that the isolation occurred anywhere from 1858 (Forno, Young, and Levitt, 1981) to 1860 (Gay et al., 1973; Schatzman, Sabbadini, and Forti, 1976; Spotts and Shontz, 1980) to 1862 (Nicholi, 1984). Dispute also exists as to the name given to the alkaloid. The *Journal of the American Medical Association* (1912) claims that "cocain" was the given name. This spelling was used throughout the early decades of the twentieth century by that journal.

7. Although usage declined in Europe after 1930, cocaine's popularity among Nazi officials from that time through World War II has been reported (Spotts and Shontz, 1980).

8. In 1902 only 3% to 8% of all cocaine sold in major metropolitan areas was found to have been used for medical or dental purposes (Gay et al., 1973).

9. Fear of cocaine has been used to further racist stereotypes. In 1900 reports of the "cocain habit in the negro," who supposedly obtained the drug in "drug stores," were reported in the *Journal of the American Medical Association* (Jones, 1900), and in 1911 a popular magazine claimed that most attacks on white women in the South were the result of the "coke-crazed Negro brain" (Moffett, 1911, p. 604). In 1918 the *New York Times* declared that cocaine use was the result of a "German plot to enslave the United States" (Young, 1987, p. 179).

10. Medical interest was maintained, however, with new articles in the literature citing additional medical uses for the drug, for example, for whooping cough (Wells and Carré, 1895), as well as reports of "the peculiar circular perforation of the cartilaginous nasal septum" (Crookshank, 1921, p. 917) and descriptions of cocaine hallucinations and acute cocaine poisoning (Tatum, Atkinson, and Collins, 1925; Zucker, 1933).

11. Amphetamines did not remain a "safe" drug for long, however. By the late 1940s reports of their dangers had already been published (Ray, 1978). Their popularity was also evident: "This was the period of charm bracelets with an attached pillbox and the advertisement: FOR 'BENZEDRINE' IF YOU'RE HAVING FUN AND GOING ON FOREVER, 'ASPIRIN' IF IT'S ALL A HEADACHE. Wearing your bracelet and singing one of the recently current pop tunes, 'Who Put the Benzedrine in Mrs. Murphy's Ovaltine' [was indicative of this popularity]" (Ray, 1978, pp. 278–279).

12. The term *abuse,* in the sense of substances of abuse, has typically been defined as any use (usually excessive and persistent), by self-administration, of a chemical substance that is inconsistent with approved medical opinion or social pattern within a culture, typically where such use carries with it the notion of social disapproval (see, for example, Jaffe, 1990; Sheridan, Patterson, and Gustafson, 1985). In this volume the term *use* is employed with some frequency, not out of any disagreement with definitions such as this of *abuse* but because of the greater precision it imparts.

13. The Drug Abuse Warning Network (DAWN) is an ongoing national survey of hospital emergency departments conducted by the Substance Abuse and Mental Health Services Administration. This survey, which has been conducted since the early 1970s, collects data on patients seeking hospital emergency treatment related to their use of an illegal drug or the nonmedical use of a drug within the contiguous United States and in 21 metropolitan areas. Data collected by DAWN are used to develop population-based estimates of current drug abuse trends, and represent a widely used index of the prevalence of drug abuse in the nation.

14. Drug Use Forecasting data are based on interview and urine specimens collected in selected booking facilities throughout the United States. For two weeks each quarter, data are collected on booked arrestees. Rather than being selected on a random basis, persons are selected for inclusion in this survey with the intent of collecting a target sample size and range of criminal charges.

15. Cocaine abuse and addiction are far from being solely an American problem. Nonetheless, this country has been the primary location of the current

cocaine epidemic, and of much of the work which has been done on the problem as well. For descriptions of the cocaine problem in other countries, the reader is referred to Strang, Johns, and Caan (1993) and Gossop et al. (1994) for the United Kingdom, Bühringer et al. (1994) and Reuband (1992) for Germany, and Grund, Adriaans, and Kaplan (1991) and Grund and Blanken (1993) for the Netherlands.

16. Synthetic estimation applies mathematical formulas to available data to infer information about data which are unavailable. In this case data about cocaine use in specific cities were used to infer the use of cocaine in all cities and then in all of the United States (Rhodes, 1993).

17. The use of another stimulant, amphetamine, increased by 62%, from 2,296 emergency room mentions in 1991 to 3,713 in 1992. Both this increase and that for cocaine were statistically significant.

18. Cyclothymic disorder is a chronic, fluctuating mood disorder characterized by periods of hypomanic symptoms alternating with depressive symptoms.

19. *Diagnostic and Statistical Manual of Mental Disorders,* 3rd ed., rev. (1987).

20. Chiu, Vaughn, and Carzoli (1990) noted that special education needs of cocaine-exposed children when they enter school would further raise the costs of care.

21. The monies for treatment actually represent a rather drastic decrease (from about 35% to about 20%) when considered as a percentage of the total federal drug abuse budget (Bureau of Justice Statistics, 1992). Of interest is a 1994 Rand Corporation study which found that reducing cocaine use by 1% would cost $783 million per year in source country control, $366 million per year in interdiction, $246 million per year in domestic enforcement, and only $34 million per year for treatment (Drug Strategies, 1995).

22. This figure is based on 1990 values of $15,823 median income, 15% federal income tax rate, 7.65% social security and Medicare tax rate, and an average of $1,662 per person in state and local taxes (U.S. Bureau of the Census, 1994).

23. Methamphetamine, also variously called "poor man's cocaine," "crack," "ice," "crystal," crystal methamphetamine, and "speed," produces many of the same central stimulating effects seen in amphetamine and cocaine use. A white, odorless, bitter powder which is soluble in alcohol, it has a long serum half-life. It is used intranasally, mixed in liquid and taken orally, or melted and injected intravenously. "Ice" is a smokable form that vaporizes when heated in a glass pipe and is then inhaled. Powdered methamphetamine, sometimes called "MAP," can be inhaled intranasally or liquefied, either by heating or by being mixed with water and injected intravenously. It can also be mixed with a liquid (frequently coffee or tea) and taken orally (Lynch and House, 1992).

2.   Administration, Action, and Pharmacology of Cocaine

1. Street names for some of these drugs, either alone or in combination, include "bennies," "beans," or "whites" (D, L-amphetamine), "dexies," "brownies" (dextroamphetamine), "black beauties" (D, L-amphetamine plus dextroamphetamine), "meth," "speed," "crystal" (methamphetamine), and "greenies" (dextroamphetamine plus amobarbitol; Goff and Ciraulo, 1991).

2. Cocaine is classified as a Schedule II drug under the Controlled Substances Act, Title II of the Comprehensive Drug Abuse Prevention and Control Act of 1970. Schedule II drugs have a high potential for abuse; either a currently accepted medical use in treatment in the United States or a currently accepted medical use with severe restrictions; and abuse potential leading to severe psychological or physical dependence.

3. A study by Paly et al. (1979) of coca leaf chewing among native Peruvians found that the chewing of approximately 10 gm of cocaine leaves produced plasma concentrations ranging from 50 to 90 ng/ml. Fifty grams of leaves chewed over three hours produced cocaine plasma levels ranging from 150 to 450 ng/ml. By comparison, the smoking of coca paste yields levels of 91 to 462 ng/ml after three minutes.

4. Benzol, or benzine, is a highly toxic petroleum derivative made from light coal tar oil. In addition to its use in the manufacture of motor fuels, detergents, and insecticides, it also used as a solvent—the reason for its use in this process.

5. It has been suggested that the term "speedball" originated during the 1860s, when competition cyclists used a cocaine-heroin mixture to enhance performance (Kaplan, Husch, and Bieleman, 1994). Other names applied to this combination of drugs are "dynamite" and "whizbang," although the latter term has also been applied to cocaine-morphine combinations (Cox et al., 1983).

6. Although pharmacological kindling has been demonstrated in animals in response to cocaine administration (see, for example, Post, Kopanda, and Black, 1976; Post, Weiss, and Pert, 1984), and this phenomenon is generally accepted as occurring in response to cocaine administration in humans, at least one investigator (Abraham, 1989) has questioned the existence of sufficient evidence for cocaine-induced kindling in humans. Both behavioral sensitization and kindling can result from repeated, intermittent application of either psychomotor stimulants, such as cocaine, or electrical stimulation of the same brain site(s). The two phenomena have in common a progressively increasing response to repeated administrations of the same stimulus (Post, Weiss, and Pert, 1984). Kindling has been demonstrated in animal studies, where the repeated administration of cocaine, over time, in subconvulsive doses, can result in dyskinesias and increased susceptibility to seizures (Post and Kopanda, 1976; Post, Kopanda, and Black, 1976).

7. Several authors have noted the confusion which often arises from use of the term "freebase." Freebase is cocaine produced by freeing the alkaloid from the hydrochloride salt in a straightforward process. Freebase is also sometimes called "base," although this latter term, deriving from the Spanish base (for "paste"), is most appropriately applied to the crude, early-stage product of the refining of coca leaves. Thus, freebase is a distinctly new compound with its own physiochemical properties, including a lower melting point, resistance to thermal degradation, and lipid solubility (Khalsa, Tashkin, and Perrochet, 1992; Siegel, 1982a).

8. Khalsa, Tashkin, and Perrochet (1992) found that 96% of their sample of crack smokers used baking soda in the refining process, while 88% most frequently used water to extract the freebase. Only 9% used ammonia and 4%

used ether. The low rates of use of ammonia and ether may reflect awareness of the risks of using volatile substances resulting from the publicity surrounding the associated dangers (that is, the publicity given celebrities who
have sustained injuries while preparing freebase).

9. Inciardi (1987) notes that in Peru, Bolivia, Ecuador, and Brazil, the combination of a marijuana cigarette laced with coca paste had been referred to
as a *pitillo*. More recently this term has been applied to a combination of
marijuana and cocaine paste residue, the dregs that remain in the processing drum after coca paste residue has been removed. This combination is
extremely toxic owing to the higher than usual concentrations of sulfuric
acid and petroleum products. Needless to say, smoking coca paste containing kerosene and other solvents may have potentially serious adverse effects
on the lung and liver in addition to those of cocaine itself (Brown, 1989).

10. The highly addictive nature of crack smoking, particularly among teenagers,
is evident in the results of a study by Schwartz, Luxenberg, and Hoffmann
(1991), who found progression from first use of cocaine to use at least once
weekly in 12% of snorters but in 60% of crack smokers who had used cocaine at least ten times.

11. One way in which crack and freebase differ is that the former is more likely
to have residual salts and other impurities present in the end product
(Cohen, 1986). The addition of baking powder, ammonia, and other bases
during the refining process also adds mass to the final product. Thus, the final combustion products resulting from crack use may differ chemically from
those resulting from use of freebase (Khalsa, Tashkin, and Perrochet, 1992;
Snyder et al., 1988).

12. The NADR program was a major nationwide study which involved 26,356
out-of-treatment injection drug users and 5,435 sexual partners. The large sample size, and the inclusion of 50 cities and 60 separate communities with
high rates of injection drug use, likely resulted in a highly representative
sample of the injection drug user population in the United States.

13. The finding by Karler et al. (1989) that haloperidol selectively blocked sensitization to cocaine-induced stereotypy but not to convulsions, while MK-
801, the NMDA antagonist, blocked the development of sensitization to locomotor stimulation, stereotypy, and convulsions, suggests that the
glutamate system is also involved in the development of sensitization to the
dopaminergic and convulsant effects of cocaine.

14. The Diagnostic Interview Schedule is a structured psychiatric interview designed for non-clinicians (see Robbins et al. 1981). Hasin and Grant (1987)
have reported that drug assessments made with the Diagnostic Interview
Schedule agree well with extensive, reliable clinical assessments of drug abuse
and/or dependence.

15. A psychological test on which the patient selects those adjectives (from a
list of 300) which are most descriptive of his or her personality, the Adjective
Check List is intended to measure basic psychological needs such as achievement, dominance, endurance, order, and so on (Gough and Heilbrun, 1983).

16. The Millon Clinical Multiaxial Inventory (Millon, 1984) is a psychological
self-report inventory consisting of 175 items intended to measure the re-
spondent's standing on 8 basic personality styles (schizoid-asocial, avoidant,

dependent-submissive, histrionic-gregarious, narcissistic, antisocial-aggressive, compulsive-conforming, passive-aggressive-negativistic), 3 pathological personality styles (schizotypal-schizoid, borderline-cycloid, and paranoid), and 9 clinical syndromes (anxiety, somatoform, hypomania, dysthymia, alcohol abuse, drug abuse, psychotic thinking, psychotic depression, and psychotic delusion).

3.   The Subjective Experience, Course, and Parameters of Cocaine Abuse

1. A variant of this hallucination, which is also called *Magnan's sign,* after the French psychiatrist who first labeled it, may take the shape of crystals moving under the skin (Magnan and Saury, 1889, cited by Siegel, 1978).
2. Gustatory responses were among those reported by Freud (1884; reprinted 1984) in his assessment of research existing at that time.
3. The Epidemiological Catchment Area study was a collaborative study of approximately 21,000 persons at five sites in the United States (Baltimore, Durham, Los Angeles, New Haven, and St. Louis) conducted between 1980 and 1984 and involving probability samples of area residents aged 18 and older.
4. In the case of opiate abusers, opiate-related stimuli elicit either drug-like or drug-opposite reactions. In the case of cocaine, physiological responses are more diffuse, representing both signs of stimulant drug effects and nonspecific arousal effects (O'Brien, Childress, et al., 1992).
5. The Beck Depression Inventory is a psychological test consisting of twenty-one items, each comprising four statements that reflect increasing severity of a specific depressive symptom (Beck et al., 1979).
6. These phenomena may result from changes in the optic system rather than being hallucinatory in nature (Cohen, 1984).
7. Convulsions may, of course, result from a large single dose as well as from a spree, which involves administration of multiple smaller doses.
8. Gawin and his associates (Gawin, 1991; Gawin and Ellinwood, 1988; Gawin and Kleber, 1986a) noted the lack of desire for more cocaine at this time in contrast with the intense desire for more of the abused substance in the case of opiates, sedatives, and alcohol.
9. American Psychiatric Association, the *Diagnostic and Statistical Manual of Mental Disorders,* 3rd ed. (1980).
10. American Psychiatric Association, the *Diagnostic and Statistical Manual of Mental Disorders,* 4th ed. (1994).

4.   Characteristics and Behavioral Patterns of Cocaine Abusers

1. Use appears to remain constant over most ages. Chitwood (1993) found that in the NADR study, IDUs between the ages of 30 and 39 were as likely to abuse crack (50.7%) as were injectors both in their twenties (52.0%) and under 20 years of age (51.6%). Crack abuse was somewhat less prevalent among IDUs over 50 years of age (34.4%).
2. In addition, of the unemployed subjects in the same study, 26% were work-

ing illegally (that is, without being officially reported), or "off the books," a not uncommon situation for substance abusers.

5.   Cocaine Abuse, Psychopathology, and Personality Disorders

1. See Platt (1986), chap. 8, and (1995a), chap. 5, for a review and discussion of this issue in heroin addicts.
2. In a study of retention in therapeutic communities, De Leon (1993) noted that among admissions to a therapeutic community, primary cocaine abusers had fewer occurrences of multiple diagnoses, and suggested that they may have less pervasive psychological problems. Crack use, however, may be destabilizing, in that its users appeared to have lower thresholds of tolerance for irritation, frustration, and provocation.
3. The Epidemiological Catchment Area study was a collaborative project conducted at five sites in the United States (Baltimore, Durham, Los Angeles, New Haven, St. Louis) between 1980 and 1984. The population studied included 21,000 individuals aged 18 and older who were selected for inclusion using probability sampling methods.
4. Anthony, Tien, and Petronis (1989) have suggested that the reason for this last finding may be related to experience with specific drug side effects. Marijuana users are accustomed to a sensation of increased cardiovascular activity in response to drugs of abuse. Thus, those with no prior experience of this sensation would be more likely to have a panic attack.
5. An alternative explanation for the development of cocaine-induced panic disorders is behavioral sensitization. Louie, Lannon, and Ketter (1989) reviewed the evidence for both mechanisms, and concluded that the existing evidence favored a kindling mechanism.
6. Siegel (1978) credits the first report of cocaine hallucinations to Paolo Mantegazza's "On the Hygienic and Medical Virtues of Coca," which appeared in 1859 (reprinted in Andrews and Solomon, 1975). See also Freud's description in his *Cocaine Papers* (Freud, 1884, reprinted 1974).
7. One study has suggested that such perfusion abnormalities are reversible with buprenorphine treatment and cessation of drug use (Holman et al., 1993).

6.   Medical and Related Consequences of Cocaine Abuse

1. Medical examiner data can be difficult to interpret, however, since a "drug abuse death" can mean "drug-induced," that is, caused by an overdose; "drug-related," that is, with drug use as a contributory factor; "in combination with medical disorder," that is, probably caused in part by drugs; and so on.
2. Cocaine "body packers" have been reported to carry up to 175 packets of cocaine. Each packet may contain some 3 to 6 grams of cocaine at 85% to 90% purity. Condoms are usually used, although finger cots, plastic bags, and balloons have also been used for this purpose. The packer will swallow the packages or insert them into the rectum before boarding an airplane in another country, later expelling them after passing through customs in-

spection (Commissaris, 1989). A constipating agent such as paregoric will frequently be taken beforehand, then, upon arrival, laxatives, enemas, and fast foods (hamburgers) will be ingested to help pass the packets through the gastrointestinal tract (Wetli, 1993).

3. A case of madarosis secondary to crack smoking was described by Tames and Goldenring (1986). The loss of eyebrows and eyelashes was attributed to their having been singed by the hot cocaine vapors rising from the pipe used to smoke the cocaine.

7. Cocaine Abuse and Sexual Behavior

1. See Platt (1995b), chap. 6, for a discussion of the epidemiology and transmission of HIV among drug users.

2. Typically the price of sex falls to correspond to the unit price of the street drug being purchased—in this case, crack.

8. Major Nonpharmacological Treatment Modalities

1. *Standards für die Durchführung von Katamnesen bei Abhängigen* (Deutsche Gesellshaft für Suchtfroschung und Suchttherapie e. V. [Hrsg.], 1994). The latest update of the *Standards, Documentationstandards 2 für die Behandlung von Abhängigen* (Documentation Standards 2 for the Treatment of Addictions), is available in English. See also Platt et al. (1996) for a discussion of the *Standards* in English.

2. While not usually mentioned as an indicator for inpatient treatment, homelessness clearly works against successful outpatient intervention.

3. This is also the case for psychiatric disorders in general (see Kiesler, 1982). For research regarding the treatment of alcoholism, see Miller and Hester (1986).

4. The operant model may be contrasted with the classic conditioning approach, which emphasizes the role of temporal contiguity in the development of associations between previously neutral cues and reinforcers which come to elicit drug taking (see, for example, O'Brien et al., 1975, 1977; Wikler, 1965, 1973).

5. Such aversive consequences were derived from the patients' own views of the consequences that could result from continued drug use. Thus, for a patient who feared arrest in the event of continued use, a letter informing the district attorney or the Drug Enforcement Administration of such use might be deposited with the program, to be sent if drug use continued.

6. This finding is confirmed by studies on nicotine analyzed according to behavioral economics techniques (Bickel, DeGrandpre, and Higgins, 1993).

9. Pharmacological Interventions in Cocaine Abuse Treatment

1. Symptoms of this syndrome include jitteriness, shakiness, increased anxiety, and insomnia. See Pohl et al. (1988) for a description of this disorder. This syndrome can develop even with low doses of tricyclic antidepressants in persons who are sensitive to these drugs.

2. Tropamine contains the enzyme inhibitor D-phenylalanine, the dopamine precursors L-phenylalanine, L-tyrosine, L-tryptophan, and L-glutamine, and vitamin B complex, ascorbate, folic acid, zinc, calcium, and magnesium, all of which are cofactors in transmitter synthesis, or promote gastrointestinal absorption of amino acids.

3. Haloperidol, a central dopamine blocker, has been shown in a rat model to have limited efficacy in preventing the toxic effects of cocaine. While haloperidol decreased the incidence of cocaine-induced seizures when administered in high doses, it did not significantly reduce cocaine-induced mortality. This effect is in contrast to that obtained with amphetamines, where haloperidol failed to reduce the incidence of amphetamine-induced seizures but did lower the mortality rate (Derlet, Albertson, and Rice, 1989).

4. Haloperidol is not recommended for the treatment of acute cocaine toxicity, according to Goldfrank and Hoffman (1993), because of a lack of experimental support for such use. Among the reasons cited by these writers is the presence of significant clinical difficulties encountered in using haloperidol in sedative-hypnotic withdrawal, particularly in the presence of agitation and hyperthermia (see, for example, Greenblatt et al., 1978), which in the acutely agitated or psychotic patient may reflect the loss of thermoregulatory control. There is also a high likelihood of acute dystonic reactions generally associated with cocaine intoxication (see, for example, Merab, 1988; Farrell and Diehl, 1991), and associated specifically with the use of haloperidol in otherwise healthy cocaine addicts.

5. Lidocaine, itself a seizure-provoking agent when administered simultaneously with cocaine, has been shown in rats to increase the incidence of both seizures and death dramatically over what would be expected with cocaine alone (Derlet, Albertson, and Tharratt, 1991).

References

Abel, F. L., Wilson, S. P., Zhao, R. R., and Fennell, W. H. (1989). Cocaine depresses the canine myocardium. *Circulatory Shock, 28,* 309–319.

Abelson, U. I. and Miller, J. D. (1985). A decade of trends in cocaine use in the household population. In N. J. Kozel and E. H. Adams (Eds.), *Cocaine use in America: Epidemiologic and clinical perspectives* (NIDA Research Monograph No. 61). Rockville, Md.: NIDA, pp. 35–49.

Abraham, H. D. (1989). Stimulants, panic, and BEAM EEG abnormalities (letter). *American Journal of Psychiatry, 146,* 947–948.

Acker, D., Sachs, B. P., Tracey, K. J., and Wise, W. E. (1983). Abruptio placentae associated with cocaine use. *American Journal of Obstetrics and Gynecology, 146(2),* 220–221.

Adebimpe, V. R. (1993). Race and crack cocaine. *Journal of the American Medical Association, 270(1),* 45.

Adrouny, A. and Magnusson, P. (1985). Pneumopericardium from cocaine inhalation. *New England Journal of Medicine, 313,* 48–49.

Agosti, V., Nunes, E., Stewart, J. W., and Quitkin, F. M. (1991). Patient factors related to early attrition from an outpatient cocaine research clinic: A preliminary report. *International Journal of the Addictions, 26(3),* 327–334.

Alldredge, B., Lowenstein, D. H., and Simon, R. P. (1989). Seizures associated with recreational drug abuse. *Neurology, 39,* 1037–39.

Alling, F. A., Johnson, B. D., and Elmoghazy, E. (1990). Cranial electrostimulation (CES) use in the detoxification of opiate-dependent patients. *Journal of Substance Abuse Treatment, 7,* 173–180.

Allred, R. J. and Ewer, S. (1981). Fatal pulmonary edema following intravenous "free-base" cocaine use. *Annals of Emergency Medicine, 10(8),* 441–442.

Alper, K. R., Chabot, R. J., Kim, A. H., Prichep, L. S., and John, R. (1990). Quantitative EEG correlates of crack cocaine dependence. *Psychiatry Research, 35,* 95–105.

Alterman, A. I., O'Brien, C. P., and Droba, M. (1993). Day hospital vs. inpatient rehabilitation of cocaine abusers: An interim report. In F. M. Tims and C. G. Leukefeld (Eds.), *Cocaine treatment: Research and clinical perspectives*

(NIDA Research Monograph Series No. 135). Rockville, Md.: NIDA, pp. 150–162.

—— O'Brien, C. P., McLellan, A. T., August, D. S., Snider, E. C., Droba, M., Cornish, J. W., Hall, C. P., Raphaelson, A. H., and Schrade, F. X. (1994). Effectiveness and costs of inpatient versus day hospital cocaine rehabilitation. *Journal of Nervous and Mental Disease, 182(3),* 157–163.

Ambre, J. J., Belknap, S. M., Nelson, J., Ruo, T. I., Shin, S. G., and Atkinson, A. J. (1988). Acute tolerance to cocaine in humans. *Clinical Pharmacology and Therapeutics, 44(1),* 1–8.

American Medical Assocation (1908). The propaganda for reform in proprietary medicines. *American Medical Association,* 82–87.

Ananth, J., Vandewater, S., Kamal, M., Brodsky, A., Gamal, R., and Miller, M. (1989). Missed diagnosis of substance abuse in psychiatric patients. *Hospital and Community Psychiatry, 40(3),* 297–299.

Anderson, W. H., O'Malley, J. E., and Lazare, A. (1972). Failure of outpatient treatment of drug abuse: II. Amphetamines, barbiturates, hallucinogens. *American Journal of Psychiatry, 128(12),* 1572–76.

Andrews, G. and Solomon, D. (Eds.) (1975). *The coca leaf and cocaine papers.* New York: Harcourt Brace Jovanovich.

Andriani, J. and Zepernick, R. (1964). Clinical effectiveness of drugs used for topical anesthesia. *Journal of the American Medical Association, 188(8),* 711–716.

Änggård, E., Jönsson, L-E., Hogmark, A-L., and Gunne, L-M. (1973). Amphetamine metabolism in amphetamine psychosis. *Clinical Pharmacology and Therapeutics, 14(5),* 870–880.

Angrist, B., Lee, H. K., and Gershon, S. (1974). The antagonism of amphetamine induced symptomatology by a neuroleptic. *American Journal of Psychiatry, 131,* 817–819.

—— Rotrosen, J. and Gershon, S. (1980). Differential effects of amphetamine and neuroleptics on negative and positive symptoms in schizophrenia. *Psychopharmacology, 72,* 17–19.

—— Sathanathan, G., Wilk, S., and Gershon, S. (1975). Amphetamine psychosis: Behavioral and biochemical aspects. In S. W. Matthysse, and S. S. Kety (Eds.), *Catecholamines and schizophrenia.* Oxford: Pergamon Press, pp. 13–23.

Angrist, B. M. and Gershon, S. (1970). The phenomenology of experimentally induced amphetamine psychosis: Preliminary observations. *Biological Psychiatry, 2,* 95–107.

Anker, A. L. and Crowley, T. J. (1982). Use of contingency contracts in specialty clinics for cocaine abuse. In L. S. Harris (Ed.), *Problems of drug dependence, 1981* (NIDA Research Monograph No. 41). Rockville, Md.: NIDA, pp. 452–459.

Anthony, J. C. and Petronis, K. R. (1989). Cocaine and heroin dependence compared: Evidence from an epidemiologic field survey. *American Journal of Public Health, 79(10),* 1409–10.

—— and Trinkoff, A. M. (1989). United States epidemiologic data on drug use and abuse: How are they relevant to testing abuse liability of drugs? In M. W. Fischman and N. K. Mello (Eds.), *Testing for abuse liability of drugs in humans* (NIDA Research Monograph No. 92). Washington, D.C.: NIDA, pp. 241–266.

———— Tien, A. Y., and Petronis, K. R. (1989). Epidemiologic evidence on cocaine use and panic attacks. *American Journal of Epidemiology, 129,* 543–549.

———— Warner, L. A., and Kessler, R. C. (1994). Comparative epidemiology of dependence on tobacco, alcohol, controlled substances, and inhalants: Basic findings from the National Comorbidity Survey. *Experimental and Clinical Psychopharmacology, 2(3),* 244–268.

Ardila, A., Rosselli, M., and Strumwasser, S. (1991). Neuropsychological deficits in chronic cocaine abusers. *International Journal of Neuroscience, 57,* 73–79.

Arndt, I., Dorozynsky, L., Woody, G., McLellan, A. T., and O'Brien, C. P. (1990). Desipramine treatment of cocaine abuse in methadone maintenance patients. In L. S. Harris (Ed.), *Problems of drug dependence, 1989* (NIDA Research Monograph No. 95). Washington, D.C.: NIDA, pp. 322–325.

Arndt, I. O., McLellan, A. T., Dorozynsky, L., Woody, G. E., and O'Brien, C. P. (1994). Desipramine treatment for cocaine dependence: Role of antisocial personality disorder. *Journal of Nervous and Mental Disease, 182(3),* 151–156.

Aroesty, D. J., Stanley, R. B., Jr., and Crockett, D. M. (1986). Pneumomediastinum and cervical emphysema from the inhalation of "free based" cocaine: Report of three cases. *Otolaryngology of Head and Neck Surgery, 94,* 372–374.

Aronson, T. A. and Craig, T. J. (1986). Cocaine precipitation of panic disorder. *American Journal of Psychiatry, 143,* 643–645.

Ascher, E., Stauffer, J., and Gaasch, W. (1988). Coronary artery spasm, cardiac arrest, transient electrocardiographic Q waves and stunned myocardium in cocaine-associated acute myocardial infarction. *American Journal of Cardiology, 61,* 939–941.

Ashley, R. (1975). *Cocaine: Its history, uses and effects.* New York: St. Martin's Press, p. 150.

Azrin, N. H. (1976). Improvements in the community reinforcement approach to alcoholism. *Behavior Research and Therapy, 14,* 339–348.

———— Sisson, W., Meyers, R., and Godley, M. (1982). Alcoholism treatment by disulfiram and community reinforcement therapy. *Journal of Behavior Therapy and Experimental Psychiatry, 13,* 105–112.

Azuma, S. D. and Chasnoff, I. J. (1993). Outcome of children prenatally exposed to cocaine and other drugs: A path analysis of three-year data. *Pediatrics, 92(3),* 396–402.

Baekeland, F. and Lundwall, L. (1975). Dropping out of treatment: A critical review. *Psychological Bulletin, 82(5),* 738–783.

Bailey, M. E., Fraire, A. E., Greenberg, S. D., Barnard, J., and Cagle, P. T. (1994). Pulmonary histopathology in cocaine abusers. *Human Pathology, 25(2),* 203–207.

Bale, R. N., Van Stone, W. W., Kuldau, J. M., Engelsing, T. M., Elashoff, R. M., and Zarcone, V. P. (1980). Therapeutic communities vs. methadone maintenance: A prospective controlled study of narcotic addiciton treatment: Design and one-year follow-up. *Archive of General Psychiatry, 37,* 179–193.

Ball, J. C. (1994). What I would most like to know: Why has it proved so difficult to match drug abuse patients to appropriate treatment? *Addiction, 89,* 263–265.

———— and Ross, A. R. (1991). *The effectiveness of methadone maintenance treatment: Patients, programs, services, and outcome.* New York: Springer Verlag.

———— Lange, W. R., Myers, C. P., and Friedman, S. R. (1988). Reducing the risk of AIDS through methadone maintenance treatment. *Journal of Health and Social Behavior, 29,* 214–226.

Barden, J. C. (1989, December 24). Crack smoking seen as a peril to the lungs. *New York Times,* p. 19.

Barglow, P. and Kotun, J. (1992). Methadone and cocaine. *Hospital and Community Psychiatry, 43(12),* 1245–46.

Barnett, G., Hawks, R., and Resnick, R. (1981). Cocaine pharmacokinetics in humans. *Journal of Ethnopharmacology, 3,* 353–366.

Barone, D. (1993). Wednesday's child: Literacy development of children prenatally exposed to crack or cocaine. *Research in the Teaching of English, 27(1),* 7–45.

Barth, C. W., Bray, M., and Roberts, W. C. (1986). Rupture of the ascending aorta during cocaine intoxication. *American Journal of Cardiology, 57,* 496.

Bastien, A., DeHovitz, J., Covino, J. M., Smith, B., Landesman, S., Stevens, R., and McCormack, W. (1990). Risk factors for HIV infection in an urban hospital based STD clinic. Presented at the Sixth International Conference on AIDS. San Francisco, June 20–24.

Batki, S. L., Manfredi, L., Jacob, P., III, Delucchi, K., Murphy, J., Washburn, A., Goldberger, L., and Jones, R. T. (1993). Double-blind fluoxetine treatment of cocaine dependence in methadone maintenance treatment patients: Interim analysis. In L. S. Harris (Ed.), *Problems of drug dependence, 1992* (NIDA Research Monograph No. 132). Rockville, Md.: NIDA, p. 102.

—— Manfredi, L. B., Jacob, P., III, and Jones, R. T. (1993). Fluoxetine for cocaine dependence in methadone maintenance: Quantitative plasma and urine cocaine/benzoylecgonine concentrations. *Journal of Clinical Psychopharmacology, 13(4),* 243–250.

—— Manfredi, L., Sorenson, J. L., Jacob, P., Dumontet, R., and Jones, R. T. (1990). Fluoxetine for cocaine abuse in methadone patients: Preliminary findings. In L. S. Harris (Ed.), *Problems of drug dependence, 1989* (NIDA Research Monograph No. 105). Rockville, Md.: NIDA, pp. 516–517.

—— Washburn, A., Manfredi, L., Murphy, J., Herbst, M. D., Delucchi, K., Jones, T., Nanda, N., Jacob, P., III, and Jones, R. T. (1994). Fluoxetine in primary and secondary cocaine dependence: Outcome using quantitative benzoylecgonine concentration. In L. S. Harris (Ed.), *Problems of drug dependence, 1993* (NIDA Research Monograph No. 141). Rockville, Md.: NIDA, p. 140.

Batlle, M. A. and Wilcox, W. D. (1993). Pulmonary edema in an infant following passive inhalation of free-base ("crack") cocaine. *Clinical Pediatrics,* 105–106.

Baxter, L. R. (1983). Desipramine in the treatment of hypersomnolence following abrupt cessation of cocaine use. *American Journal of Psychiatry, 140(11),* 1525–26.

Bean-Bayog, M. (1986). Psychopathology produced by alcoholism. In R. E. Meyer (Ed.), *Psychopathology and addictive disorders.* New York: Guilford Press, pp. 334–345.

—— (1991). The lay treatment community. In P. E. Nathan, J. W. Langebucher, W. Frankenstein, and B. S. McCrady (Eds.), *Annual review of addictions research and treatment, 1,* 343–351.

Beck, A. T., Rush, A. J., Shaw, B. F., and Emery, G. (1979). *Cognitive therapy of depression.* New York: Guilford Press.

—— Wright, F. D., and Newman, C. F. (1992). Cocaine abuse. In A. Freeman and F. Dattilio (Eds.), *Comprehensive casebook of cognitive therapy.* New York: Plenum Press, pp. 185–192.

—— Wright, F. D., Newman, C. F., and Liese, B. S. (1993). *Cognitive therapy of substance abuse.* New York: Guilford Press.

Beck, N. E. and Hale, J. E. (1993). Cocaine "body packers." *British Journal of Surgery, 80(12),* 1513–16.

Beeram, M. R., Abedin, M., Young, M., Leftridge, C., and Dhanidreddy, R. (1994). Effect of intrauterine cocaine exposure on respiratory distress syndrome in very low birthweight infants. *Journal of the National Medical Association, 86(5),* 370–372.

Bell, D. S. (1973). The experimental reproduction of amphetamine psychosis. *Archives of General Psychiatry, 29,* 35–40.

Bellis, D. J. (1993). Reduction of AIDS risk among 41 heroin addicted female street prostitutes: Effects of free methadone maintenance. *Journal of Addictive Disease, 12(1),* 7–23.

Benchimol, A., Bartall, H., and Desser, K. B. (1978). Accelerated ventricular rhythm and cocaine abuse. *Annals of Internal Medicine, 88,* 519–520.

Benjamin-Bauman, J., Reiss, M. L., and Bailey, J. S. (1984). Increasing appointment keeping by reducing the call-appointment interval. *Journal of Applied Behavior Analysis, 17,* 295–301.

Berger, P., Gawin, F. H., and Kosten, T. R. (1989). Treatment of cocaine abuse with mazindol. *Lancet, 1,* 283.

Berry, J., van Gorp, W. G., Herzberg, D. S., Hinkin, C., Boone, K., Steinman, L., and Wilkins, J. N. (1993). Neuropsychological deficits in abstinent cocaine abusers: Preliminary findings after two weeks of abstinence. *Drug and Alcohol Dependence, 32(3),* 231–237.

Bickel, W. K., DeGrandpre, R. J., and Higgins, S. T. (1993). Behavioral economics: A novel experimental approach to the study of drug dependence. *Drug and Alcohol Dependence, 33,* 173–192.

—— Stitzer, M. L., Bigelow, G. E., Liebson, I. A., Jasinski, D. R., and Johnson, R. E. (1988). Buprenorphine: Dose-related blockade of opioid challenge effects in opioid dependent humans. *Journal of Pharmacology and Experimental Therapeutics, 247,* 47–53.

Bilsky, E. J., Montegut, M. J., Delong, C. L., and Reid, L. D. (1992). Opioidergic modulation of cocaine conditioned place preferences. *Life Sciences, 50(14),* 85–90.

Bingol, N., Fuchs, M., Diaz, V., Stone, R. K., and Gromisch, D. S. (1987). Teratogenicity of cocaine in humans. *Journal of Pediatrics, 110,* 93–96.

Black, J. L., Dolan, M. P., Penk, W. E., Robinowitz, R., and DeFord, H. A. (1987). The effect of increased cocaine use on drug treatment. *Addictive Behaviors, 12(3),* 289–292.

Blum, K., Allison, D., Trachtenberg, M. C., Williams, R. W., and Loeblich, L. A. (1988). Reduction of both drug hunger and withdrawal against advice rate of cocaine abusers in a 30-day inpatient treatment program by the neuronutrient tropamine. *Current Therapeutic Research, 43(6),* 1204–14.

Booth, R. E., Watters, J. K., and Chitwood, D. D. (1993). HIV risk-related sex behaviors among injection drug users, crack smokers, and injection drug users who smoke crack. *American Journal of Public Health, 83(8),* 1144–48.

———— Koester, S., Brewster, J. T., et al. (1991). Intravenous drug users and AIDS: Risk behaviors. *American Journal of Drug and Alcohol Abuse, 17*, 337–353.

Borowsky, B. and Kuhn, C. M. (1991). Monoamine mediation of cocaine-induced hypothalamo-pituitary-adrenal activation. *Journal of Pharmacology and Experimental Therapeutics, 256(1)*, 204–210.

Bourgois, P. (1989). In search of Horatio Alger: Culture and ideology in the crack economy. *Contemporary Drug Problems, 16*, 619–649.

Bowser, B. P. (1989). Crack and AIDS: An ethnographic impression. *Journal of the National Medical Association, 81(5)*, 538–540.

Boyd, C. and Mieczkowski, T. (1990). Drug use, health, family and social support in "crack" cocaine users. *Addictive Behaviors, 15*, 481–485.

Bozarth, M. A. and Wise, R. A. (1981). Intracranial self-administration of morphine into the ventral tegmental area in rats. *Life Sciences, 28*, 551–555.

———— and Wise, R. A. (1985). Toxicity associated with long-term intravenous heroin and cocaine self-administration in the rat. *Journal of the American Medical Association, 254(1)*, 81–83.

———— and Wise, R. A. (1986). Involvement of the ventral tegmental dopamine system in opioid and psychomotor reinforcement. In L. S. Harris (Ed.), *Problems of drug dependence, 1985* (NIDA Research Monograph No. 67). Washington, DC: NIDA, pp. 190–196.

Brady, K., Anton, R., Ballenger, J. C., Lydiard, B., Adinoff, B., and Selander, J. (1990). Cocaine abuse among schizophrenic patients. *American Journal of Psychiatry, 147(9)*, 1164–67.

Brady, K. T., Lydiard, R. B., Malcolm, R., and Ballenger, J. C. (1991). Cocaine-induced psychosis. *Journal of Clinical Psychiatry, 52*, 509–512.

Breakey, W. R., Goodell, H., Lorenz, P. C., and McHugh, P. R. (1974). Hallucinogenic drugs as precipitants of schizophrenia. *Psychological Medicine, 4*, 225–261.

Brecher, E. M. (1972). *Licit and illicit drugs*. Boston: Little, Brown.

Brewer, C. (1993). Treatment of cocaine abuse with monoamine oxidase inhibitors. *British Journal of Psychiatry, 163*, 815–816.

Brody, S. L., Slovis, C. M., and Wrenn, K. D. (1990). Cocaine-related medical problems: Consecutive series of 233 patients. *American Journal of Medicine, 88*, 325–331.

———— Wrenn, K. D., Wilber, M. M., and Slovis, C. M. (1990). Predicting the severity of cocaine-associated rhabdomyolysis. *Annals of Emergency Medicine, 19(10)*, 1137–43.

Brookoff, D., Campbell, E. A., and Shaw, L. M. (1993). The underreporting of cocaine-related trauma: Drug Abuse Warning Network reports vs. hospital toxicology tests. *American Journal of Public Health, 83(3)*, 369–371.

———— Cook, C., Williams, C., and Mann, C. (1994). Testing reckless drivers for cocaine and marijuana. *New England Journal of Medicine, 331(8)*, 518–522.

Brothwell, D. and Spigelman, M. (1993). Drugs in ancient populations (reply). *Lancet, 341(1)*, 1157.

Brotman, A. W., Witkie, S. M., Gelenberg, A. J., Falk, W. E., Wojcik, J., and Leahy, L. (1988). An open trial of maprotiline for the treatment of cocaine abuse: A pilot study. *Journal of Clinical Psychopharmacology, 8(2)*, 125–127.

Brower, K. (1988). Self-medication of migraine headaches with freebase cocaine. *Journal of Substance Abuse Treatment, 5*, 23–26.

Brower, K. J. and Paredes, A. (1987). Cocaine withdrawal. *Archives of General Psychiatry, 44*, 297–298.

Brown, B. S. (1992). A report on the National AIDS Demonstration Research Program. In G. Bühringer and J. J. Platt (Eds.), *Drug addiction treatment research: German and American perspectives*. Malabar, Fla.: Krieger, pp. 519–528.

—— and Beschner, G. M. (1993). At risk for AIDS-injection drug users and their sexual partners. In B. S. Brown, G. M. Beschner, and the National AIDS Research Consortium (Eds.), *Handbook on risk of AIDS: Injection drug users and sexual partners*. Westport, Conn.: Greenwood Press, pp. xxxi–xlil (introduction).

—— Rose, M. R., Weddington, W. W., and Jaffe, J. H. (1989). Kids and cocaine: A treatment dilemma. *Journal of Substance Abuse Treatment, 6*, 3–8.

Brown, D. N., Rosenholtz, M. J., and Marshall, J. B. (1994). Ischemic colitis related to cocaine abuse (review). *American Journal of Gastroenterology, 89*(9), 1558–61.

Brown, E., Prager, J., Lee, H. Y., and Ramsey, R. G. (1992). CNS complications of cocaine abuse: Prevalence, pathophysiology, and neuroradiology. *American Journal of Roentgenology, 159*, 137–147.

Brown, E. E., Finlay, J. M., Wong, J. T., Damsma, G., and Fibiger, H. C. (1991). Behavioral and neurochemical interactions between cocaine and buprenorphine: Implications for the pharmacotherapy of cocaine abuse. *Journal of Pharmacology and Experimental Therapeutics, 256*, 119–126.

Brown, R. M. (1989). Pharmacology of cocaine abuse. In K. K. Redda, C. A. Walker, and G. Barnett (Eds.), *Cocaine, marijuana, designer drugs: Chemistry, pharmacology, and behavior*. Boca Raton, Fla.: CRC Press, pp. 39–52.

Brown, T. G., Seraganian, P., and Tremblay, J. (1993). Alcohol and cocaine abusers 6 months after traditional treatment: Do they fare as well as problem drinkers? *Journal of Substance Abuse Treatment, 10*(6), 545–552.

Brown, W. A., Corriveau, P., and Ebert, M. H. (1978). Acute psychologic and neuroendocrine effects of dextroamphetamine and methylphenidate. *Psychopharmacology, 58*, 189–195.

Brust, J. C. and Richter, R. W. (1977). Stroke associated with cocaine abuse? *New York State Journal of Medicine, 77*, 1473–75.

Budde, D., Rounsaville, B., and Bryant, K. (1992). Inpatient and outpatient cocaine abusers: Clinical comparisons at intake and one-year follow-up. *Journal of Substance Abuse Treatment, 9*, 337–342.

Budney, A. J., Higgins, S. T., Bickel, W., and Kent, L. (1993). Relationship between intravenous use and achieving initial cocaine abstinence. *Drug and Alcohol Dependence, 32*(2), 133–142.

—— Higgins, S. T., Delaney, D. D., Kent, L., and Bickel, W. K. (1991). Contingent reinforcement of abstinence with individuals abusing cocaine and marijuana. *Journal of Applied Behavior Analyses, 24*, 657–665.

Buffum, J. (1982). Pharmacosexology: The effects of drugs on sexual function: A review. *Journal of Psychoactive Drugs, 14*(1–2), 5–44.

—— (1988). Substance abuse and high-risk sexual behavior: Drugs and sex— the dark side. *Journal of Psychoactive Drugs, 20*(2), 165–168.

Bühringer, G., Kraus, L., Herbst, K., and Simon, R. (1994). Epidemiologic research on substance abuse in Germany and recent trends. In National Institute on Drug Abuse (Ed.), *Epidemiologic trends in drug abuse*. Rockville, Md.: NIDA, pp. 328–341.

Bunt, G., Galanter, M., Lifshutz, H., and Castaneda, R. (1990). Cocaine/"crack" dependence among psychiatric inpatients. *American Journal of Psychiatry, 147(11),* 1542–46.

Bureau of Justice Statistics (1992). What are the costs to society of illegal drug use? *Drugs, crime and the justice system.* Washington, D.C.: U.S. Department of Justice, pp. 126–165.

Burkett, G., Yasin, S. Y., Palow, D., LaVoie, L., and Martinez, M. (1994). Patterns of cocaine binging: Effect on pregnancy. *American Journal of Obstetrics and Gynecology, 171(2),* 372–378.

Bush, M. N., Rubenstein, R., Hoffman, I., and Bruno, M. S. (1984). Spontaneous pneumomediastinum as a consequence of cocaine use. *New York State Journal of Medicine, 84,* 618–619.

Bux, D. A., Lamb, R. J., and Iguchi, M. Y. (1995). Cocaine use and HIV risk behavior in methadone maintenance patients. *Drug and Alcohol Dependence, 37(1),* 29–35.

―――― Iguchi, M. Y., Lidz, V., Baxter, R. C., and Platt, J. J. (1993). Participation in an outreach-based coupon distribution program for free methadone detoxification. *Hospital and Community Psychiatry, 44(11),* 1066–72.

Cabral, H., Timperi, R., and Buchner, H. (1989). Effects of maternal marijuana and cocaine use on fetal growth. *New England Journal of Medicine, 320,* 762–768.

Cacciola, J. S., Rutherford, M. J., Altman, A. I., and Snider, E. C. (1994). An examination of the diagnostic criteria for antisocial personality disorder in substance abuse. *Journal of Nervous and Mental Disease, 182(9),* 517–523.

Callaway, C. W. and Clark, R. F. (1994). Hyperthermia in psychostimulant overdose (review). *Annals of Emergency Medicine, 24(1),* 68–76.

Calsyn, D. A. and Saxon, A. J. (1990). Personality disorder subtypes among cocaine and opioid addicts using the Millon Clinical Multiaxial Inventory. *International Journal of the Addictions, 25,* 1037–49.

Campbell, A., Baldessarini, R. J., Cremens, C., Teicher, M. H., March, E., and Kula, N. S. (1989). Bromocriptine antagonizes behavioral effects of cocaine in the rat. *Neuropsychopharmacology, 2(3),* 209–221.

Cannon, D. S., Rubin, A., Keefe, C. K., Black, J. L., Leeka, J. K., and Phillips, L. A. (1992). Affective correlates of alcohol and cocaine use. *Addictive Behaviors, 17,* 517–524.

Caplan, L. R., Hier, D. B., and Banks, G. (1982). Current concepts of cerebrovascular disease—stroke: Stroke and drug abuse. *Stroke, 13(6),* 869–872.

Carlson, R. G. and Siegal, H. A. (1991). The crack-life: An ethnographic overview of crack use and sexual behavior among African-Americans in a midwest metropolitan city. *Journal of Psychoactive Drugs, 23(1),* 11–20.

Carr, R. R. and Meyers, E. J. (1988). Marijuana and cocaine: The process of change in drug policy. In Drug Abuse Council (Ed.), *The facts about "drug abuse."* New York: Free Press, pp. 153–189.

Carrera, M. R. A., Ashley, J. A., Parsons, L. H., Wirschling, P., Koob, G. F., and Janda, K. D. (1995). Suppression of psychoactive effects of cocaine by active immunization. *Nature, 378,* 727–730.

Carroll, K. M. (1993). Psychotherapeutic treatment of cocaine abuse: Models for its evaluation alone and in combination with pharmacotherapy. In F. M.

Tims and C. G. Leukefeld (Eds.), *Cocaine treatment: Research and clinical perspectives* (NIDA Research Monograph No. 135). Rockville, Md.: NIDA, pp. 116–132.

—— and Rounsaville, B. J. (1992). Contrast of treatment-seeking and untreated cocaine abusers. *Archives of General Psychiatry, 49,* 464–471.

—— and Rounsaville, B. J. (1993). History and significance of childhood attention deficit disorder in treatment: Seeking cocaine abusers. *Comprehensive Psychiatry, 34*(2), 75–82.

—— Ball, S. A., and Rounsaville, B. J. (1993). A comparison of alternate systems for diagnosing antisocial personality disorder in cocaine abusers. *Journal of Nervous and Mental Disease, 181*(7), 436–443.

—— Rounsaville, B. J., and Bryant, K. (1993). Alcoholism in treatment-seeking cocaine abusers: Clinical and prognostic significance. *Journal of Studies on Alcohol, 54*(2), 199–208.

—— Rounsaville, B. J., and Gawin, F. H. (1991). A comparative trial of psychotherapies for ambulatory cocaine abusers: Relapse prevention and interpersonal psychotherapy. *American Journal of Drug and Alcohol Abuse, 17*(3), 229–247.

—— Rounsaville, B. J., and Keller, D. S. (1991). Relapse prevention strategies for the treatment of cocaine abuse. *American Journal of Drug and Alcohol Abuse, 17*(3), 249–265.

—— Power, M. D., Bryant, K., and Rounsaville, B. J. (1993). One-year follow-up status of treatment-seeking cocaine abusers: Psychopathology and dependence severity as predictors of outcome. *Journal of Nervous and Mental Disease, 181*(2), 71–79.

—— Rounsaville, B. J., Gordon, L. T., Nich, C., Jatlow, P., Bisighini, R. M., and Gawin, F. H. (1994). Psychotherapy and pharmacotherapy for ambulatory cocaine abusers. *Archives of General Psychiatry, 51,* 177–187.

Carroll, M. E., Lac, S. T., Asencio, M., Halikas, J. A., and Kragh, R. (1990). Effects of carbamazepine on self-administration of intravenously delivered cocaine in rats. *Pharmacology, Biochemistry, and Behavior, 37,* 551–556.

—— Lac, S. T., Walker, M. J., Kragh, R., and Newman, T. (1986). Effects of naltrexone on intravenous cocaine self-administration in rats during food satiation and deprivation. *Journal of Pharmacology and Experimental Therapeutics, 238*(1), 1–7.

Caruana, D. S., Weinbach, B., Goerg, D., and Gardner, L. B. (1984). Cocaine-packet ingestion: Diagnosis, management and natural history. *Annals of Internal Medicine, 100,* 73–74.

Cesarec, Z. and Nyman, A. K. (1985). Differential response to amphetamine in schizophrenia. *Acta Psychiatrica Scandinavica, 71,* 523–538.

Chadwick, M. J., Gregory, D. L., and Wendling, G. (1990). A double-blind amino acids, L-tryptophan and L-tyrosine, and placebo, study with cocaine-dependent subjects in an inpatient chemical dependency treatment center. *American Journal of Drug and Alcohol Abuse, 16,* 275–286.

Chaisson, R. E., Bacchetti, P., Osmond, D., Brodie, B., Sande, M. A., and Moss, A. R. (1989). Cocaine use and HIV infection in intravenous drug users in San Francisco. *Journal of the American Medical Association, 261*(4), 561–565.

Chait, L. D., Uhlenhuth, E. H., and Johanson, C. E. (1987). Reinforcing and subjective effects of several anorectics in normal human volunteers. *Journal of Pharmacology and Experimental Therapeutics, 242(3)*, 777–783.

Chambers, C. D., Taylor, W. J. R., and Moffett, A. D. (1972). The incidence of cocaine abuse among methadone maintenance patients. *International Journal of the Addictions, 7(3)*, 427–441.

Chan, K. M., Matthews, W. S., Saxena, S., and Wong, E. T. (1993). Frequency of cocaine and phencyclidine detection at a large urban public teaching hospital. *Journal of Analytical Toxicology, 17(5)*, 299–303.

Chasnoff, I. J. (1985). Fetal alcohol syndrome in twin pregnancy. *Acta Geneticae Medicae et Gemellologiae, 34*, 229–232.

—— (1986). Cocaine- and methadone-exposed infants: A comparison. In L. S. Harris (Ed.), *Problems of drug dependence, 1986* (NIDA Research Monograph No. 76). Rockville, Md.: NIDA, pp. 278.

—— (1991). Cocaine and pregnancy: Clinical and methodologic issues. *Clinics in Perinatology, 18(1)*, 113–123.

—— and Chisum, G. (1987). Genitourinary tract dysmorphology and maternal cocaine use. *Pediatric Research, 21*, 225A.

—— and MacGregor, S. (1988). Cocaine in pregnancy: Trimester abuse pattern and perinatal outcome. *Pediatric Research, 4*, 403A.

—— Chisum, G. M., and Kaplan, W. E. (1988). Maternal cocaine use and genitourinary tract malformations. *Teratology, 37*, 201–204.

—— Landress, H. J., and Barrett, M. E. (1990). The prevalence of illicit-drug or alcohol use during pregnancy and discrepancies in mandatory reporting in Pinellas County, Florida. *New England Journal of Medicine, 322*, 1202–06.

—— Bussey, M. E., Savich, R., and Stack, C. M. (1986). Perinatal cerebral infraction and maternal cocaine use. *Journal of Pediatrics, 108*, 456–459.

—— Burns, W. J., Schnoll, S. H., and Burns, K. A. (1985). Cocaine use in pregnancy. *New England Journal of Medicine, 313(11)*, 666–669.

—— Griffith, D. R., MacGregor, S., Dirkes, K., and Burns, K. (1989). Temporal patterns in cocaine use in pregnancy. *Journal of the American Medical Association, 261(12)*, 1741–44.

Chávez, G. F., Mulinare, J., and Cordero, J. F. (1989). Maternal cocaine use and the risk for genitourinary tract defects. *Journal of the American Medical Association, 262(6)*, 795–798.

Chavkin, W. (1990). Drug addiction and pregnancy: Policy crossroads. *American Journal of Public Health, 80*, 483–487.

Cherek, D., Steinberg, J., Kelly, T., and Robinson, D. E. (1986). Effects of d-amphetamine on human aggressive behavior. *Psychopharmacology, 88*, 381–386.

Cherukuri, R., Minkoff, H., Feldman, J., Parekh, A., and Glass, L. (1988). A cohort study of alkaloid cocaine ("crack") in pregnancy. *Obstetrics and Gynecology, 72*, 147–151.

Chiasson, M. A., Stoneburner, R. L., Hildebrandt, D. S., Ewing, W. E., Telzak, E. E., and Jaffe, H. W. (1991). Heterosexual transmission of HIV-1 associated with the use of smokable freebase cocaine (crack). *AIDS, 5(9)*, 1121–26.

Childress, A. R., Ehrman, R., McLellan, A. T., and O'Brien, C. P. (1988a). Conditioned craving and arousal in cocaine addiction: A preliminary report. In L. S. Harris (Ed.), *Problems of drug dependence, 1987* (NIDA Research Monograph No. 81). Washington, D.C.: NIDA, pp. 74–80.

——— Ehrman, R., McLellan, A. T., and O'Brien, C. P. (1988b). Update on behavioral treatments for substance abuse. In L. Harris (Ed.), *Problems of drug dependence, 1988* (NIDA Research Monograph No. 90). Rockville, Md.: NIDA, pp. 183–192.

——— McLellan, A. T., and O'Brien, C. P. (1986a). Conditioned responses in a methadone population: A comparison of laboratory, clinic and natural settings. *Journal of Substance Abuse Treatment, 3,* 173–179.

——— McLellan, A. T., and O'Brien, C. P. (1986b). Nature and incidence of conditioned responses in a methadone population: A comparison of laboratory, clinic, and naturalistic settings. In L. S. Harris (Ed.), *Problems of drug dependence, 1985* (NIDA Research Monograph No. 67). Rockville, Md.: NIDA, pp. 366–372.

——— McLellan, A. T., Ehrman, R., and O'Brien, C. P. (1988). Classically conditioned responses in opioid and cocaine dependence: A role in relapse? In B. A. Ray (Ed.), *Learning factors in substance abuse* (NIDA Research Monograph No. 84). Washington, D.C.: NIDA, pp. 25–43.

——— McLellan, A. T., Woody, G. E., and O'Brien, C. P. (1991). Are there minimum conditions necessary for methadone maintenance to reduce intravenous drug use and AIDS risk behaviors? In R. W. Pickens, C. G. Leukefeld, and C. R. Schuster (Eds.), *Improving drug treatment.* (NIDA Research Monograph No. 106). Rockville, Md.: NIDA, pp. 167–177.

Chirgwin, K., DeHovitz, J. A., Dillon, S., and McCormack, W. M. (1991). HIV infection, genital ulcer disease, and crack cocaine use among patients attending a clinic for sexually transmitted diseases. *American Journal of Public Health, 81(12),* 1576–79.

Chitwood, D. D. (1985). Patterns and consequences of cocaine use. In N. J. Kozel and E. H. Adams (Ed.), *Cocaine use in America: Epidemiologic and clinical perspectives.* (NIDA Research Monograph No. 61). Rockville, Md.: NIDA, pp. 111–129.

——— (1993). Epidemiology of crack use among injection drug users and sex partners of injection drug users. In B. S. Brown, G. M. Beschner, and the National AIDS Research Consortium (Eds.), *Handbook on risk of AIDS: Injection drug users and sexual partners.* Westport, Conn.: Greenwood Press, pp. 155–169.

——— and Morningstar, P. C. (1985). Factors which differentiate cocaine users in treatment from nontreatment users. *International Journal of the Addictions, 20,* 449–459.

——— Inciardi, J. A., McBride, D. C., McCoy, C. B., McCoy, H. V., and Trapido, E. J. (1991). *A community approach to AIDS intervention: Exploring the Miami Outreach Project for injecting drug users and other high risk groups.* Westport, Conn.: Greenwood Press.

Chiu, T. T. W., Vaughn, A. J., and Carzoli, R. P. (1990). Hospital costs for cocaine-exposed infants. *Journal of the Florida Medical Association, 77(10),* 897–900.

Chouteau, M., Namerow, P. B., and Leppert, P. (1988). The effect of cocaine abuse on birth weight and gestational age. *Obstetrics and Gynecology, 72,* 351–354.

Chow, M. J., Ambre, J. J., Ruo, T. I., Atkinson, A. J., Bowsher, D. J., and Fischman, M. W. (1985). Kinetics of cocaine distribution elimination and chronotropic effects. *Clinical Pharmacology and Therapeutics, 38,* 318–324.

Cimbura, G., Lucas, D. M., Bennett, R. C., Warren, R. A., and Simpson, H. M. (1982). Incidence and toxicological aspects of drugs detected in 484 fatally injured drivers and pedestrians in Ontario. *Journal of Forensic Science, 27,* 855–867.

Clayton, R. R. (1985). Cocaine use in the United States: In a blizzard or just being snowed? In N. J. Kozel and E. H. Adams (Eds.), *Cocaine use in America: Epidemiological and clinical perspectives* (NIDA Research Monograph No. 61). Rockville, Md.: NIDA, pp. 8–33.

Cocaine Fatalities (1892). *Druggists' circular and chemical gazette;* reprinted in *New York Medical Journal,* 55, 457.

Cocores, J. A., Dackis, C. A., and Gold, M. S. (1986). Sexual dysfunction secondary to cocaine abuse in two patients. *Journal of Clinical Psychiatry, 47,* 384–385.

Cohen, E. and Henkin, I. (1993). Prevalence of substance abuse by seriously mentally ill patients in a partial hospital program. *Hospital and Community Psychiatry, 44(2),* 178–180.

Cohen, S. (1984). Cocaine: Acute medical and psychiatric complications. *Psychiatric Annals, 14(10),* 747–749.

—— (1986). The implications of crack. *Drug Abuse and Alcoholism Newsletter, 15(6),* 1–3.

Cohen, W. R., Piasecki, G. J., Cohn, H. E., Young, J. B., and Jackson, B. T. (1984). Adrenal secretion of catecholamines during hypoxemia in fetal lambs. *Endocrinology, 114,* 383–390.

Coleman, D. L., Ross, T. F., and Naughton, J. L. (1982). Myocardial ischemia and infarction related to recreational cocaine use. *Western Journal of Medicine, 136(5),* 444–446.

Collins, G. B., Watson, E. W., and Zrimec, G. L. (1980). A hospital day care program for alcoholics. *General Hospital Psychiatry, 2(1),* 20–22.

Collins, K. A., Davis, G. J., and Lantz, P. E. (1994). An unusual case of maternal-fetal death due to vaginal insufflation of cocaine. *American Journal of Forensic Medicine and Pathology, 15(4),* 335–339.

Comer, S. D., Lac, S. T., Curtis, L. K., and Carroll, M. E. (1993). Effects of buprenorphine and naltrexone on reinstatement of cocaine-reinforced responding in rats. *Journal of Pharmacology and Experimental Therapeutics, 267(3),* 1470–77.

Commissaris, R. L. (1989). Cocaine pharmacology and toxicology. In K. K. Redda, C. A. Walker, and G. Barnett (Eds.), *Cocaine, marijuana, designer drugs, chemistry, pharmacology, and behavior.* Boca Raton, Fla.: CRC Press, pp. 71–82.

Conan Doyle, A. (1888). The sign of the four; reprinted in W. S. Baring-Gould (Ed.), *The annotated Sherlock Holmes.* Vol. 1 (1967). New York: Clarkson N. Potter, pp. 610–688.

Condelli, W. S., Fairbank, J. A., Dennis, M. L., and Rachal, J. V. (1991). Cocaine use by clients in methadone programs: Significance, scope, and behavioral interventions. *Journal of Substance Abuse Treatment, 8,* 203–212.

Conners, C. K., Rothschild, G., Eisenberg, L., et al. (1969). Dextroamphetamine sulfate in children with learning disorders. *Archives of General Psychiatry, 21,* 182–190.

Cook, C. C. (1988a). The Minnesota Model in the management of drug and alcohol dependency: Miracle, method, or myth? Part I. The philosophy and the programme. *British Journal of Addiction, 83,* 625–634.

—— (1988b). The Minnesota Model in the management of drug and alcohol dependency: Miracle, method, or myth? Part II. Evidence and conclusions. *British Journal of Addiction, 83,* 735–748.

Corby, N. H., Wolitski, R. J., Thornton-Johnson, S., and Tanner, W. M. (1991). AIDS knowledge, perception of risk, and behaviors among female sex partners of injection drug users. *AIDS Education and Prevention, 3(4),* 353–366.

Courtwright, D. T. (1993). Should we legalize drugs? History Answers: No. *American Heritage (Feb./March),* 43–56.

Coven, C. R. (1981). Ongoing group treatment with severely disturbed medical outpatients: The group formation process. *International Journal of Group Psychotherapy, 31(1),* 99–116.

Covi, L., Hess, J. M., Kreiter, N. A., and Haertzen, C. A. (1994). Three models for the analysis of a fluoxetine placebo controlled treatment in cocaine abuse. In L. S. Harris (Ed.), *Problems of drug dependence, 1993* (NIDA Research Monograph No. 141). Rockville, Md.: NIDA, pp. 138.

Cox, T., Jacobs, M., LeBlanc, A., and Marshman, J. (Eds.) (1983). *Drugs and drug abuse: A reference text.* Toronto: Addiction Research Foundation Press.

Craig, R. J. (1988). Psychological functioning of cocaine free-basers derived from objective psychological tests. *Journal of Clinical Psychology, 44(4),* 599–606.

—— and Olson, R. E. (1990). MCMI comparisons of cocaine abusers and heroin addicts. *Journal of Clinical Psychology, 46(2),* 230–237.

Creed, F., Black, D., and Anthony, P. (1989). Day-hospital and community treatment for acute psychiatric illness: A critical appraisal. *British Journal of Psychiatry, 154,* 300–310.

Cregler, L. L. and Mark, H. (1986a). Medical complications of cocaine abuse (special report). *New England Journal of Medicine, 315,* 1495–1500.

—— and Mark, H. (1986b). Cardiovascular dangers of cocaine abuse. *American Journal of Cardiology, 57,* 1185–86.

Cronson, A. J. and Flemenbaum, A. (1978). Antagonism of cocaine highs by lithium. *American Journal of Psychiatry, 135(7),* 856–857.

Crookshank, F. G. (1921). Perforation of the nasal septum in cocaine takers. *British Medical Journal,* 917.

Croughan, J. L. (1985). The contributions of family studies to understanding drug abuse. In L. N. Robins (Ed.), *Studying drug abuse.* New Brunswick, NJ: Rutgers University Press.

Culhane, C. (1990). Patients sell methadone for illicit drugs. *U.S. Journal of Drug and Alcohol Dependence, 14(2),* 5.

Cunningham, S. C., Corrigan, S. A., Malow, R. M., and Smason, I. H. (1993). Psychopathology in inpatients dependent on cocaine or alcohol and cocaine. *Psychology of Addictive Behaviors, 7(4),* 246–250.

Cushman, P. (1988). Cocaine use in a population of drug abusers on methadone. *Hospital and Community Psychiatry, 39(11),* 1205–7.

Dackis, C. A. and Gold, M. S. (1985a). Bromocriptine as a treatment of cocaine abuse (letter). *Lancet, 2,* 1151–52.

—— and Gold, M. S. (1985b). Pharmacological approaches to cocaine addiction. *Journal of Substance Abuse Treatment, 2,* 139–145.

—— and Gold, M. S. (1985c). New concepts in cocaine addiction: The dopamine depletion hypothesis. *Neuroscience and Biobehavioral Reviews, 9,* 469–477.

—— Gold, M. S., and Estroff, T. W. (1989). Inpatient treatment of addiction. In T. B. Karasu (Ed.), *Treatment of psychiatric disorders.* Vol. 2. Washington, D.C.: American Psychiatric Press, pp. 1359–79.

—— Gold, M. S., Davies, R. K., and Sweeney, D. R. (1985–86). Bromocriptine treatment for cocaine abuse: The dopamine depletion hypothesis. *International Journal of Psychiatry in Medicine, 15(2),* 125–135.

—— Gold, M. S., Estroff, T. W., and Sweeney, D. R. (1984). Hyperprolactinemia in cocaine abuse. *Society Neuroscience Abstract, 10,* 1099.

—— Gold, M. S., Sweeney, D. R., Byron, J. P., Jr., and Climko, R. (1987). Single-dose bromocriptine reverses cocaine craving. *Psychiatry Research, 20,* 261–264.

—— Pottash, A. L. C., Annitto, W., and Gold, M. S. (1982). Persistence of urinary marijuana levels after supervised abstinence. *American Journal of Psychiatry, 139(9),* 1196–98.

Daras, M., Tuchman, A. J., and Marks, S. (1991). Central nervous system infarction related to cocaine abuse. *Stroke, 22,* 1320–25.

Das, G. (1993). Cocaine abuse in North America: A milestone in history. *Journal of Clinical Pharmacology, 33(4),* 296–310.

Davis, J. M. and Glassman, A. H. (1989). Antidepressant drugs. In H. I. Kaplan and B. J. Sadock (Eds.), *Comprehensive textbook of psychiatry.* Baltimore: Williams & Wilkins, pp. 1627–55.

De Leon, G. (1984). *The therapeutic community: Study of effectiveness* (NIDA Services Research Monograph ADM, 84–1286). Rockville, Md.: Government Printing Office.

—— (1986). Therapeutic community research: Overview and implications. In G. De Leon and J. T. Ziegenfuss (Eds.), *Therapeutic communities for addictions.* Springfield, Ill.: Charles C. Thomas, pp. 85–95.

—— (1991). Retention in drug-free therapeutic communities. In R. W. Pickens, C. G. Leukefeld, and C. R. Schuster (Eds.), *Improving drug abuse treatment* (NIDA Research Monograph No. 106). Rockville, Md.: NIDA, pp. 218–244.

—— (1993). Cocaine abusers in therapeutic community treatment. In F. M. Tims and C. G. Leukefeld (Eds.), *Cocaine treatment: Research and clinical perspectives* (NIDA Research Monograph No. 135). Rockville, Md.: NIDA, pp. 163–189.

—— and Jainchill, N. (1981–82). Male and female drug abusers: Social and psychological status 2 years after treatment in a therapeutic community. *American Journal of Drug and Alcohol Abuse, 8,* 465–497.

—— and Jainchill, N. (1991). Residential therapeutic communities for female substance abusers. *Bulletin of the New York Academy of Medicine, 67,* 277–290.

de Wit, H. and Stewart, J. (1981). Reinstatement of cocaine-reinforced responding in the rat. *Psychopharmacology, 75,* 134–143.

—— and Wise, R. A. (1977). Blockade of cocaine reinforcement in rats with dopamine receptor blocker pimozide but not with the noradrenergic blockers phentolamine or phenoxybenzamine. *Canadian Journal of Psychology, 31,* 195–203.

Delafuente, J. C. and DeVane, C. L. (1991). Immunologic effects of cocaine and related alkaloids. *Immunopharmacology and Immunotoxicology, 13(1–2),* 11–23.

Delavan, D. B. (1894). The use and abuse of cocaine. *Journal of the American Medical Association, 23(12),* 452.

Delay, J. and Deniker, P. (1968). Drug-induced extrapynidal syndromes. In P. J. Vinken and G. W. Bruyn (Eds.), *Handbook of clinical neurology: Diseases of the basal ganglia.* Vol. 6. Amsterdam: North Holland Publishing, pp. 248–266.

DelBono, E. A., O'Brien, K., and Murphy, R. L. H., Jr. (1989). Lung sound abnormalities in cocaine freebasers. *Substance Abuse, 10,* 201–208.

Dennis, M. L., Fairbank, J. A., Bonito, A. J., and Rachal, J. V. (1990). *Methadone enhanced treatment trials: Treatment process study design* (NIDA Contract No. 271–88–8230). Research Triangle Park, N.C.: Research Triangle Institute.

Deren, S., Davis, R., Tortu, S., and Ahluwalia, I. (1993). Characteristics of female sexual partners. In B. S. Brown and G. M. Beschner (Eds.), *Handbook on risk of AIDS: Injection drug users and sexual partners.* Westport, Conn.: Greenwood Press, pp. 195–210.

Derlet, R. W. and Albertson, T. E. (1989a). Emergency department presentation of cocaine intoxication. *Annals of Emergency Medicine, 18(2),* 182–186.

—— and Albertson, T. E. (1989b). Potentiation of cocaine toxicity with calcium channel blockers. *American Journal of Emergency Medicine, 7(5),* 464–468.

—— Albertson, T. E., and Rice, P. (1989). The effect of haloperidol in cocaine and amphetamine intoxication. *Journal of Emergency Medicine, 7,* 633–637.

—— Albertson, T. E., and Tharratt, R. S. (1991). Lidocaine potentiation of cocaine toxicity. *Annals of Emergency Medicine, 20,* 135–138.

—— Tseng, C. C., and Albertson, T. E. (1994). Cocaine toxicity and the calcium channel blockers nifedipine and nimodipine in rats. *Journal of Emergency Medicine, 12(1),* 1–4.

Des Jarlais, D. C. (1990). AIDS impact in the 1990s. Plenary address presented at the Second Annual NADAR National Meeting, Bethesda, Md, November.

—— Wenston, J., Friedman, S. R., Sotheran, J. L., Maslansky, R., and Marmor, M. (1992). Crack cocaine use in a cohort of methadone maintenance patients. *Journal of Substance Abuse Treatment, 9,* 319–325.

Devenyi, P. (1989). Cocaine complications and pseudocholinesterase. *Annals of Internal Medicine, 110,* 167–168.

Dhopesh, V., Maany, I., and Herring, C. (1991). The relationship of cocaine to headache in polysubstance abusers. *Headache,* 17–19.

Diakogiannis, I. A., Steinberg, M., and Kosten, T. R. (1991). Mazindol treatment of cocaine abuse: A double-blind investigation. In L. S. Harris (Ed.), *Problems of drug dependence, 1990* (NIDA Research Monograph No. 105). Washington, D.C.: NIDA, p. 514.

Diaz, T. and Chu, S. Y. (1993). Crack cocaine use and sexual behavior among people with AIDS. *Journal of the American Medical Association, 269(22),* 2845–46.

DiMaio, V. J. and Garriott, J. C. (1978). Four deaths due to intravenous injection of cocaine. *Forensic Science International, 12,* 119–125.

Dinsmoor, M. J., Irons, S. J., and Christmas, J. T. (1994). Preterm rupture of the membranes associated with recent cocaine use. *American Journal of Obstetrics and Gynecology, 171(2),* 305–308.

Dixon, L., Haas, G., Weiden, P., Sweeney, J., and Frances, A. (1990). Acute effects of drug abuse in schizophrenic patients: Clinical observations and patients' self-reports. *Schizophrenia Bulletin, 16,* 69–79.

———— Haas, G. H., Weiden, P. J., Sweeney, J., and Frances, A. J. (1991). Drug abuse in schizophrenic patients: Clinical correlates and reasons for use. *American Journal of Psychiatry, 148(2),* 224–230.

Dolan, M. P., Black, J. L., Malow, R. M., and Penk, W. E. (1991). Clinical differences among cocaine, opioid, and speedball users in treatment. *Psychology of Addictive Behavior, 5(2),* 78–84.

———— Black, J. L., Penk, W. E., Robinowitz, R., and DeFord, H. A. (1985). Contracting for treatment termination to reduce illicit drug use among methadone maintenance treatment failures. *Journal of Consulting and Clinical Psychology, 53(4),* 549–551.

Dole, V. P. and Nyswander, M. E. (1965). A medical treatment for diacetylmorphine (heroin) addiction. *Journal of the American Medical Association, 193(8),* 80–84.

———— and Nyswander, M. E. (1967). Heroin addiction—a metabolic disease. *Archives of Internal Medicine, 120(1),* 19–24.

Dominguez, R., Vila-Coro, A. A., Slopis, J. M., and Bohan, T. P. (1991). Brain and ocular abnormalities in infants with in utero exposure to cocaine and other street drugs. *American Journal of Diseases of Children, 145,* 688–695.

Dorus, W. and Senay, E. C. (1980). Depression, demographic dimensions, and drug abuse. *American Journal of Psychiatry, 137(6),* 699–704.

Dougherty, R. J. and Lesswing, N. J. (1989). Inpatient cocaine abusers: An analysis of psychological and demographic variables. *Journal of Substance Abuse Treatment, 6,* 45–47.

Dowdeswell, G. F. (1876). The coca leaf: Observations on the properties and action of the leaf of the coca plant (erythloxylon coca), made in the physiological laboratory of University College. *Lancet,* 631–633 (part 1), 664–667 (part 2).

Dressler, F. A., Malekzadeh, S., and Roberts, W. C. (1990). Quantitative analysis of amounts of coronary arterial narrowing in cocaine addicts. *American Journal of Cardiology, 65,* 303–308.

Drug Strategies (1995). *What we are getting for our federal drug control dollars.* New York: Carnegie Corporation.

Dunlap, E. and Johnson, B. D. (1992). The setting for the crack era: Macro forces, micro consequences (1960–1992). *Journal of Psychoactive Drugs, 24(4),* 307–321.

Dunteman, G. H., Condelli, W. S., and Fairbank, J. A. (1992). Predicting cocaine use among methadone patients: Analysis of findings from a national study. *Hospital and Community Psychiatry, 43(6),* 608–611.

DuPont, R. L. (Ed.) (1991). *Crack cocaine: A challenge for prevention* (OSAP Prevention Monograph No. 9). Rockville, Md.: Office for Substance Abuse Prevention.

Dykstra, L. A., Doty, P., Johnson, A. B., and Picker, M. J. (1992). Discriminative stimulus properties of cocaine, alone and in combination with buprenorphine, morphine and naltroxene. *Drug and Alcohol Dependence, 30(3),* 227–234.

Edlin, B. R., Irwin, K. L., Ludwig, D. D., McCoy, H. V., Serrano, Y., Word, C., Bowser, B. P., Faruque, S., McCoy, C. B., Schilling, R. F., Holmberg, S. D., and the Multicenter Crack Cocaine and HIV Infection Study Team (1992). High-risk sex behavior among young street-recruited crack cocaine smokers in three American cities: An interim report. *Journal of Psychoactive Drugs* *24(4)*, 363–371.

Edwards, G., Arif, A., and Hodgson, R. (1981). Nomenclature and classification of drug- and alcohol-related problems: A WHO Memorandum. *Bulletin of the World Health Organization, 59(2)*, 225–242.

—— Arif, A., and Hodgson, R. (1982). Nomenclature and classification of drug- and alcohol-related problems: A shortened version of a WHO memorandum. *British Journal of Addiction, 77*, 3–20.

Ehrman, R., Robbins, S., Childress, A. R., and O'Brien, C. P. (1992). Conditioned responses to cocaine-related stimuli in cocaine abuse patients. *Psychopharmacology, 107*, 523–529.

Ehrman, R. N. and Robbins, S. J. (1994). Reliability and validity of 6-month timeline reports of cocaine and heroin use in a methadone population. *Journal of Consulting and Clinical Psychology, 62(4)*, 843–850.

Ellinwood, E. H. (1974). The epidemiology of stimulant abuse. In F. Josephson and E. Carroll (Eds.). *Drug use: Epidemiological and sociological approaches.* Washington, D.C.: Hemisphere, pp. 303–329.

Ellinwood, E. H. Jr., (1967). Amphetamine psychosis, I: Description of the individuals and process. *Journal of Nervous and Mental Diseases, 144*, 273–283.

—— Smith, W. G., and Vaillant, G. E. (1966). Narcotic addiction in males and females: A comparison. *International Journal of the Addictions, 1(2)*, 33–45.

—— Sudilovsky, A., and Nelson, L. M. (1973). Evolving behavior in the clinical and experimental amphetamine (model) psychosis. *American Journal of Psychiatry, 130*, 1088–93.

Ellis, J. E., Byrd, L. D., Sexson, W. R., and Patterson-Barnett, C. A. (1993). In utero exposure to cocaine: A review. *Southern Medical Journal, 86(7)*, 725–731.

Emrick, C. D. (1987). Alcoholics Anonymous: Affiliation processes and effectiveness as treatment. *Alcoholism: Clinical and Experimental Research, 11(5)*, 416–423.

Erickson, P. G. and Alexander, B. K. (1989). Cocaine and addictive liability. *Social Pharmacology, 3*, 249–270.

—— and Murray, G. F. (1989). The undeterred cocaine user: Intention to quit and its relationship to perceived legal and health threats. *Contemporary Drug Problems, 16*, 141–156.

—— Adlaf, E. M., Murray, G. F., and Smart, R. G. (1987). *The steel drug: Cocaine in perspective.* Lexington, Mass.: D. C. Heath and Co.

Estroff, T. W. and Gold, M. S. (1986). Medical and psychiatric complications of cocaine abuse with possible points of pharmacological treatment. *Advances in Alcohol and Substance Abuse, 5*, 61–76.

—— and Gold, M. S. (1987). Chronic medical complications of drug abuse. *Psychiatric Medicine, 3*, 267–286.

Ettenberg, A., Pettit, H. O., Bloom, F. E., and Koob, G. F. (1982). Heroin and cocaine intravenous self-administration in rats: Mediation by separate neural systems. *Psychopharmacology, 78(3)*, 204–209.

Ettinger, N. A. and Albin, R. J. (1989). A review of the respiratory effects of smoking cocaine. *American Journal of Medicine, 87*, 664–668.

Evans, M. A., Martz, R., Rodda, B. E., Lemberger, L., and Forney, R. B. (1976). Effects of marihuana-dextroamphetamine combination. *Clinical Pharmacology and Therapeutics, 20*, 350–358.

Executive Office of the President (1995). *National Drug Control Strategy.* Washington, D.C.

Eyler, F. D., Behnke, M., Conlon, M., Stewart, N., Frentzen, B., and Cruz, A. (1990). Perinatal outcome of cocaine-using mothers compared to controls matched on prental risk factors. *Pediatric Research, 24(4),* 243A.

Eyre, S. L., Rounsaville, B. J., and Kleber, H. D. (1982). History of childhood hyperactivity in a clinic population of opiate addicts. *Journal of Nervous and Mental Diseases, 170,* 522–529.

Fagan, J. (1989). Myths and realities about crack. *Contemporary Drug Problems, 16,* 527–532.

——— (1992). Drug selling and licit income in distressed neighborhoods: The economic lives of street-level drug users and dealers. In A. V. Harrell and G. E. Peterson (Eds.), *Drugs, crime, and social isolation: Barriers to urban opportunity.* Washington, D.C.: Urban Institute Press, pp. 99–146.

——— and Chin, K. (1989). Initiation into crack and cocaine: A tale of two epidemics. *Contemporary Drug Problems, 16 (Winter),* 579–617.

——— and Chin, K. (1991). Social processes of initiation into crack. *Journal of Drug Issues, 21,* 313–343.

Farley, T. A., Hadler, J. L., and Gunn, R. A. (1990). The syphilis epidemic in Connecticut: Relationship to drug use and prostitution. *Sexually Transmitted Diseases (Oct./Dec.),* 163–168.

Farré, M., De La Torre, R., Llorente, M., Lamas, X., Ugena, B., Segura, J., and Cami, J. (1993). Alcohol and cocaine interactions in humans. *Journal of Pharmacology and Experimental Therapeutics, 266(3),* 1364–73.

——— Llorente, M., Ugena, B., Lamas, X., and Cami, J. (1991). Interaction of cocaine with ethanol. In L. Harris (Ed.), *Problems of drug dependence, 1990.* (NIDA Research Monograph No. 105). Rockville, Md.: NIDA, pp. 570–571.

Farrell, P. E. and Diehl, A. K. (1991). Acute dystonic reaction to crack cocaine. *Annals of Emergency Medicine, 20,* 322.

Fendrich, M. and Vaughn, C. (1994). Diminished lifetime substance use over time: An inquiry into differential underreporting. *Public Opinion Quarterly, 58,* 96–123.

Ferriero, D., Partridge, J., and Wong, D. (1988). Congenital defects and stroke in cocaine exposed neonates. *Annals of Neurology, 24(2),* 348–349.

Festinger, D. S., Lamb, R. J., Kirby, K. C., and Marlowe, D. B. (1996). Accelerated intake as a method of reducing initial appointment no-show. *Journal of Applied Behavior Analysis, 29,* 387–390.

——— Lamb, R. J., Kountz, M., Kirby, K. C., and Marlowe, D. B. (1995). Pretreatment dropout as a function of treatment delay and client variables. *Addictive Behaviors, 20(1),* 111–115.

Feucht, T. E. (1993). Prostitutes on crack cocaine: Addiction, utility, and marketplace economics. *Deviant Behavior, 14,* 91–108.

——— Stephens, R. C., and Gibbs, B. H. (1991). Knowledge about AIDS among intravenous drug users: An evaluation of an education program. *AIDS Education and Prevention, 3(1),* 10–20.

——— Stephens, R. C., and Roman, S. W. (1990). The sexual behavior of intravenous drug users: Assessing the risk of sexual transmission of HIV. *Journal of Drug Issues, 20(2),* 195–213.

———— Stephens, R. C., and Sullivan, T. S. (1993). Drug use patterns among injection drug users and their sex partners. In B. S. Brown and G. M. Beschner (Eds.), *Handbook on risk of AIDS: Injection drug users and sexual partners.* Westport, Conn.: Greenwood Press, pp. 91–115.

Fibiger, H. C. and Phillips, A. G. (1981). Increased intracranial self-stimulation in rats after long-term administration of desipramine. *Science, 214,* 683–685.

Finelli, L., Budd, J., and Spitalny, K. C. (1993). Early syphilis. Relationship to sex, drugs, and changes in high-risk behavior from 1987–1990. *Sexually Transmitted Diseases, 20(2),* 89–95.

Finnegan, L. P. (1994). Perinatal morbidity and mortality in substance using families: Effects and intervention strategies. *Bulletin on Narcotics, 46(1),* 19–43.

Fischman, M. W. (1978). Cocaine and amphetamine effects on repeated acquisition in humans. *Federation Proceedings, 37,* 618.

———— (1984). The behavioral pharmacology of cocaine in humans. In J. Grabowski (Ed.), *Cocaine: Pharmacology, effects, and treatment of abuse* (NIDA Research Monograph No. 50). Rockville, Md.: NIDA, pp. 72–91.

———— (1988). Behavioral pharmacology of cocaine. *Journal of Clinical Psychiatry, 49 (suppl.),* 7–10.

———— and Schuster, C. R. (1980). Cocaine effects in sleep-deprived humans. *Psychopharmacology, 72,* 1–8.

———— and Schuster, C. R. (1981). Acute tolerance to cocaine in humans. In L. S. Harris (Ed.), *Problems of drug dependence, 1980* (NIDA Research Monograph No. 34). Washington, D.C.: NIDA, pp. 241–242.

———— and Schuster, C. R. (1982). Cocaine self-administration in humans. *Federation Proceedings, 41(2),* 241–246.

———— Foltin, R. W., Nestadt, G., and Pearlson, G. D. (1990). Effects of desipramine maintenance on cocaine self-administration by humans. *Journal of Pharmacology and Experimental Therapeutics, 253(2),* 760–770.

———— Schuster, C. R., Javaid, J., Hatano, Y., and Davis, J. (1985). Acute tolerance development to the cardiovascular and subjective effects of cocaine. *Journal of Pharmacology and Experimental Therapeutics, 235(3),* 677–682.

———— Schuster, C. R., Resnekov, L., Shick, J. F. E., Krasnegor, N. A., Fennell, W., and Freedman, D. X. (1976). Cardiovascular and subjective effects of intravenous cocaine administration in humans. *Archives of General Psychiatry, 33,* 983–989.

Fish, F. and Wilson, W. D. C. (1969). Excretion of cocaine and its metabolites in man. *Journal of Pharmacy and Pharmacology, 21 (suppl.),* 135S–85.

Fishbain, D. A. and Wetli, C. V. (1981). Cocaine intoxication, delirium, and death in a body packer. *Annals of Emergency Medicine, 10(10),* 531–532.

Fishel, R., Hamamoto, G., Barbul, A., Jiji, V., and Efron, G. (1985). Cocaine colitis: Is this a new syndrome? *Diseases of the Colon and Rectum, 28(4),* 264–266.

Flaherty, E. W., Kotranski, L., and Fox, E. (1984). Frequency of heroin use and drug users' lifestyle. *American Journal of Drug and Alcohol Abuse, 10(2),* 285–314.

Flemenbaum, A. (1974). Does lithium block the effects of amphetamine? A report of three cases. *American Journal of Psychiatry, 131(7),* 820–821.

———— (1977). Antagonism of behavioral effects of cocaine by lithium. *Pharmacology, Biochemistry, and Behavior, 7,* 83–85.

Flowers, Q., Elder, I. R., Voris, J., Sebastian, P. S., Blevins, O., and Dubois, J. (1993). Daily cocaine craving in a 3-week inpatient treatment program. *Journal of Clinical Psychology, 49(2)*, 292–297.

Foltin, R. W. and Fischman, M. W. (1988). Ethanol and cocaine interactions in humans: Cardiovascular consequences. *Pharmacology, Biochemistry, and Behavior, 31*, 877–883.

——— and Fischman, M. W. (1990). The effects of combinations of intranasal cocaine, smoked marijuana and task performance on heart rate and blood pressure. *Pharmacology, Biochemistry, and Behavior, 36*, 311–315.

——— Fischman, M. W., Nestadt, G., Stromberger, H., Cornell, E. E., and Pearlson, G. D. (1990). Demonstration of naturalistic methods for cocaine smoking by human volunteers. *Drug and Alcohol Dependence, 26*, 145–154.

——— Fischman, M. W., Pedroso, J. J., and Pearlson, G. D. (1987). Marijuana and cocaine interactions in humans: Cardiovascular consequences. *Pharmacology, Biochemistry, and Behavior, 28*, 459–464.

——— Fischman, M. W., Pedroso, J. J. , and Pearlson, G. D. (1988). Repeated intranasal cocaine administration: Lack of tolerance to pressor effects. *Drug and Alcohol Dependence, 22*, 169–177.

——— Fischman, M. W., Pippen, P. A., and Kelly, T. H. (1993). Behavioral effects of cocaine alone and in combination with ethanol or marijuana in humans. *Drug and Alcohol Dependence, 32*, 93–106.

Forno, J. J., Young, R. T., and Levitt, C. (1981). Cocaine abuse. The evolution from coca leaves to freebase. *Journal of Drug Education, 11(4)*, 311–315.

Fowler, R. C., Rich, C. L., and Young, D. (1986). San Diego Suicide Study, II: Substance abuse in young cases. *Archives of General Psychiatry, 43*, 962–965.

Fox, V. and Lowe, G. D. (1967). Day-hospital treatment of the alcoholic patient. *Quarterly Journal of Studies on Alcohol, 29*, 634–641.

Frawley, P. J. (1987). Neurobehavioral model of addiction. *Journal of Drug Issues, 17*, 29–46.

——— and Smith, J. W. (1992). One-year follow-up after multimodal inpatient treatment for cocaine and methamphetamine dependencies. *Journal of Substance Abuse Treatment, 9*, 271–286.

Freud, S. (1884). Über Coca, Secundararzt im k.k. Allgemeinen Krankenhause in Wien. *Centralblatt für die Gesellschaft Therapie, 2*, 289–314; reprinted in English (1984), *Journal of Substance Abuse Treatment, 1*, 206–217.

——— (1974). Contributions about the applications of cocaine, second series, 1: Remarks on craving for and fear of cocaine with reference to a lecture by W. A. Hammond (1887), in Sigmund Freud, *Cocaine Papers*, edited by R. Byck. New York: Stonehill, pp. 171–176.

Freudenberger, R. S., Cappell, M. S., and Hutt, D. A. (1990). Intestinal infarction after intravenous cocaine administration. *Annals of Internal Medicine, 113(9)*, 715–716.

Friedland, G. H. and Klein, R. S. (1987). Transmission of the human immunodeficiency virus. *New England Journal of Medicine, 317*, 1125–35.

Friedman, S. R., Stepherson, B., Woods, J., Des Jarlais, D. C., and Ward, T. P. (1992). Society, drug injectors, and AIDS. *Journal of Health Care for the Poor and Underserved, 3(1)*, 73–89.

Fries, M. H., Kuller, J. A., Norton, M. E., Yankowitz, J., Kobori, J., Good, W. V.,

Ferriero, D., Cox, V., Donlin, S. S., and Golabi, M. (1993). Facial features of infants exposed prenatally to cocaine. *Teratology, 48,* 413–420.

Fritz, P., Galanter, M., Lifshutz, H., and Egelko, S. (1993). Developmental risk factors in postpartum women in urine tests positive for cocaine. *American Journal of Drug and Alcohol Abuse, 19(2),* 187–197.

Frowein, H. W. (1981). Selective effects of barbiturates and amphetamine on information processing and response execution. *Acta Psychologia, 47,* 105–115.

Fudala, P. J., Johnson, R. E. and Jaffe, J. H. (1991). Outpatient comparison of buprenorphine and methadone maintenance. II: Effects on cocaine usage, retention time in study and missed clinic visits. In L. Harris (Ed.). *Problems of drug dependence, 1990* (NIDA Research Monograph No. 105). Rockville, Md.: NIDA, pp. 587–588.

Fullilove, M. T., Golden, E., Fullilove, R. E., III, Lennon, R., Porterfield, D., Schwarcz, S., and Bolan, G. (1993). Crack cocaine use and high-risk behaviors among sexually active black adolescents. *Journal of Adolescent Health, 14,* 295–300.

Fullilove, R. E., Fullilove, M. T., Bowser, B. P., and Gross, S. A. (1990). Risk of sexually transmitted disease among black adolescent crack users in Oakland and San Francisco, California. *Journal of the American Medical Association, 263(6),* 851–855.

Gainey, R. R., Wells, E. A., Hawkins, J. D., and Catalano, R. F. (1993). Predicting treatment retention among cocaine users. *International Journal of the Addictions, 28(6),* 487–505.

Galanter, M. (1985). Use of the social and family network in individual therapy. In S. Zimberg (Ed.), *Practical approaches to alcoholism psychotherapy.* New York: Plenum, 173–186.

——— (1986). Social network therapy for cocaine dependence. *Advances in Alcohol and Substance Abuse, 6(2),* 159–175.

——— Castaneda, R., and Ferman, J. (1988). Substance abuse among general psychiatric patients: Place of presentation, diagnosis, and treatment. *American Journal of Drug and Alcohol Abuse, 14,* 211–235.

——— Egelko, S., DeLeon, G., and Rohrs, C. (1993). A general hospital day program combining peer-led and professional treatment of cocaine abusers. *Hospital and Community Psychiatry, 44(7),* 644–649.

——— Egelko, S., De Leon, G., Rohrs, C., and Franco, H. (1992). Crack/cocaine abusers in the general hospital: Assessment of initiation of care. *American Journal of Psychiatry, 149(6),* 810–815.

Gambarana, C., Ghiglieri, O., Tagliamonte, A., D'Alessandro, N., and de Montis, M. G. (1995). Crucial role of D1 dopamine receptors in mediating the antidepressant effect of imipramine. *Pharmacology, Biochemistry, and Behavior, 50(2),* 147–151.

Gariti, P., Auriacombe, M., Incmikoski, R., McLellan, A. T., Patterson, L., Dhopesh, V., Mezochow, J., Patterson, M., and O'Brien, C. (1992). A randomized double-blind study of neuroelectric therapy in opiate and cocaine detoxification. *Journal of Substance Abuse, 4,* 299–308.

Gastfriend, D. R., Mendelson, J. H., Mello, N. K., and Teoh, S. K. (1992). Preliminary results of an open trial of buprenorphine in the outpatient treatment of combined heroin and cocaine dependence. In L. Harris (Ed.),

Problems of drug dependence, 1991 (NIDA Research Monograph No. 119). Rockville, Md.: NIDA, pp. 461.

—— Mendelson, J. H., Mello, N. K., Teoh, S. K., and Reif, S. (1993). Buprenorphine pharmacotherapy for concurrent heroin and cocaine dependence. *American Journal of Addictions, 2(4),* 269–278.

Gawin, F. and Kleber, M. (1984). Cocaine abuse treatment: Open pilot trial with desipramine and lithium carbonate. *Archives of General Psychiatry, 41,* 903–909.

Gawin, F. H. (1986a). New uses of antidepressants in cocaine abuse. *Psychosomatics, 27,* S24–S29.

—— (1986b). Neuroleptic reduction of cocaine-induced paranoia but not euphoria? *Psychopharmacology, 90,* 142–143.

—— (1988). Chronic neuropharmacology of cocaine: Progress in pharmacotherapy. *Journal of Clinical Psychiatry, 49 (suppl. 2),* 11–16.

—— (1991). Cocaine addiction: Psychology and neurophysiology. *Sciences, 251,* 1580–86.

—— and Ellinwood, E. H. (1988). Cocaine and other stimulants: Actions, abuse, and treatment. *New England Journal of Medicine, 318,* 1173–82.

—— and Ellinwood, E. H. (1989). Cocaine dependence. *Annual Review of Medicine, 40,* 149–161.

—— and Kleber, H. (1987). Issues in cocaine abuse treatment research. In S. Fisher, A. Raskin, and E. H. Uhlenhuth (Eds)., *Cocaine: Clinical and behavioral aspects.* New York: Oxford University Press, pp. 174–192.

—— and Kleber, H. D. (1984). Cocaine abuse treatment: An open trial with lithium and desipramine. *Archives of General Psychiatry, 41,* 903–910.

—— and Kleber, H. D. (1985a). Neuroendocrine findings in chronic cocaine abusers: A preliminary report. *British Journal of Psychiatry, 147,* 569–573.

—— and Kleber, H. D. (1985b). Cocaine abuse in treatment population: Patterns and diagnostic distractions. In *Cocaine use in America: Epidemiologic and clinical perspectives* (NIDA Research Monograph No. 61). Rockville, Md.: NIDA, pp. 182–192.

—— and Kleber, H. D. (1986a). Abstinence symptomatology and psychiatric diagnosis in cocaine abusers. *Archives of General Psychiatry, 43,* 107–113.

—— and Kleber, H. D. (1986b). Pharmacologic treatments of cocaine abuse. *Psychiatric Clinics in North America, 9,* 573–583.

—— Allen, D., and Humblestone, B. (1989). Outpatient treatment of "crack" cocaine smoking with flupenthixol decanoate. *Archives of General Psychiatry, 46,* 322–325.

—— Khalsa, M. E., and Ellinwood, E. (1994). Stimulants. In M. Galanter and H. D. Kleber (Eds.). *Textbook of substance abuse treatment.* Washington, D.C.: American Psychiatric Press, pp. 11–140.

—— Riordan, C., and Kleber, H. (1985). Methylphenidate treatment of cocaine abusers without attention deficit disorder: A negative report. *American Journal of Drug and Alcohol Abuse, 11(3&4),* 193–197.

—— Kleber, H. D., Byck, R., Rounsaville, B. J., Kosten, T. R., Jatlow, P. I., and Morgan, C. (1989). Desipramine facilitation of initial cocaine abstinence. *Archives of General Psychiatry, 46,* 117–121.

—— Morgan, C., Kosten, T. R., and Kleber, H. D. (1989). Double-blind evaluation of the effect of acute amantadine on cocaine craving. *Psychopharmacology, 97,* 402–403.

Gay, G. R. (1981). You've come a long way baby! Coke time for the new American lady of the eighties. *Journal of Psychoactive Drugs, 13,* 287–318.

—— (1982). Clinical management of acute and chronic cocaine poisoning. *Annals of Emergency Medicine, 11(10),* 562–572.

—— (1983). The deadly delights of cocaine. *Emergency Medicine, 2,* 67–81.

—— and Sheppard, C. W. (1973). "Sex-crazed dope fiends"—myth or reality? *Drug Forum, 2(2),* 125–140.

—— Sheppard, C. W., Inaba, D. S., and Newmeyer, J. A. (1973). Cocaine perspective: Gift from the sun god to the rich man's drug. *Drug Forum, 2,* 409–430.

General Accounting Office [GAO] (1993). *Drug Use Measurement: Strengths, limitations, and recommendations for improvement.* Washington, D.C.: U.S. General Accounting Office.

Geracioti, T. D., Jr. and Post, R. M. (1991). Onset of panic disorder associated with rare use of cocaine. *Biological Psychiatry, 29,* 403–406.

Gfroerer, J., Flewelling, R., Rachal, J. V., and Folsom, R. (1993). Race and crack cocaine. *Journal of the American Medical Association, 270(1),* 45–46.

Gfroerer, J. C. and Brodsky, M. D. (1993). Frequent cocaine users and their use of treatment. *American Journal of Public Health, 83(8),* 1149–54.

Giannini, A. J. and Billett, W. (1987). Bromocriptine-desipramine protocol in treatment of cocaine addiction. *Journal of Clinical Pharmacology, 27,* 549–554.

—— Baumgartel, P., and Dimarzio, L. R. (1987). Bromocriptine therapy in cocaine withdrawal. *Journal of Clinical Pharmacology, 27,* 267–270.

—— Folts, D. J., Feather, J. N., and Sullivan, B. S. (1989). Bromocriptine and amantadine in cocaine detoxification. *Psychiatry Research, 29,* 11–16.

—— Loiselle, R. H., Graham, B. H., and Folts, D. J. (1993). Behavioral response to buspirone in cocaine and phencyclidine withdrawal. *Journal of Substance Abuse Treatment, 10(6),* 523–527.

—— Malone, D. A., Giannini, J. C., Price, W. A., and Loiselle, R. H. (1986). Treatment of depression in chronic cocaine and phencyclidine abuse with desipramine. *Journal of Clinical Pharmacology, 26,* 211–214.

—— Miller, N. S., Loiselle, R. H., and Turner, C. E. (1993). Cocaine-associated violence and relationship to route of administration. *Journal of Substance Abuse Treatment, 10,* 67–69.

Gillin, J. C., Pulvirenti, L., Withers, N., Golshan, S., and Koob, G. (1994). The effects of lisuride on mood and sleep during acute withdrawal in stimulant abusers: A preliminary report. *Society of Biological Psychiatry, 35,* 843–849.

Gingras, J. L., Weese-Mayer, D. E., Hume, R. F., Jr., and O'Donnell, K. J. (1992). Cocaine and development: Mechanisms of fetal toxicity and neonatal consequences of prenatal cocaine exposure. *Early Human Development, 31,* 1–24.

Goddard, G. V., McIntire, D. C., and Leech, C. K. (1969). A permanent change in brain function resulting from daily electrical stimulation. *Experimental Neurology, 25,* 295–330.

Goeders, N. E. and Smith, J. E. (1983). Cortical dopaminergic involvement in cocaine reinforcement. *Science, 221(4612),* 773–775.

Goff, D. C. and Ciraulo, D. A. (1991). Stimulants. In D. A. Ciraulo and R. I. Shader

(Eds.), *Clinical manual of chemical dependence*. Washington, D.C.: American Psychiatric Press, pp. 195–231.

Gold, M. S. (1984). *800-COCAINE*. New York: Bantam Books.

——— (1992). Cocaine (and crack): Clinical aspects. In J. H. Lowinson, P. Ruiz, R. B. Millman, and J. G. Langrod (Eds.), *Substance abuse: A comprehensive textbook*. Baltimore, Md.: Williams & Wilkins, pp. 205–221.

——— and Byck, R. (1978). Lithium, naloxone, endorphins and opiate receptors: Possible revelance to pathological and drug-induced manic-euphoric states in man. In R. C. Petersen (Ed.), *The international challenge of drug abuse* (NIDA Research Monograph No. 19). Rockville, Md.: NIDA, pp. 192–209.

——— and Dackis, C. A. (1984). New insights and treatments: Opiate withdrawal and cocaine addiction. *Clinical Therapy, 7,* 6–21.

——— and Verebey, K. (1984). The psychopharmacology of cocaine. *Psychiatric Annals, 14(10),* 714–723.

——— Washton, A. M., and Dackis, C. A. (1985). Cocaine abuse: Neurochemistry, phenomenology, and treatment. In N. J. Kozel and E. H. Adams (Eds.), *Cocaine use in America: Epidemiologic and clinical perspectives* (NIDA Research Monograph No. 61). Washington, D.C.: Government Printing Office, pp. 130–150.

——— Pottash, A. L. C., Annitto, W. J., Verebey, K., and Sweeney, D. R. (1983). Cocaine withdrawal: Effect of tyrosine. *Social Neuroscience Abstracts, 9,* 157.

Goldfrank, L. R. and Hoffman, R. S. (1991). The cardiovascular effects of cocaine. *Annals of Emergency Medicine, 20(2),* 165–175.

——— and Hoffman, R. S. (1993). The cardiovascular effects of cocaine—update, 1992. In H. Sorer, (Ed.), *Acute cocaine intoxication: Current methods of treatment* (NIDA Research Monograph No. 123). Rockville, Md.: NIDA, pp. 70–109.

Goldsmith, M. F. (1988). Sex tied to drugs = STD spread. *Journal of the American Medical Association, 260(14),* 2009.

Goldstein, A. and Kalant, H. (1990). Drug policy: Striking the right balance. *Science, 249,* 1513–21.

Goldstein, P. J., Ouellet, L. J., and Fendrich, M. (1992). From bag brides to skeezers: A historical perspective on sex-for-drugs behavior. *Journal of Psychoactive Drugs, 24(4),* 349–361.

——— Brownstein, H. H., Ryan, P. J., and Bellucci, P. A. (1989). Crack and homicide in New York City, 1988: A conceptually based event analysis. *Contemporary Drug Problems (Winter),* 651–686.

Golub, A. and Johnson, B. D. (1994). A recent decline in cocaine use among youthful arrestees in Manhattan, 1987 through 1993. *American Journal of Public Health, 84(8),* 1250–54.

Golwyn, D. H. (1988). Cocaine abuse treated with phenelzine. *International Journal of the Addictions, 23(9),* 897–905.

Gordon, A. S., Moran, D. T., Jafek, V. W., Eller, P. M., and Strahan, C. R. (1990). The effect of chronic cocaine abuse on human olfaction. *Archives of Otolaryngology—Head and Neck Surgery, 116,* 1415–1418.

Gorelick, D. A. (1992). Pathophysiological effects of cocaine in humans: Review of scientific issues. In A. Paredes, D. A. Gorelick, and B. Stimmel (Eds.), *Cocaine: Physiological and physiopathological effects,* 97–110.

—— and Paredes, A. (1992). Effect of fluoxetine on alcohol consumption in male alcoholics. *Alcoholism, Clinical and Experimental Research, 16(2),* 261–265.

Gossop, M., Bradley, B., Strang, J., and Connell, P. (1984). Clinical effectiveness of electrostimulation versus oral methadone in managing opiate withdrawal. *British Journal of Psychiatry, 144,* 203–208.

—— Griffiths, P., Powis, B., and Strang, J. (1994). Cocaine: Patterns of use, routes of administration, and severity of dependence. *British Journal of Psychiatry, 164,* 660–664.

Gough, H. G. and Heilbrun, A. B. (1983). *The Adjective Checklist manual.* Palo Alto, Calif.: Consulting Psychologists Press.

Grabowski, J. and Dworkin, S. I. (1985). Cocaine: An overview of current issues. *International Journal of the Addictions, 20,* 1065–88.

—— Higgins, S. T., and Kirby, K. C. (1993). Behavioral treatments of cocaine dependence. In F. M. Tims and C. G. Leukefeld (Eds.), *Cocaine treatment: Research and clinical perspectives* (NIDA Research Monograph No. 135). Rockville, Md.: NIDA, pp. 133–149.

—— Rhoades, H., Elk, R., Schmitz, J., and Creson, D. (1993). Methadone dosage, cocaine and opiate abuse. *American Journal of Psychiatry, 150(4),* 675.

Gram, L. F. (1994). Fluoxetine (review). *New England Journal of Medicine, 331(20),* 1354–61.

Grant, B. F. and Harford, T. C. (1990). Concurrent and simultaneous use of alcohol with cocaine: Results of a national survey. *Drug and Alcohol Dependence, 25,* 97–104.

Green, R. M., Kelly, K. M., Gabrielsen, T., Levine, S. R., and Vanderzant, C. (1990). Multiple intracerebral hemorrhages after smoking "crack" cocaine. *Stroke, 21(6),* 957–962.

Greenberg, J., Schnell, D., and Conlon, R. (1992). Behaviors of crack cocaine users and their impact on early syphilis intervention. *Sexually Transmitted Diseases, 19(6),* 346–350.

Greenberg, M. S. Z., Singh, T., Htoo, M., and Schultz, S. (1991). The association between congenital syphilis and cocaine/crack use in New York City: A case-control study. *American Journal of Public Health, 81,* 1316–18.

Greenblatt, D. J., Gross, P. L., Harris, J., Shader, R. I., and Ciraulo, D. A. (1978). Fatal hyperthermia following haloperidol therapy of sedative-hypnotic withdrawal. *Journal of Clinical Psychiatry, 39(8),* 673–675.

Greenstein, R. A., Arndt, I. C., McLellan, A. T., O'Brien, C. P., and Evans, B. (1984). Naltrexone: A clinical perspective. *Journal of Clinical Psychiatry, 45(9),* 25–28.

Griffin, M. L., Weiss, R. D., Mirin, S. M., and Lange, U. (1989). A comparison of male and female cocaine abusers. *Archives of General Psychiatry, 46,* 122–126.

Griffiths, R. R., Bigelow, G. E., and Henningfield, J. E. (1980). Similarities in animal and human drug-taking behavior. In N. K. Mello (Ed.), *Advances in substance abuse.* Vol. 1. Greenwich, Conn.: JAI Press, pp. 1–90.

—— and Bakalar, J. B. (1976). *Cocaine: A drug and its social evolution.* New York: Basic Books.

Grinspoon, L. and Bakalar, J. B. (1980). Drug dependence: Non-narcotic agents: In H. I. Kaplan, A. M. Freedman, and B. J. Sadock (Eds.), *Comprehensive textbook of psychiatry.* 3rd ed. Baltimore: Williams & Wilkins, pp. 1621–22.

——— Bakalar, J. B. (1985). *Cocaine: A drug and its social evolution.* Rev. ed. New York: Basic Books.

Grund, J. P. C. and Blanken, P. (1993). *From chasing the dragon to chinezen: The diffusion of heroin smoking in the Netherlands.* Rotterdam: IVO.

——— Adriaans, N. F. P., and Kaplan, C. D. (1991). Changing cocaine smoking rituals in the Dutch heroin addict population. *British Journal of Addiction, 86,* 439–448.

Gunne, L. M., Änggård, E., and Jönsson, L. E. (1972). Clinical trials with amphetamine-blocking drugs. *Psychiatria, Neurologia, Neurochirurgia, 75,* 225–226.

Gutierrez-Esteinou, R., Baldessarini, R. J., Cremens, M. C., Campbell, A., and Teicher, M. H. (1988). Interactions of bromocriptine with cocaine. *American Journal of Psychiatry, 145(9),* 1173.

Guydish, J., Bucardo, J., Chan, M., Nebelkopf, E., Acampora, A., and Werdegar, D. (1993). Drug abuse day treatment using the therapeutic community model. In J. A. Inciardi, F. M. Tims, and B. W. Fletcher (Eds.), *Innovative approaches in the treatment of drug abuse: Program models and strategies.* Westport, Conn.: Greenwood Press, pp. 179–190.

Haberman, P. W., French, J. F., and Chin, J. (1993). HIV infection and IV drug use: Medical examiner cases in Essex and Hudson Counties, New Jersey. *American Journal of Drug and Alcohol Abuse, 19(3),* 299–307.

Hadeed, A. J. and Siegel, S. R. (1989). Maternal cocaine use during pregnancy: Effect on the newborn infant. *Pediatrics, 84,* 205–210.

Hale, S. L., Alker, K. J., Rezkalla, S. H., Eisenhauer, A. C., and Kloner, R. A. (1991). Nifedipine protects the heart from the acute deleterious effects of cocaine if administered before but not after cocaine. *Circulation, 83(4),* 1437–43.

Halikas, J., Kemp, K., Kuhn, K., Carlson, G., and Crea, F. (1989). Carbamazepine for cocaine addiction? *Lancet, 1,* 623–624.

Halikas, J. A. and Kuhn, K. L. (1990). A possible neurophysiological basis of cocaine craving. *Annals of Clinical Psychiatry, 2,* 79–83.

——— Kuhn, K. L., and Maddux, T. L. (1990). Reduction of cocaine use among methadone maintenance patients using concurrent carbamazepine maintenance. *Annals of Clinical Psychiatry, 2,* 3–6.

——— Crosby, R. D., Carlson, G. A., Crea, F., Graves, N. M., and Bowers, L. D. (1991). Cocaine reduction in unmotivated crack users using carbamazepine versus placebo in a short-term, double-blind crossover design. *Clinical Pharmacology and Therapeutics, 50(1),* 81–95.

——— Crosby, R. D., Pearson, V. L., Nugent, S. M., and Carlson, G. A. (1994). Psychiatric comorbidity in treatment-seeking cocaine abusers. *American Journal on Addictions, 3,* 25–35.

——— Kuhn, K. L., Carlson, G., Crea, F., and Crosby, R. (1992). The effect of carbamazepine on cocaine use. *American Journal of Addiction, 1,* 30–39.

——— Nugent, S. M., Crosby, R. D., and Carlson, G. A. (1993). 1990–1992 survey of pharmacotherapies used in the treatment of cocaine abuse. *Journal of Addictive Diseases, 12(2),* 129–139.

——— Nugent, S. M., Pearson, V. L., Crosby, R. D., Carlson, G., and Crea, F. (1993). The effect of carbamazepine on the white blood cell count in cocaine abusers. *Psychopharmacology Bulletin, 29(3),* 383–388.

Hall, S., Tunis, S., Banys, D., Tusel, D., and Clark, H. W. (1993). The interaction of enhanced continuity of care and desipramine in early cocaine treatment.

In L. S. Harris (Ed.), *Problems of drug dependence, 1992* (NIDA Research Monograph No. 132). Rockville, Md.: NIDA, pp. 207.

Hall, S. M., Havassy, B. E., and Wasserman, D. A. (1991). Effects of commitment to abstinence, positive moods, stress, and coping on relapse to cocaine use. *Journal of Consulting and Clinical Psychology, 59,* 526–532.

—— Tunis, S., Banys, P., Tusel, D., Clark, H. W., Presti, D., and Stewart, P. (1994). Enhanced continuity of care and desipramine in crack cocaine abusers. In L. S. Harris (Ed.), *Problems of drug dependence, 1993* (NIDA Research Monograph No. 141). Rockville, Md.: NIDA, p. 3.

—— Tunstall, C., Ginsberg, D., Benowitz, N. L., and Jones, R. T. (1987). Nicotine gum and behavioral treatment: A placebo controlled trial. *Journal of Consulting and Clinical Psychology, 55,* 603–605.

Hall, W. C., Talbert, R. L., and Ereshefsky, L. (1990). Cocaine abuse and its treatment. *Pharmacotherapy, 10,* 47–65.

Hamid, A. (1992). The developmental cycle of a drug epidemic: The cocaine smoking epidemic of 1981–1991. *Journal of Psychoactive Drugs, 24(4),* 337–348.

Hammerseley, R., Lavelle, T., and Forsyth, A. (1990). Buprenorphine and temazepam—abuse. *British Journal of Addictions, 85(2),* 301–303.

Hammond, W. A. (1974). Coca: Its preparations and their therapeutical qualities with some remarks on so-called "cocaine habit." In R. Byck (Ed.), *Cocaine papers.* New York: Stonehill, pp. 179–193.

Hanbury, R., Sturiano, V., Cohen, M., Stimmel, B., and Aguillaume, C. (1986). Cocaine use in persons on methadone maintenance. *Advances in Alcohol and Substance Abuse, 6(2),* 97–106.

Handelsman, L., Chordia, P. L., Escovar, I. M., Marion, I. J., and Lowinson, J. H. (1988). Amantadine for the treatment of cocaine dependence in methadone-maintained patients. *American Journal of Psychiatry, 145,* 533.

Handler, A. S., Mason, E. D., Rosenberg, D. L., and Davis, F. G. (1994). The relationship between exposure during pregnancy to cigarette smoking and cocaine use and placenta previa. *American Journal of Obstetrics and Gynecology, 170(3),* 884–889.

Hansen, H. J., Caudill, S. P., and Boone, D. J. (1985). Crisis in drug testing. Results of CDC blind study. *Journal of the American Medical Association, 253(16),* 2382–87.

Harruff, R. C., Francisco, J. T., Elkins, S. K., Phillips, A. M., and Fernandez, G. S. (1988). Cocaine and homicide in Memphis and Shelby County: An epidemic of violence. *Journal of Forensic Science, 33,* 1231–37.

Harsham, J., Keller, J. H., and Disbrow, D. (1994). Growth patterns of infants exposed to cocaine and other drugs in utero. *Journal of the American Dietetic Association, 94(9),* 999–1007.

Hartel, D. M., Schoenbaum, E. E., Selwyn, P. A., Kline, J., Davenny, K., Klein, R. S., and Friedland, G. H. (1995). Heroin use during methadone maintenance treatment: The importance of methadone dose and cocaine use. *American Journal of Public Health, 85,* 83–88.

Hasin, D. S. and Grant, B. F. (1987). Assessing specific drug disorders in a sample of substance abuse patients: A comparison of the DIS and the SADS-L procedures. *Drug and Alcohol Dependence, 19,* 165–176.

—— Grant, B. F., Endicott, J., and Harford, T. C. (1988). Cocaine and heroin dependence compared in poly-drug abusers. *American Journal of Public Health, 78(5)*, 567–569.

Hatsukami, D., Keenan, R., Halikas, J., Pentel, P. R., and Brauer, L. H. (1991). Effects of carbamazepine on acute responses to smoked cocaine-base in human cocaine users. *Psychopharmacology 104(1)*, 120–124.

Hatsukami, D. K., Morgan, S. F., Pickens, R. W., and Champagne, S. E. (1990). Situational factors in cigarette smoking. *Addictive Behaviors, 15*, 1–12.

——— Pentel, P. R., Glass, J., Nelson, R., Brauer, L. H., Crosby, R., and Hanson, K. (1994). Methodological issues in the administration of multiple doses of smoked cocaine-base in humans. *Pharmacology, Biochemistry, and Behavior, 47(3)*, 531–540.

Hauger, R. L., Huliham-Giblin, B., Janowsky, A., Angel, I., Berger, P., Luu, M. D., Schweir, M. M., Skolnick, P., and Paul, S. M. (1986). Central recognition sites for psychomotor stimulants: Methylphenidate and amphetamine. In R. A. O'Brien (Ed.), *Receptor binding in drug research*. New York: Dekker, pp. 167–182.

Havassy, B. E., Wasserman, D. A., and Hall, S. M. (1993). Relapse to cocaine abuse: Conceptual issues. In F. M. Tims and C. G. Leukefeld (Eds.), *Cocaine treatment: Research and clinical perspectives* (NIDA Research Monograph No. 135). Rockville, Md.: NIDA, pp. 203–217.

Hawkins, J. D. and Catalano, R. F., Jr. (1985). Aftercare in drug abuse treatment. *International Journal of the Addictions, 20*, 917–945.

——— Catalano, R. F., and Wells, E. A. (1986). Measuring effects of a skills training intervention for drug abusers. *Journal of Consulting and Clinical Psychology, 54*, 661–669.

——— Lishner, D. M., and Catalano, R. F. (1986). Childhood predictors of adolescent substance abuse. In C. L. Jones and R. J. Battjes (Eds.), *Etiology of drug abuse: Implications for prevention* (NIDA Research Monograph No. 56). Rockville, Md.: NIDA, pp. 75–126.

Hearn, W. L., Flynn, D. D., Hime, G. W., Rose, S., Cofino, J. C., Mantero-Atienza, E., Wetli, C. V., and Mash, D. C. (1991). Cocaethylene: A unique cocaine metabolite displays high affinity for the dopamine transporter. *Journal of Neurochemistry, 56*, 698–701.

——— Rose, S., Wagner, J., Ciarleglio, A., and Mash, D. C. (1991). Cocaethylene is more potent than cocaine in mediating lethality. *Pharmacology, Biochemistry, and Behavior, 39*, 531–533.

Helfrich, A. A., Crowley, T. J., Atkinson, C. A., and Post, R. D. (1983). A clinical profile of 136 cocaine abusers. In L. S. Harris (Ed.), *Problems of drug dependence, 1982* (NIDA Research Monograph No. 43). Washington, D.C.: NIDA, pp. 343–350.

Hellinger, F. J. (1992). Forecasts of the costs of medical care for persons with HIV: 1992–1995. *Inquiry, 29*, 356–365.

Helzer, J. E. and Pryzbeck, T. R. (1988). The co-occurrence of alcoholism with other psychiatric disorders in the general population and its impact on treatment. *Journal of Studies on Alcohol, 49*, 219–224.

Herning, R. I., Glover, B. J., Koeppl, B., Weddington, W., and Jaffe, J. H. (1990). Cognitive deficits in abstaining cocaine abusers. In J. W. Spencer and J. J. Boren (Eds.), *Residual effects of abused drugs on behavior* (NIDA Research Monograph No. 101). Rockville, Md.: NIDA, pp. 167–178.

——— Jones, R. T., Hooker, W. D., and Tulunay, F. C. (1985). Information processing components of the auditory event related potential are reduced by cocaine. *Psychopharmacology, 87,* 178–185.

Hesselbrock, M. N., Meyer, R. E., and Keener, J. J. (1985). Psychopathology in hospitalized alcoholics. *Archives of General Psychiatry, 42(11),* 1050–55.

Higgins, S. T., Bickel, W. K., and Hughes, J. R. (1994). Influence of an alternative reinforcer on human cocaine self-administration. *Life Sciences, 55(3),* 179–187.

——— Bickel, W. K., Hughes, J. R., Lynn, M., Capeless, M. A., and Fenwick, J. W. (1990). Effects of intranasal cocaine on human learning, performance and physiology. *Psychopharmacology, 102(4),* 451–458.

——— Budney, A. J., Bickel, W. K., and Badger, G. J. (1994). Participation of significant others in outpatient behavioral treatment predicts greater cocaine abstinence. *American Journal of Drug and Alcohol Abuse, 20(1),* 47–56.

——— Budney, A. J., Bickel, W. K., Foerg, F. E., Donham, R., and Badger, G. J. (1994). Incentives improve outcome in outpatient behavioral treatment of cocaine dependence. *Archives of General Psychiatry, 51(7),* 568–576.

——— Budney, A. J., Bickel, W. K., Hughes, J. R., and Foerg, F. (1993a). Disulfiram therapy in patients abusing cocaine and alcohol (letter). *American Journal of Psychiatry, 150(4),* 675–676.

——— Budney, A. J., Bickel, W. K., Hughes, J. R., Foerg, F., and Badger, G. (1993b). Achieving cocaine abstinence with a behavioral approach. *American Journal of Psychiatry, 150(5),* 763–769.

——— Delaney, D. D., Budney, A. J., Bickel, W. K., Hughes, J. R., Foerg, F., and Fenwick, J. W. (1991). A behavioral approach to achieving initial cocaine abstinence. *American Journal of Psychiatry, 148(9),* 1218–24.

——— Rush, C. R., Hughes, J. R., Bickel, W. K., Lynn, M., and Capeless, M. A. (1992). Effects of cocaine and alcohol, alone and in combination, on human learning and performance. *Journal of the Experimental Analysis of Behavior, 58,* 87–105.

Hindin, R., McCusker, J., Vickers-Lahti, M., Bigelow, C., Garfield, F., and Lewis, P. (1994). Radioimmunoassay of hair for determination of cocaine, heroin, and marijuana exposure: Comparison with self-report. *International Journal of the Addictions, 29(6),* 771–789.

Hoegsberg, B., Dotson, T., Abulafia, O., Tross, S., Des Jarlais, D., Landesman, S., and Minkoff, H. (1989). Social, sexual and drug use profile of HIV+ and HIV- women with PID. Presented at the Fifth International Conference on AIDS, Montreal, June 4–9.

Hoffman, J. A., Caudill, B. D., and Koman, J. J., III (1993). Craving for cocaine and retention of crack addicts in cocaine abuse treatment. In L. Harris (Ed.), *Problems of Drug Dependence, 1992* (NIDA Research Monograph No. 132). Washington, D.C.: NIDA, p. 211.

——— Wish, E. D., Koman, J. J., III, Schneider, S. J., Flynn, P. M., and Luckey, J. W. (1993). Hair, urine, and self-reported drug use concordance at treatment admission. Paper presented at the October 1993 annual meeting of the American Society of Criminology, Phoenix, Ariz.

Hoffman, R. S. and Reimer, B. I. (1993). "Crack" cocaine-induced bilateral amblyopia. *American Journal of Emergency Medicine, 11(1),* 35–37.

——— Henry, G. C., Howland, M. A., Weisman, R. S., Weil, L., and Goldfrank, L. R. (1992). Association between life-threatening cocaine toxicity and plasma cholinesterase activity. *Annals of Emergency Medicine, 21(3),* 247–253.

Holland, R. W., Marx, J. A., Earnest, M. P., and Ranniger, S. (1992). Grand mal seizures temporally related to cocaine use: Clinical and diagnostic features. *Annals of Emergency Medicine, 21(7)*, 772–776.

Hollander, J. E., Lozano, M., Fairweather, P., Goldstein, E., Gennis, P., Brogan, G. X., Cooling, D., Thode, H. C., and Gallagher, E. J. (1994). "Abnormal" electrocardiograms in patients with cocaine-associated chest pain are due to "normal" variants. *Journal of Emergency Medicine, 12(2)*, 199–205.

Hollister, L. E., Krajewski, K., Rustin, T., and Gillespie, H. (1992). Drugs for cocaine dependence: Not easy (letter; comment). *Archives of General Psychiatry, 49(11)*, 905–906.

Holman, B. L., Mendelson, J., Garada, B., Teoh, S. K., Hallgring, E., Johnson, K. A., and Mello, N. K. (1993). Regional cerebral blood flow improves with treatment in chronic cocaine polydrug users. *Journal of Nuclear Medicine, 34(5)*, 723–727.

Homer, J. B. (1993). A system dynamics model for cocaine prevalence estimation and trend projection. *Journal of Drug Issues, 23(2)*, 251–279.

Honer, W. G., Gewirtz, G., and Turey, M. (1987). Psychosis and violence in cocaine smokers (letter). *Lancet, 2*, 451.

Horton, A. M., Fiscella, R. A., O'Connor, K., Jackson, M., and Slone, D. (1987). Revised criteria for detecting alcoholic patients with attention deficit disorder, residual type. *Journal of Nervous and Mental Diseases, 175*, 371–372.

Howard, R. E., Hueter, D. C., and Davis, J. G. (1985). Acute myocardial infarction following cocaine abuse in a young woman with normal coronary arteries. *Journal of the American Medical Association, 254(1)*, 95–96.

Hoyme, H. E., Jones, K. L., Dixon, S. D., Jewett, T., Hanson, J. W., Robinson, L. K., Msall, M. E., and Allanson, J. E. (1990). Prenatal cocaine exposure and fetal vascular disruption. *Pediatrics, 85*, 743–747.

Hubbard, R. L., Marsden, M. E., Cavanaugh, E., Rachal, J. V., and Ginzburg, H. M. (1988). Role of drug-abuse treatment in limiting the spread of AIDS. *Review of Infectious Diseases, 10(2)*, 377–384.

——— Marsden, M. E., Rachal, J. V., Harwood, H. J., Cavanaugh, E. R., and Ginzburg, H. M. (1989). *Drug abuse treatment: A national study of effectiveness.* Chapel Hill: University of North Carolina Press.

Hubner, C. B. and Koob, G. F. (1990). Bromocriptine produces decreases in cocaine self-administration in the rat. *Neuropsychopharmacology, 3(2)*, 101–108.

Huessy, R., Cohen, S. M., Blair, C. L., and Rood, P. (1979). Clinical explorations in adult minimal brain dysfunction. In L. Bellak (Ed.), *Psychiatric aspects of minimal brain dysfunction in adults.* New York: Grune and Stratton, pp. 19–35.

Huey, L., Janowsky, D., Judd, L. L., Abrams, A., Parker, D., and Clopton, P. (1981). Effects of lithium carbonate on methylphenidate and induced mood, behavior, and cognitive processes. *Psychopharmacology, 73*, 161–164.

Hunt, D., Spunt, B., Lipton, D., Goldsmith, D. S., and Strug, D. (1986). The costly bonus: Cocaine related crime among methadone treatment clients. *Advances in Alcohol and Substance Abuse, 6(2)*, 107–122.

Hunt, D. E., Lipton, D. S., Goldsmith, D. S., Strug, D. L., and Spunt, B. (1985–86). "It takes your heart": The image of methadone maintenance in the addict world and its effect on recruitment into treatment. *International Journal of the Addictions, 20(11&12)*, 1751–71.

—— Strug, D. L., Goldsmith, D. S., Lipton, D. S., Spunt, B., Truitt, L., and Robertson, K. A. (1984). An instant shot of "aah": Cocaine use among methadone clients. *Journal of Psychoactive Drugs, 16(3),* 217–227.

Hunt, G. M. and Azrin, N. H. (1973). A community-reinforcement approach to alcoholism. *Behavior Research and Therapy, 11,* 91–104.

Hunt, W. A., Barnett, L. W., and Branch, L. G. (1971). Relapse rates in addiction programs. *Journal of Clinical Psychology, 27,* 455–456.

Hursh, S. R. and Bauman, R. A. (1987). The behavioral analysis of demand. In L. Green and J. H. Kagel (Eds.), *Advances in behavioral economics.* Vol. 1. Norwood, N.J.: Ablex, pp. 117–165.

Hurst, P. M., Radlow, R., Chubb, N. C., and Bagley, S. K. (1969). Effects of *d*-amphetamine on acquisition, persistence, and recall. *American Journal of Psychology, 82(3),* 307–319.

Hurt, H., Brodsky, N., and Giannetta, J. (1990). Maternal cocaine use (COC) in women of low socioeconomic status (SES): A major factor adversely affecting prenatal care (PNC) (abstract). *Pediatric Research, 27,* 246A.

Hutchings, D. E. (1993). The puzzle of cocaine's effects following maternal use during pregnancy: Are there reconcilable differences? *Neurotoxicology and Teratology, 15,* 281–286.

Iguchi, M. Y., Husband, S. D., Marlowe, D. B., Kirby, K. C., Lamb, R. J., and Platt, J. J. (1994). Early decline of self-reported dysphoria in inner-city cocaine addicts beginning treatment. Poster presentation at the annual College on Problems of Drug Dependence Meeting, Palm Beach, Fla., June.

Imperato, P. J. (1992). Commentary: Syphilis, AIDS and crack cocaine. *Journal of Community Health, 17,* 69–71.

Inaba, T., Stewart, D. J., and Kalow, W. (1978). Metabolism of cocaine in man. *Clinical Pharmacology and Therapeutics, 23,* 547–552.

Inciardi, J. A. (1987). Beyond cocaine: Basuco, crack, and other coca products. *Contemporary Drug Problems (Fall),* 461–492.

—— (1990). Trading sex for crack among juvenile drug users: A research note. *Contemporary Drug Problems (Winter),* 689–700.

—— (1992). The crack epidemic revisited. *Journal of Psychoactive Drugs, 24(4),* 305–306.

—— and McBride, D. C. (1989). Legalization: A high-risk alternative in the war on drugs. *American Behavioral Scientist, 32(3),* 259–260.

—— Lockwood, D., and Pottieger, A. E. (1991). Crack-dependent women and sexuality: Implications for STD acquisition and transmission. *Addiction and Recovery,* 25–28.

Institute of Medicine (1989). *Prevention and treatment of alcohol problems: Research opportunities.* Washington, D.C.: National Academy Press.

Iriye, B. K., Bristow, R. E., Hsu, C. D., Bruni, R., and Johnson, T. R. B. (1994). Uterine rupture associated with recent antepartum cocaine abuse. *Obstetrics and Gynecology, 83(5, pt.2),* 840–841.

Isenschmidt, D. S., Fischman, M. W., Foltin, R. W., and Caplan, Y. H. (1992). Concentration of cocaine metabolites in plasma of humans following intravenous administration and smoking of cocaine. *Journal of Analytical Toxicology, 16,* 311–314.

Isner, J. M, Estes, N. A. M., III, Thompson, P. D., Costanzo-Nordin, M. R.,

Subramanian, R., Miller, G., Katsas, G., Sweeney, K., and Sturner, W. Q. (1986). Acute cardiac events temporally related to cocaine abuse. *New England Journal of Medicine, 315(23),* 1438–43.

Itkonen, J., Schnoll, S., and Glassroth, J. (1984). Pulmonary dysfunction in "freebase" cocaine users. *Archives of Internal Medicine, 144,* 2195–97.

Jackson, H. C., Ball, D. M., and Nutt, D. J. (1990). Noradrenergic mechanisms appear not to be involved in cocaine-induced seizures and lethality. *Life Sciences, 47,* 353–359.

Jackson, J. F., Rotkiewicz, L. G., Quinones, M. A., and Passannante, M. R. (1989). A coupon program—drug treatment and AIDS education. *International Journal of the Addictions, 24(11),* 1035–51.

Jaffe, J. (1985). Drug addiction and drug abuse. In A. G. Goodman, L. S. Goodman, T. W. Rall, and F. Murad (Eds.), *The pharmacological basis of therapeutics.* New York: Macmillan, pp. 522–540.

Jaffe, J. H. (1990). Drug addiciton and drug abuse. A. G. Goodman, L. S. Gilman, and A. Goodman (Eds.), *The pharmacological basis of therapeutics.* New York: Macmillan, p. 539.

———— Cascella, N. G., Kumor, K. M., and Sherer, M. A. (1989). Cocaine-induced cocaine craving. *Psychopharmacology, 97,* 59–64.

Janak, P. H. and Martinez, J. L., Jr. (1992). Cocaine and amphetamine facilitate retention of jump-up responding in rats. *Pharmacology, Biochemistry, and Behavior, 41(4),* 837–840.

Janowsky, D. S. and Davis, J. M. (1976). Methylphenidate, dextroamphetamine, and levamfetamine: Effects of schizophrenic symptoms. *Archives of General Psychiatry, 33,* 304–308.

Järbe, T. U. C. (1978). Cocaine as a discriminative cue in rats: Interactions with neuroleptics and other drugs. *Psychopharmacology, 59,* 183–187.

———— (1984). Discriminative stimulus properties of cocaine: Effects of apomorphine, haloperidol, procaine, and other drugs. *Neuropharmacology, 23,* 899–907.

Jarvik, M. E. (1990). The drug dilemma: Manipulating the demand. *Science, 250,* 387–392.

Jasinski, D. R., Pevnick, J. S., and Griffith, J. D. (1978). Human pharmacology and abuse potential of the analgesic buprenorphine: A potential agent for treating narcotic addiction. *Archives of General Psychiatry, 35(4),* 501–516.

Jatlow, P. (1993). Cocaethylene: Pharmacologic activity and clinical significance. *Therapeutic Drug Monitoring, 15,* 533–536.

———— Hearn, W. L., Elsworth, J. D., Roth, R. H., Bradberry, C. W., and Taylor, J. R. (1990). Cocaethylene inhibits uptake of dopamine and can reach high plasma concentrations following combined cocaine and ethanol use. In L. Harris (Ed.), *Problems of Drug Dependence, 1990* (NIDA Research Monograph No. 105). Rockville, Md.: NIDA, pp. 572–573.

Javaid, J. I., Musa, M. N., Fischman, M., Schuster, C. R., and Davis, J. M. (1983). Kinetics of cocaine in humans after intravenous and intranasal administration. *Biopharmaceutics and Drug Disposition, 4(1),* 9–18.

Javaid, J. I., Fischman, M. W., Schuster, C. R., Dekirmenjian, H., and Davis, J. M. (1978). Cocaine plasma concentration: Relation to physiological and subjective effects in humans. *Science, 202,* 227–228.

Johanson, C. E. (1984). Assessment of the dependence potential of cocaine in animals. In J. Grabowski (Ed.), *Cocaine: Pharmacology, effects, and treatment of abuse* (NIDA Research Monograph No. 50). Rockville, Md.: NIDA, pp. 54–71.

——— and Fischman, M. W. (1989). The pharmacology of cocaine related to its abuse. *Pharmacological Reviews, 41(1)*, 3–52.

Johns, M. E., Berman, A. R., Price, J. C., Pillsbury, R. C., and Henderson, R. L. (1977). Metabolism of intranasally applied cocaine. *Annals of Otology, rhinology and laryngology, 86*, 342–347.

Johnson, D. N. and Vocci, F. J. (1993). Medications development at the National Institute on Drug Abuse: Focus on cocaine. In F. M. Tims and C.G. Leukefeld (Eds.) *Cocaine treatment: Research and clinical perspectives* (NIDA Research Monograph no. 135). Rockville, Md.: NIDA, pp. 57–70.

Johnson, R. E., Fudala, P. J., and Jaffe, J. H. (1991). Outpatient comparison of buprenorphine and methadone maintenance. I: Effects on opiate use and self-reported adverse effects and withdrawal sypmtomatology (NIDA Research Monograph No. 105). Rockville, Md.: NIDA, pp. 585–586.

——— Jaffe, J. H., and Fudala, P. J. (1992). A controlled trial of buprenorphine treatment for opioid dependence. *Journal of the American Medical Association, 267*, 2750–55.

——— Fudala, P. J. Collins, C. C., and Jaffe, J. H. (1990). Outpatient maintenance/detoxification comparison of methadone and buprenorphine. In L. S. Harris (Ed.), *Problems of drug dependence, 1989* (NIDA Research Monograph No. 95). Washington, D.C.: NIDA, pp. 384.

Johnson, R. S., Tobin, J. W., and Cellucci, T. (1992). Personality characteristics of cocaine and alcohol abusers: More alike than different. *Addictive Behaviors, 17(2)*, 159–166.

Johnston, J. F. W. (1853). The narcotics we indulge in. Part II. *Blackwood's Edinburgh Magazine, 74 (357)*, 605–628.

Jonas, J. M. and Gold, M. S. (1986). Cocaine abuse and eating disorders. *Lancet, 1*, 390–391.

Jonas, S. (1992). Public health approach to the prevention of substance abuse. In J. H. Lowinson, P. Ruiz, R. B. Millman, and J. G. Langrod (Eds.), *Substance abuse: A comprehensive textbook*. Baltimore: Williams & Wilkins, pp. 928–943.

Jones, A., Lewis, C., and Shorty, V. J. (1993). African American injection drug users. In B. S. Brown and G. M. Beschner (Eds.), *Handbook on risk of AIDS: Injection drug users and sexual partners*. Westport, Conn.: Greenwood Press, pp. 275–296.

Jones, F. A. (1900). Cocain habit among the negroes. *Journal of the American Medical Association, 175*.

Jones, R. T. (1984). The pharmacology of cocaine. In J. Grabowski (Ed.), *Cocaine: Pharmacology, effects, and treatment of abuse* (NIDA Research Monograph No. 50). Rockville, Md.: NIDA, pp. 34–52.

——— (1987). Psychopharmacology of cocaine. In A. M. Washton and M. S. Gold, (Eds.), *Cocaine: A clinician's handbook*. New York: Guilford, pp. 55–72.

Jonsson, S., O'Meara, M., and Young, J. B. (1983). Acute cocaine poisoning: Importance of treating seizures and acidosis. *American Journal of Medicine, 75*, 1061–64.

Kaku, D. A. and Lowenstein, D. H. (1989). Recreational drug use: A growing risk factor for stroke in young people. *Neurology, 39,* 161.

Kalivas, P. W. and Duffy, P. (1990). Effect of acute and daily cocaine treatment on extracellular dopamine in the nucleus accumbens. *Synapse, 5,* 48–58.

Kalix, P., Geisshusler, S., Brenneisen, R., Koelbing, V., and Fisch, H. U. (1991). Cathinone, a phenylpropylamine alkaloid from khat leaves that has amphetamine effects in humans. In L. Harris (Ed.), *Problems of drug dependence, 1991* (NIDA Research Monograph No. 105). Rockville, Md.: NIDA, pp. 289–290.

Kandel, D. and Yamaguchi, K. (1993). From beer to crack: Developmental patterns of drug involvement. *American Journal of Public Health, 83(6),* 851–855.

————— Simcha-Fagan, O., and Davies, M. (1986). Risk factors for deliquency and illicit drug use from adolescence to young adulthood. *Journal of Drug Issues, 16,* 67–90.

————— (1975). Stages in adolescent involvement in drug use. *Science, 190,* 912–914.

————— (1982). Epidemiological and psychosocial perspectives in adolescent drug use. *Journal of the American Academy of Child Psychiatry, 21,* 328–347.

————— and Faust, R. (1975). Sequence and stages in patterns of adolescent drug use. *Archives of General Psychiatry, 32,* 923–932.

————— Murphy, D. B., and Karus, D. (1985). Cocaine use in young adulthood: Patterns of use and psychosocial correlates. In N. J. Kozel and E. H. Adams (Eds.), *Cocaine use in America: Epidemiologic and clinical perspectives* (NIDA Research Monograph No. 61). Rockville, Md.: NIDA, pp. 76–110.

————— Simcha-Fagan, O., and Davies, M. (1986). Risk factors for deliquency and illicit drug use from adolescence to young adulthood. *Journal of Drug Issues, 60,* 67–90.

————— Yamaguchi, K., and Chen, K. (1992). Stages of progression in drug involvement from adolescence to adulthood: Further evidence for the gateway theory. *Journal of Studies on Alcohol, 53(5),* 447–457.

Kang, S.-Y. and De Leon, G. (1993). Criminal involvement of cocaine users enrolled in a methadone treatment program. *Addiction, 88,* 395–404.

————— Kleinman, P. H., Woody, G. E., Millman, R. B., Todd, T. C., Kemp, J., and Lipton, D. S. (1991). Outcomes for cocaine abusers after once-a-week psychosocial therapy. *American Journal of Psychiatry, 148(5),* 630–635.

Kaplan, C. D. (1992). Drug craving and drug use in the daily life of heroin addicts. In M. W. deVries (Ed.), *The experience of psychopathology: Investigating mental disorders in their natural settings.* Cambridge: Cambridge University Press, pp. 193–218.

————— Bieleman, B., and TenHouten, W. D. (1992). Are there casual users of cocaine? *Cocaine: Scientific and social dimensions* (Ciba Foundation Symposium 166). Chichester: Wiley, pp. 57–80.

————— Husch, J. A., and Bieleman, B. (1994). The prevention of stimulant misuse. *Addiction, 89,* 1517–21.

Karch, S. B. (1993). *The pathology of drug abuse.* Boca Raton, Fla.: CRC Press.

————— and Billingham, M. E. (1988). The pathology and etiology of cocaine-induced heart disease. *Archives of Pathology and Laboratory Medicine, 112,* 225–230.

Karler, R., Calder, L. D., Chaudhry, I. A., and Turkanis, S. A. (1989). Blockade of "reverse tolerance" to cocaine and amphetamine by MK-801. *Life Sciences, 45,* 599–606.

Katz, J. L., Terry, P., and Witkin, J. M. (1992). Comparative behavioral pharmacology and toxicology of cocaine and its ethanol-derived metabolite, cocaine ethyl-ester (cocaethylene). *Life Sciences, 50(18),* 1351–61.

Kaye, B. R. and Fainstat, M. (1987). Cerebral vasculitis associated with cocaine abuse. *Journal of the American Medical Association, 258,* 2104–6.

Kemper, V. (1993). Drug treatment on demand. *Common Case Magazine, 19(4),* 5–6.

Khalsa, E., Jatlow, P., and Gawin, F. (1994). Flupenthixol and desipramine treatment of crack users: Double blind results. In L. S. Harris (Ed.), *Problems of drug dependence, 1993* (NIDA Research Monograph No. 141). Rockville, Md.: NIDA, pp. 438.

Khalsa, H., Paredes, A., and Anglin, M. D. (1992). The role of alcohol in cocaine dependence. In M. Galanter (Ed.), *Recent developments in alcoholism.* Vol. 10. New York: Plenum, pp. 7–35.

Khalsa, M. E., Paredes, A., and Anglin, M. D. (1992). Cocaine abuse: Outcomes of therapeutic interventions. *Substance Abuse, 13,* 165–179.

———— Paredes, A., and Anglin, M. D. (1993). Cocaine dependence: Behavioral dimensions and patterns of progression. *American Journal on Addictions, 2(4),* 330–345.

———— Tashkin, D. P., and Perrochet, B. (1992). Smoked cocaine: Patterns of use and pulmonary consequences. *Journal of Psychoactive Drugs, 24(3),* 265–272.

———— Anglin, M. D., Paredes, A., Potepan, P., and Potter, C. (1993). Pretreatment natural history of cocaine addiction: Preliminary 1-year followup results. In F. M. Tims and C. G. Leukefeld (Eds.), *Cocaine treatment: Research and clinical perspectives* (NIDA Research Monograph No. 135). Rockville, Md.: NIDA, pp. 218–236.

———— Gawin, F. H., Rawson, R., Carrol, K., and Jatlow, P. (1993). A desipramine ceiling in cocaine abusers. In L. S. Harris (Ed.), *Problems of drug dependence, 1992* (NIDA Research Monograph No. 132). Rockville, Md.: NIDA, p. 318.

———— Paredes, A., Anglin, M. D., Potepan, P., and Potter, C. (1993). Combinations of treatment modalities and therapeutic outcome for cocaine dependence. In F. M. Tims and C. G. Leukefeld (Eds.), *Cocaine treatment: Research and clinical perspectives* (NIDA Research Monograph No. 135). Rockville, Md.: NIDA, pp. 237–259.

Khantzian, E. J. (1972). A preliminary dynamic formulation of the psychopharmacologic action of methadone. In *Proceedings, Fourth National Methadone Conference (January).* San Francisco.

———— (1974). Opiate addiction: A critique of theory and some implications for treatment. *American Journal of Psychotherapy, 28,* 59–70.

———— (1975). Self-selection and progression in drug dependence. *Psychiatry Digest, 10,* 19–22.

———— (1979). Impulse problems in addiction: Cause and effect relationships. In H. Wishine (Ed.), *Working with the impulsive person.* New York: Plenum, pp. 97–112.

———— (1981). Self-selection and progression in drug dependence. In H. Shaffer and M. E. Burglass (Eds.), *Classic contributions in the addictions.* New York: Brunner/Mazel, pp. 154–160.

────── (1983). An extreme case of cocaine dependence and marked improvement with methylphenidate treatment. *American Journal of Psychiatry, 140,* 784–785.

────── (1985). The self-medication hypothesis of addictive disorders: Focus on heroin and cocaine dependence. *American Journal of Psychiatry, 142(11),* 1259–64.

────── and Khantzian, N. J. (1984). Cocaine addiction: Is there a psychological predisposition? *Psychiatric Annals, 14(10),* 753–759.

────── Mack, J. E., and Schatzberg, A. F. (1974). Heroin use as an attempt to cope: Clinical observations. *American Journal of Psychiatry, 131,* 160–164.

────── Gawin, F. H., Kleber, H. D., and Riordan, C. E. (1984). Methylphenidate (Ritalin) treatment of cocaine dependence—a preliminary report. *Journal of Substance Abuse Treatment, 1,* 107–112.

Kidorf, M. and Stitzer, M. L. (1993). Descriptive analysis of cocaine use of methadone patients. *Drug and Alcohol Dependence, 32,* 267–275.

Kiesler, C. A. (1982). Mental hospitals and alternative care: Noninstitutionalization as potential public policy for mental patients. *American Psychologist, 37(4),* 349–360.

Kirby, K. C., Marlowe, D. B., and Platt, J. J. (1994). Predictors of initial treatment retention in cocaine abusers. Poster presentation at the 55th Annual Meeting of the College on Problems of Drug Dependence, Palm Beach, Fla., June.

────── Marlowe, D. B., and Platt, J. J. (1995). Preliminary comparison of three voucher systems for cocaine abstinence: Dimensions to consider. Poster presentation at the 1995 College on Problems of Drug Dependence Conference, Scottsdale, Ariz. June.

────── Lamb, R. J., Iguchi, M. Y., Husband, S. D., and Platt, J. J. (1995). Situations occasioning cocaine use and cocaine abstinence strategies. *Addiction, 90(9),* 1241–52.

────── Marlowe, D. B., Lamb, R. J., Husband, S. D., and Platt, J. J. (1995). Cognitive-behavioral cocaine treatment with and without contingency management. In L. Harris (Ed.), *Problems of drug dependence, 1994* (NIDA Research Monograph No. 153). Washington, D.C.: NIDA, p. 346.

Klahr, A. L., Gold, M. S., Sweeney, K., Cocores, J. A., and Sweeney, D. R. (1990). Cannabis diagnosis of patients receiving treatment for cocaine dependence. *Journal of Substance Abuse, 2,* 107–111.

Kleber, H. D. (1988). Epidemic cocaine abuse: America's present, Britain's future? *British Journal of Addiction, 83,* 1359–71.

────── (1989). Treatment of drug dependence: What works. *International Review of Psychiatry, 1,* 81–100.

────── and Gawin, F. H. (1984). Cocaine abuse: A review of current and experimental treatments. In J. Grabowski (Ed.), *Cocaine: Pharmacology, effects, and treatment of abuse.* (NIDA Research Monograph No. 50). Washington, D.C.: NIDA, pp. 111–129.

────── and Gawin, F. H. (1987). Cocaine Abuse: In reply. *Archives of General Psychiatry 44,* 298.

────── Kosten, T. R., Gaspari, J., and Topazian, M. (1985). Nontolerance to the opioid antagonism of naltrexone. *Biological Psychiatry, 20,* 66–72.

Klein, T. W., Newton, C. A., and Friedman, H. (1988). Suppression of human and mouse lymphocyte proliferation by cocaine. In T. P. Bridge, A. F. Mirsky, and F. K. Goodwin (Eds.), *Psychological, neuropsychiatric and substance abuse aspects of AIDS*. New York: Raven Press, pp. 139–143.

—— Matsui, K., Newton, C. A., Young, J., Widen, R. E., and Friedman, H. (1993). Cocaine suppresses proliferation of phytohemagglutinin-activated human peripheral blood T-cells. *International Journal of Immunopharmacology, 15(1)*, 77–86.

Kleinman, P. H., Kang, S. Y., Lipton, D., Woody, G., Kemp, J., and Millman, R. B. (1992). Retention of cocaine abusers in outpatient psychotherapy. *American Journal of Drug and Alcohol Abuse, 18(1)*, 29–43.

—— Miller, A. B., Millman R. B., Woody, G. E., Todd, T., Kemp, J., and Lipton, D. S. (1990). Psychopathology among cocaine abusers entering treatment. *Journal of Nervous and Mental Disease, 178(7)*, 442–447.

Klerman, G. L., Weissman, M. M., Rounsaville, B. J., and Chevron, E. (1984). *The theory and practice of interpersonal psychotherapy for depression*. New York: Basic Books.

Kliegman, R. M., Madura, D., Kiwi, R., Eisenberg, I., and Yamashita, T. (1994). Relation of maternal cocaine use to the risks of prematurity and low birth weight. *Journal of Pediatrics, 124(5, pt.1)*, 751–756.

Klonoff, D. C., Andrews, B. C., and Obana, W. G. (1989). Stroke associated with cocaine use. *Archives of Neurology, 46*, 989–993.

Koffler, A., Friedler, R. M., and Massry, S. G. (1976). Acute renal failure due to nontraumatic rhabdomyolysis. *Annals of Internal Medicine, 85*, 23–28.

Kogan, M. J., Verebey, K. G., DePace, A. C., Resnick, R. B., and Mulé, S. J. (1977). Quantitative determination of benzoylecgonine and cocaine in human biofluids by gas-liquid chromatography. *Analytical Chemistry, 49(13)*, 1965–68.

Kolar, A. F., Brown, B. S., Weddington, W. W., and Ball, J. C. (1990). A treatment crisis: Cocaine use by clients in methadone maintenance programs. *Journal of Substance Abuse Treatment, 7*, 101–107.

Köller, C. (1884). On the use of cocaine for producing anaesthesia on the eye. *Lancet*, 990–992.

Kosten, T. A., Gawin, F. H., Kosten, T. R., and Rounsaville, B. J. (1993). Gender differences in cocaine use and treatment response. *Journal of Substance Abuse Treatment, 10*, 63–66.

Kosten, T. R. (1989). Pharmacotherapeutic interventions for cocaine abuse: Matching patients to treatments. *Journal of Nervous and Mental Disease, 177(7)*, 379–389.

—— (1990). Neurobiology of abused drugs: Opioids and stimulants. *Journal of Nervous and Mental Disease, 178(4)*, 217–227.

—— (1991). Client issues in drug abuse treatment: Addressing multiple drug abuse. In R. W. Pickens, C. G. Leukefeld, and C. R. Schuster (Eds.), *Improving drug abuse treatment* (NIDA Research Monograph No. 106). Rockville, Md.: NIDA, pp. 136–151.

—— (1993). Clinical and research perspectives on cocaine abuse: The pharmacotherapy of cocaine abuse. In F. M. Tims and C. G. Leukefeld (Eds.), *Cocaine treatment: Research and clinical perspectives* (NIDA Research Monograph No. 135). Rockville, Md.: NIDA, pp. 48–56.

————— and Kleber, H. D. (1988). Rapid death during cocaine abuse: A variant of the neuroleptic malignant syndrome. *American Journal of Drug and Alcohol Abuse, 14.* 335–346.

————— Kleber, H. D., and Morgan, C. (1989a). Treatment of cocaine abuse with buprenorphine. *Biological Psychiatry, 26,* 637–639.

————— Kleber, H. D., and Morgan, C. (1989b). Role of opioid antagonists in treating intravenous cocaine abuse. *Life Sciences, 44,* 887–892.

————— Morgan, C. J., and Schottenfeld, R. (1990). Amantadine and desipramine treatment of cocaine abusing methadone maintained patients. In L. Harris (Ed.), *Problems of drug dependence, 1990* (NIDA Research Monograph No. 105). Rockville, Md.: NIDA, pp. 510–511.

————— Rounsaville, B. J., and Kleber, H. D. (1985). Ethnic and gender differences among opiate addicts. *International Journal of the Addictions, 20,* 1143–1162.

————— Rounsaville, B. J., and Kleber, H. D. (1986). A 2.5-year follow-up of depression, life crises, and treatment effects on abstinence among opioid addicts. *Archives of General Psychiatry, 44,* 281–285.

————— Rounsaville, B. J., and Kleber, H. D. (1987). Multidimensionality and prediction of treatment outcome in opioid addicts: 2.5-year follow-up. *Comprehensive Psychiatry, 28,* 3–13.

————— Rounsaville, B. J., and Kleber, H. D. (1988). Antecedents and consequences of cocaine abuse among opioid addicts: A 2.5-year follow-up. *Journal of Nervous and Mental Disease, 176(3),* 176–181.

————— Gawin, F. H., Rounsaville, B. J., and Kleber, H. D. (1986). Cocaine abuse among opioid addicts: Demographic and diagnostic factors in treatment. *American Journal of Drug and Alcohol Abuse, 12(1&2),* 1–16.

————— Gawin, F. H., Silverman, D. G., Fleming, J., Compton, M., Jatlow, P., and Byck, R. (1992). Intravenous cocaine challenges during desipramine maintenance. *Neuropsychopharmacology, 7(3),* 169–176.

————— Morgan, C. M., Falcione, J., and Schottenfeld, R. S. (1992). Pharmacotherapy for cocaine-abusing methadone-maintained patients using amantadine or desipramine. *Archives of General Psychiatry, 49,* 894–898.

————— Schottenfeld, R. S., Morgan, C. H., Falcione, J., and Ziedonis, D. (1992). Buprenorphine vs. methadone for opioid and cocaine dependence. In L. S. Harris (Ed.), *Problems of drug dependence, 1991* (NIDA Research Monograph No. 119). Rockville, Md.: NIDA, p. 359.

————— Schumann, B., Wright, D., Carney, M. K., and Gawin, F. H. (1987). A preliminary study of desipramine in the treatment of cocaine abuse in methadone maintenance patients. *Journal of Clinical Psychiatry, 48(11),* 442–444.

Kowatch, R. A., Schnoll, S. S., Knisely, J. S., Green, D., and Elswick, R. K. (1992). Electroencephalographic sleep and mood during cocaine withdrawal. *Journal of Addictive Diseases, 11(4),* 21–45.

Kozel, N. J. and Adams, E. H. (1986). Epidemiology of drug abuse: An overview. *Science, 234,* 970–974.

Krajicek, D. J. (1988, December 30). "Crack whips killing toll." *New York Daily News,* p. C13.

Kramer, J. C., Fischman, V. S., and Littlefield, D. C. (1967). Amphetamine abuse: Pattern and effects of high doses taken intravenously. *Journal of the American Medical Association, 201,* 305–309.

Kramer, R. K. and Turner, R. C. (1993). Renal infarction associated with cocaine use and latent protein C deficiency. *Southern Medical Journal, 86(12),* 1436–38.

Kramer, T. H., Fine, J., Bahari, B., and Ottomanelli, G. (1990). Chasing the dragon: The smoking of heroin and cocaine (letter). *Journal of Substance Abuse Treatment, 7(1),* 65.

Kranzler, H. R. and Bauer, L. O. (1990). Effects of bromocriptine on subjective and autonomic responses to cocaine-associated stimuli. In L. S. Harris (Ed.), *Problem of drug dependence* (NIDA Research Monograph No. 105). Rockville, Md.: NIDA, pp. 505–506.

Krendel, D. A., Ditter, S. M., Frankel, M. R., and Ross, W. K. (1990). Biopsy-proven cerebral vasculitis associated with cocaine abuse. *Neurology, 40,* 1092–94.

Krohn, K. D., Slowman-Kovacs, S., and Leapman, S. B. (1988). Cocaine and rhabdomyolysis. *Annals of Internal Medicine, 208,* 639–640.

Kuhar, M. J. (1992). Molecular pharmacology of cocaine: A dopamine hypothesis and its implications (review). *Ciba Foundation Symposium, 166,* 81–89.

—— Ritz, M. C., and Boja, J. W. (1991). The dopamine hypothesis of the reinforcing properties of cocaine. *Trends in Neurosciences, 14(7),* 299–302.

Kuhn, K. L., Halikas, J. A., and Kemp, K. D. (1990). Carbamazepine treatment of cocaine dependence in methadone maintenance patients with dual opiate-cocaine addiction. In L. S. Harris (Ed.), *Problems of drug dependence, 1989* (NIDA Research Monograph No. 95). Rockville, Md.: NIDA, pp. 316–317.

Kumor, K., Sherer, M., and Jaffe, J. (1989). Effects of bromocryptine pretreatment on subjective and physiological responses to IV cocaine. *Pharmacology, Biochemistry, and Behavior, 33,* 829–837.

Kumor, K. M., Sherer, M. A., Gomez, J., Cone, E., and Jaffe, J. H. (1989). Subjective response during continuous infusion of cocaine. *Pharmacology, Biochemistry, and Behavior, 33,* 443–452.

Lam, D. and Goldschlager, N. (1988). Myocardial injury associated with polysubstance abuse. *American Heart Journal, 115,* 675–680.

Lamb, R. J., Kirby, K. C., and Platt, J. J. (1996). Treatment retention, occupational role, and cocaine use in methadone maintenance. *American Journal on Addictions, 5(1),* 12–17.

—— Marlowe, D., Festinger, D., and Kirby, K. (1994). Predictors of initial treatment retention in cocaine abusers. In L. S. Harris (Ed.), *Problems of drug dependence, 1993* (NIDA Research Monograph No. 141). Rockville, Md.: NIDA, p. 339

Lange, R. A., Cigarroa, R. G., Yancy, C. W., Willard, J. E., Pompa, J. J., Sills, M. N., McBride, W., Kim, A. S., and Hillis, L. D. (1989). Cocaine-induced coronary-artery vasoconstriction. *New England Journal of Medicine, 321,* 1557–62.

Langer, R. O., Perry, L. E., and Bement, C. L. (1989). Cocaine-induced blood vessel injury in rabbits. *Research Communications in Substance Abuse, 10,* 209–223.

Laposata, E. A. and Mayo, G. L. (1993). A review of pulmonary pathology and mechanisms associated with inhalation of freebase cocaine ("crack"). *American Journal of Forensic Medicine and Pathology, 14(1),* 1–9.

Leal, J., Ziedonis, D., and Kosten, T. (1994). Antisocial personality disorder as a prognostic factor for pharmacotherapy of cocaine dependence. Paper presented at the 55th annaul scientific meeting of the College on Problems of Drug Dependence, Toronto, June.

Lee, C. Y., Mohammadi, H., and Dixon, R. A. (1991). Medical and dental implications of cocaine abuse. *Journal of Oral Maxillofacial Surgery, 49,* 290–293.

Lee, D. (Ed.) (1983). *Cocaine handbook: An essential reference.* Novato, Calif.: What If?

Lee, H. S., LaMaute, H. R., Pizzi, W. F., Picard, D. L., and Luks, F. I. (1990). Acute gastroduodenal perforations associated with the use of crack. *Annals of Surgery, 211(1),* 15–17.

Lehrer, M. and Gold, M. S. (1987). Laboratory diagnosis of cocaine: Intoxication and withdrawal. *Advances in Alcohol and Substance Abuse, 6,* 123–141.

Leith, N. J. and Barrett, R. J. (1976a). Amphetamine and the reward system: Evidence for tolerance and post-drug depression. *Psychopharmacology, 46* (Berlin), 19–25.

———— and Barrett, R. J. (1976b). Self-stimulation and amphetamine: Tolerance to *d* and *l* isomers and cross-tolerance to cocaine and methylphenidate. *Psychopharmacology, 74* (Berlin), 23–28.

Lesko, L. M., Fischman, M. W., Javaid, J. I., and Davis, J. M. (1982). Iatrogenous cocaine psychosis (letter). *New England Journal of Medicine, 307(18),* 1153.

Lesswing, N. J. and Dougherty, R. J. (1993). Psychopathology in alcohol- and cocaine-dependent patients: A comparison of findings from psychological testing. *Journal of Substance Abuse Treatment, 10,* 53–77.

Lettieri, D. J., Sayes, M., and Pearson, H. W. (Eds.) (1980). *Theories on drug abuse: Selected contemporary perspectives* (NIDA Research Monograph No. 30). Rockville, Md.: NIDA.

Leukefeld, C. G. and Tims, F. M. (1993). Treatment of cocaine abuse and dependence: Directions and recommendations. In F. M. Tims and C. G. Leukefeld (Eds.), *Cocaine treatment: Research and clinical perspectives* (NIDA Research Monograph No. 135). Rockville, Md.: NIDA, pp. 260–266.

Levenson, J. L. (1985). Neuroleptic malignant syndrome. *American Journal of Psychiatry, 142(10),* 1137–45.

Levine, S. R., Brust, J. C. M., Futrell, N., Ho, K.-L., Blake, D., Millikan, C. H., Brass, L. M., Fayad, P., Schultz, L. R., Selwa, J. F., and Welch, K. M. Z. (1990). Cerebrovascular complications of the use of the "crack" form of alkaloidal cocaine. *New England Journal of Medicine, 323(11),* 699–704.

Lewis, B. F. and Galea, R. P. (1986). A survey of the perceptions of drug abusers concerning the Acquired Immunodeficiency Syndrome (AIDS). *Health Matrix, 4(2),* 14–17.

Lewis, J. W. (1985). Buprenorphine (review). *Drug and Alcohol Dependence, 14(3–4),* 363–372.

———— and Walter, D. (1992). Buprenorphine: Background to its development as a treatment for opiate dependence. In J. D. Baline (Ed.), *Buprenorphine: An alternative treatment for opioid dependence* (NIDA Research Monograph No. 121). Rockville, Md.: NIDA, pp. 5–11.

Licata, A., Taylor, S., Berman, M., and Cranston, J. (1993). Effects of cocaine on human aggression. *Pharmacology, Biochemistry, and Behavior, 45,* 549–552.

Lichtenfeld, P. J., Rubin, D. B., and Feldman, R. S. (1984). Subarachnoid hemorrhage precipitated by cocaine snorting. *Archives of Neurology, 41,* 223–224.

Lillie-Blanton, M., Anthony, J. C., and Schuster, C. R. (1993). Probing the meaning of racial/ethnic group comparisons in crack cocaine smoking. *Journal of the American Medical Association, 269(8)*, 993–997.

Lindsay, M. K., Peterson, H. B., Boring, J., Gramling, J., Willis, S., and Klein, L. (1992). Crack-cocaine: A risk factor for human immunodeficiency virus infection type 1 among inner-city parturients. *Crack Cocaine and HIV-1, 80(6)*, 981–984.

Lipton, D. S. and Maranda, M. J. (1983). Detoxification from heroin dependency: An overview of method and effectiveness. *Advances in Alcohol and Substance Abuse, 2(1)*, 31–55.

Lipton, R. B., Choy-Kwong, M., and Solomon, S. (1989). Headaches in hospitalized cocaine users. *Headache, 29*, 225–228.

Lisse, J. R. and Davis, C. P. (1989). Cocaine abuse with deep venous thrombosis. *Annals of Internal Medicine, 110*, 571.

Little, B. B., Snell, L. M., Klein, V. M., and Gilstrap, L. C. (1989). Cocaine abuse during pregnancy: Maternal and fetal implications. *Obstetrics and Gynecology, 73(2)*, 157–160.

Little, K. Y., Kirkman, J. A., Carroll, F. I., Clark, T. B., and Duncan, G. E. (1993). Cocaine use increases [3H]WIN 35428 binding sites in human striatum. *Brain Research, 628(1–2)*, 17–25.

Longshore, D., Hsieh, S., Danila, B., and Anglin, M. D. (1993). Methadone maintenance and needle/syringe sharing. *International Journal of the Addictions, 28(10)*, 983–996.

Lopez, M. C. and Watson, R. R. (1994). Effect of cocaine and murine AIDS on lamina propria T and B cells in normal mice. *Life Science, 54(9)*, 147–151.

Louie, A. K., Lannon, R. A., and Ketter, T. A. (1989). Dr. Louie and associates reply (Stimulants, panic, and BEAM EEG abnormalities). *American Journal of Psychiatry, 146(7)*, 948.

Lowenstein, D. H., Collins, S. D., Massa, S. M., McKinney, H. E., Jr., Benowitz, N., and Simon, R. P. (1987a). The neurologic complication of cocaine abuse (abstract). *Neurology, 37*, 195.

—— Massa, S. M., Rowbotham, M. C., Collins, S. D., McKinney, H. E., and Simon, R. P. (1987b). Acute neurologic and psychiatric complications associated with cocaine abuse. *American Journal of Medicine, 83(5)*, 841–846.

Lundberg, G. D., Garriott, J. C., Reynolds, P. C., Cravey, R. H., and Shaw, R. F. (1977). Cocaine-related death. *Journal of Forensic Sciences, 22*, 402–408.

Luthar, S. S. and Rounsaville, B. J. (1993). Substance misuse and comorbid psychopathology in a high-risk group: A study of siblings of cocaine misusers. *International Journal of the Addictions, 28(5)*, 415–434.

—— Anton, S. F., Merikangas, K. R., and Rounsaville, B. J. (1992). Vulnerability to substance abuse and psychopathology among siblings of opioid abusers. *Journal of Nervous and Mental Disease, 180*, 153–161.

Lyman, W. D. (1993). Perinatal AIDS: Drugs of abuse and transplacental infection. *Advances in Experimental Medicine and Biology, 335*, 211–217.

Lynch, J. and House, M. A. (1992). Cardiovascular effects of methamphetamine. *Journal of Cardiovascular Nursing, 6(2)*, 12–18.

Macdonald, P. T., Waldorf, D., Reinarman, C., and Murphy, S. B. (1988). Heavy cocaine use and sexual behavior. *Journal of Drug Issues, 18*, 437–455.

Madden, J. D, Payne, T. F., and Miller, S. (1986). Maternal cocaine use and effect on the newborn. *Pediatrics, 77,* 209–211.

Magura, S., Casriel, C., Goldsmith, D. S., Strug, D. L., and Lipton, D. S. (1988). Contingency contracting with polydrug-abusing metahdone patients. *Addictive Behaviors, 13(1),* 113–118.

―――― Freeman, R. C., Siddiqi, Q., and Lipton, D. S. (1992). The validity of hair analysis for detecting cocaine and heroin use among addicts. *International Journal of the Addictions, 27(1),* 51–69.

―――― Goldsmith, D., Casriel, C., Goldstein, P. J., and Lipton, D. S. (1987). The validity of methadone clients' self-reported drug use. *International Journal of the Addictions, 22,* 727–749.

―――― Grossman, J. I., Lipton, D. S., Siddiqi, Q., Shapiro, J., Marion, I., and Amann, K. (1989). Determinants of needle sharing among intravenous drug users. *American Journal of Public Health, 79(4),* 459–462.

―――― Siddiqi, Q., Freeman, R. C., and Lipton, D. S. (1991). Changes in cocaine use after entry to methadone treatment. *Journal of Addictive Diseases, 10(4),* 31–45.

Mahalik, M. P., Gautiere, R. F., and Mann, D. E. (1980). Teratogenic potential of cocaine hydrochloride in CF-1 mice. *Journal of Pharmaceutical Sciences, 69,* 703–706.

Maier, T. J. (1989, June 11). A failing drug treatment. *Newsday, 7,* 32–33.

Malbrain, M. L., Neels, H., Vissers, K., Demedts, P., Verbraeken, H., Daelemans, R., and Wauters, A. (1994). A massive, near-fatal cocaine intoxication in a body-stuffer: Case report and review of the literature. *Acta Clinica Belgica, 49(1),* 12–18.

Malow, R. M., West, J. A., Corrigan, S. A., Pena, J. M., and Lott, W. C. (1992). Cocaine and speedball users: Differences in psychopathology. *Journal of Substance Abuse Treatment, 9,* 287–291.

―――― West, J. A., Williams, J. L., and Sutker, P. B. (1989). Personality disorders classification and symptoms in cocaine and opioid addicts. *Journal of Consulting and Clinical Psychology, 57(6),* 765–767.

Man, P. L. and Chuang, M. Y. (1980). Acupuncture in methadone withdrawal. *International Journal of the Addictions, 15,* 921–926.

Manschreck, T. C., Laughery, J. A., Weisstein, C., Allen, D., Humblestone, B., Neville, M., Podlewski, H., and Mitra, N. (1988). Characteristics of freebase cocaine psychosis. *Yale Journal of Biological Medicine, 61,* 115–122.

―――― Schneyer, M. L., Weisstein, C. C., Laughery, J., Rosenthal, J., Celada, T., and Berner, J. (1990). Freebase cocaine and memory. *Comprehensive Psychiatry, 31,* 369–375.

Mantegazza, P. (1975). On the hygienic and medicinal virtues of coca (1859). In G. Andrews and D. Solomon (Eds.), *The coca leaf and cocaine papers.* New York: Harcourt Brace Jovanovich, pp. 38–42.

Maranto, G. (1985). Coke, the random killer. *Discover, 6,* 16.

Margolin, A., Kosten, T. R., and Avants, S. K. (1992). Reply to Hollister et al. Drugs for cocaine dependence: Not easy. *Archives of General Psychiatry, 49,* 905–906.

―――― Kosten, T., Petrakis, I., Avants, S. K., and Kosten, T. (1990). An open pilot study of bupropion and psychotherapy for the treatment of cocaine abuse in methadone-maintained patients. In L. S. Harris (Ed.), *Problems of drug dependence, 1989* (NIDA Research Monograph No. 105). Rockville, Md.: NIDA, pp. 367–368.

Marlatt, G. A. (1985). Relapse prevention: Theoretical rationale and overview of the model. In G. A. Marlatt and J. R. Gordon (Eds.), *Relapse prevention: Maintenace strategies in the treatment of addictive behaviors.* New York: Guilford, pp. 3–70.

—— and Gordon, J. R. (1980). Determinants of relapse: Implications for the maintenance of behavior change. In P. O. Davidson and S. M. Davidson (Eds.), *Behavioral medicine: Changing health lifestyles.* New York: Guilford, pp. 410–452.

—— and Gordon, J. R. (Eds.) (1985). *Relapse prevention: Maintenance strategies in the treatment of addictive behaviors.* New York: Guilford.

—— Baer, J. S., Donovan, D. M., and Kivlahan, D. R. (1988). Addictive behavior: Etiology and treatment. In J. W. Langebucher, B. S. McCrady, W. Frankenstein, and P. E. Nathan (Eds.), *Annual Review of Psychology, 39,* 223–252.

Marlowe, D. B., Husband, S. D., Lamb, R. J., Kirby, K. C., Iguchi, M. Y., and Platt, J. J. (1995). Psychiatric comorbidity in cocaine dependence: Diverging trends, Axis II spectrum, and gender differentials. *American Journal on Addictions, 4(1),* 1–12.

Marques, P. R., Tippetts, A. S., and Branch, D. G. (1993). Cocaine in the hair of mother-infant pairs: Quantitative analysis and correlations with urine measures and self-report. *American Journal of Drug and Alcohol Abuse, 19(2),* 159–175.

Marsh, K. L., Joe, G. W., Simpson, D. D., and Lehman, W. E. K. (1990). Treatment history. In D. D. Simpson and S. B. Sells (Eds.), *Opioid addiction and treatment: A 12-year follow-up.* Malabar, Fla.: Krieger, pp. 137–156.

Marx, R., Aral, S. O., Rolfs, R. T., Sterk, C. E., and Kahn, J. G., (1991). Crack, sex, and sexually transmitted disease. *Sexually Transmitted Diseases, 18,* 92–101.

Marzuk, P. M., Tardiff, K., Leon, A. C., Stajic, M., Morgan, E. B., and Mann, J. (1990). Prevalence of recent cocaine use among motor vehicle fatalities in New York City. *Journal of the American Medical Association, 263,* 250–256.

—— Tardiff, K., Leon, A. C., Stajic, M., Morgan, E. B., and Mann, J. J. (1992). Prevalence of cocaine use among residents of New York City who committed suicide during a one-year period. *American Journal of Psychiatry, 149(3),* 371–375.

Mattison, J. B. (1887). Cocaine dosage and cocaine addiction. *Lancet,* 1024–26.

Mayes, L. C., Granger, R. H., Bornstein, M. H., and Zuckerman, B. (1992). The problem of prenatal cocaine exposure. A rush to judgment (review). *Journal of the American Medical Association, 267(3),* 406–408.

McAuliffe, W. E. (1990). A randomized controlled trial of recovery training and self-help for opioid addicts in New England and Hong Kong. *Journal of Psychoactive Drugs, 22(2),* 197–209.

—— and Ch'ien, J. M. N. (1986). Recovery training and self-help: A relapse-prevention program for treated opiate addicts. *Journal of Substance Abuse Treatment, 3,* 9–20.

—— Albert, J., Cordill-London, G., and McGarraghy, T. K. (1990–91).

Contributions to a social conditioning model of cocaine recovery. *International Journal of the Addictions, 25(9A&10A)*, 1141–77.

McBride, D. C., Inciardi, J. A., Chitwood, D. D., McCoy, C. B., and the National AIDS Research Consortium (1992). Crack use and correlates of use in a national population of street heroin users. *Journal of Psychoactive Drugs, 24(4)*, 411–416.

McCance-Katz, E. F., Price, L. H., McDougle, C. J., Kosten, T. R., and Jatlow, P. I. (1993). Concurrent cocaine-ethanol ingestion in humans: Pharmacology, physiology, behavior, and the role of cocaethylene. In L. Harris (Ed.), *Problems of drug dependence, 1992* (NIDA Research Monograph No. 132). Rockville, Md.: NIDA, p. 345.

McCarron, M. M. and Wood, J. D. (1983). The cocaine "body packer" syndrome: Diagnosis and treatment. *Journal of the American Medical Association, 250(11)*, 1417–20.

McCarthy, J. J. and Borders, O. T. (1985). Limit setting on drug abuse in methadone maintenance patients. *American Journal of Psychiatry, 142(12)*, 1419–23.

McCoy, C. B., Rivers, J. E., and Chitwood, D. D. (1993). Community outreach for injection drug users and the need for cocaine treatment. In F. M. Tims and C. G. Leukefeld (Eds.), *Cocaine treatment: Research and clinical perspectives* (NIDA Research Monograph No. 135). Rockville, Md.: NIDA, pp. 190–202.

McCoy, H. V. and Inciardi, J. A. (1993). Women and AIDS: Social determinants of sex-related activities. *Women and Health, 20*, 69–86.

—— and Miles, C. (1992). A gender comparison of health status among users of crack cocaine. *Journal of Psychoactive Drugs, 24(4)*, 389–397.

McCusker, J., Stoddard, A. M., Zapka, J. G., Morrison, C. S., Zorn, M., and Lewis, B. F. (1992). AIDS education for drug abusers: Evaluation of short-term effectiveness. *American Journal of Public Health, 82(4)*, 533–540.

McDougle, C. J., Black, J. E., Malison, R. T., Zimmerman, R. C., Kosten, T. R., Heninger, G. R., and Price, L. H. (1994). Noradrenergic dysregulation during discontinuation of cocaine use in addicts. *Archives of General Psychiatry, 51(9)*, 713–719.

McHenry, J. G., Zeiter, J. H., Madion, M. P., and Cowden, J. W. (1989). Corneal epithelial defects after smoking crack cocaine (letter). *American Journal of Ophthalmology, 108*, 732.

McKay, J. R., Alterman, A. I., McLellan, A. T., and Snider, E. C. (1994). Treatment goals, continuity of care, and outcome in a day hospital substance abuse rehabilitation program. *American Journal of Psychiatry, 151(2)*, 254–259.

McLachlan, J. F. and Stein, R. L. (1982). Evaluation of a day clinic for alcoholics. *Journal of Studies on Alcohol, 43(3)*, 261–272.

McLarin, K. J. (1994, January 2). Camden's renaissance is touted and doubted. *New York Times*, pp. 19, 26–27.

McLellan, A. T. and Druley, K. A. (1977). Non-random relation between drugs of abuse and psychiatric diagnosis. *Journal of Psychiatric Research, 13*, 179–184.

—— Druley, K. A., and Carson, J. E. (1978). Evaluation of substance abuse problems in a psychiatric hospital. *Journal of Clinical Psychiatry, 39*, 425–430.

———— Woody, G. E., and O'Brien, C. P. (1979). Development of psychiatric illness in drug abusers. *New England Journal of Medicine, 301(24)*, 1310–14.

———— Arndt, I. O., Metzger, D. S., Woody, G. E., and O'Brien, C. P. (1993). The effects of psychosocial services in substance abuse treatment. *Journal of the American Medical Association, 269(15)*, 1953–59.

———— Luborsky, L., O'Brien, C. P., Barr, H. L., and Evans, F. (1986). Alcohol and drug abuse treatment in three different populations: Is it predictable? *American Journal of Drug and Alcohol Abuse, 12*, 101–120.

———— Luborsky, L., O'Brien, C. P., Woody, G. E., and Druley, K. A. (1982). Is treatment for substance abuse effective? *Journal of the American Medical Association, 247*, 1423–28.

———— Luborsky, L., Woody, G. E., and O'Brien, C. P. (1981). Are the "addiction-related" problems of substance abusers really related? *Journal of Nervous and Mental Disease, 169*, 232–239.

———— Luborsky, L., Woody, G. E., O'Brien, C. P., and Druley, K. A. (1983). Predicting response to alcohol and drug abuse treatments: Role of psychiatric severity. *Archives of General Psychiatry, 40*, 620–625.

McLenan, D. A., Ajayi, O. A., Rydman, R. J., and Pildes, R. S. (1994). Evaluation of the relationship between cocaine and intraventricular hemorrhage. *Journal of the National Medical Association, 86(4)*, 281–287.

McMahon, R. C., Malow, R. M., Kouzekanani, K., and Ireland, S. J. (1994). Stress and social support in predicting cocaine relapse. In L. S. Harris (Ed.), *Problems of drug dependence, 1993.* (NIDA Research Monograph No. 141). Rockville, Md.: NIDA, p. 158.

McNagny, S. E. and Parker, R. M. (1992). High prevalence of recent cocaine use and the unreliability of patient self-report in an inner-city walk-in clinic. *Journal of the American Medical Assocation, 267(8)*, 1106–8.

Means, L. B., Small, M., Capone, D. M., Capone, T. J., Condren, R., Peterson, M., and Hayward, B. (1989). Client demographics and outcome in outpatient cocaine treatment. *International Journal of the Addictions, 24*, 765–783.

Meisels, I. S. and Loke, J. (1993). The pulmonary effects of free-base cocaine: A review. *Cleveland Clinic Journal of Medicine, 60(4)*, 325–329.

Melamed, J. I. and Bleiberg, J. (1986). Neuropsychological deficits in freebase cocaine abusers after cessation of use. Presented at the annual meeting of the American Psychiatric Association, Washington, D.C., August.

Meldrum, B. and Garthwaite, J. (1990). Excitatory amino acid neurotoxicity and neurodegenerative disease. *Trends of Pharmacological Science, 11*, 379–387.

Mello, N. K. (1991). Pre-clinical evaluation of the effects of buprenorphine, naltrexone and desipramine on cocaine self-administration. In L. S. Harris (Ed.), *Problems of drug dependence, 1990* (NIDA Research Monograph No. 105). Rockville, Md.: NIDA, pp. 189–195.

———— and Mendelson, J. H. (1980). Buprenorphine reduces heroin self-administration in humans. *Science, 207*, 657–661.

———— and Mendelson, J. H. (1985). Behavioral pharmacology of buprenorphine. *Drug and Alcohol Dependence, 14*, 283–303.

———— Bree, M. P., and Mendelson, J. H. (1983). Comparison of buprenorphine and methadone effects on opiate self-administration in primates. *Journal of Pharmacology and Experimental Therapeutics, 225*, 378–386.

———— Kamien, J. B., Lukas, S. E., Mendelson, J. H., Drieze, J. M., and Sholar, J. W. (1993). Effects of intermittent buprenorphine administration on cocaine self-administration by rhesus monkeys. *Journal of Pharmacology and Experimental Therapeutics, 264(2),* 530–541.

———— Kamien, J. B., Mendelson, J. H., and Lukas, S. E. (1991). Effects of naltrexone on cocaine self-administration by rhesus monkey. In L. S. Harris (Ed.), *Problems of drug dependence, 1990* (NIDA Research Monograph No. 105). Rockville, Md.: NIDA, pp. 617–618.

———— Lukas, S. E., Kamien, J. B., Mendelson, J. H., Drieze, J., and Cone, E. J. (1992). The effects of chronic buprenorphine treatment on cocaine and food self-administration by rhesus monkeys. *Journal of Pharmacology and Experimental Therapeutics, 260(3),* 1185–93.

———— Lukas, S. E., Mendelson, J. H., and Drieze, J. (1993). Naltrexone-buprenorphine interactions: Effects on cocaine self-administration. *Neuropsychopharmacology, 9(3),* 211–224.

———— Mendelson, J. H., Bree, M. P., and Lukas, S. E. (1990a). Buprenorphine suppresses cocaine self-administration by rhesus monkeys. *Science, 245,* 859–862.

———— Mendelson, J. H., Bree, M. P., and Lukas, S. E. (1990b). Buprenorphine and naltrexone effects on cocaine self-administration by rhesus monkeys. *Journal of Pharmacology and Experimental Therapeutics, 254,* 926–939.

———— Mendelson, J. H., Kuehnle, J. C., and Sellers, M. L. (1981). Operant analysis of human heroin self-administration and the effects of naltrexone. *Journal of Pharmacology and Experimental Therapeutics, 216,* 45–54.

Memo, M., Pradhan, S., and Hanbauer, I. (1981). Cocaine-induced supersensitivity of striatal dopamine receptors: Role of endogenous calmodulin. *Neuropharmacology, 20,* 1145–50.

Mendelson, J., Teoh, S., Lange, U., Mello, N., Weiss, R., and Skupny, A. (1988). Hyperprolactinemia during cocaine withdrawal. In L. S. Harris (Ed.), *Problems of drug dependence, 1987* (NIDA Research Monograph No. 81). Rockville, Md.: NIDA, pp. 67–73.

Mendelson, J. H., Teoh, S. K., Mello, N. K., Ellingboe, J., and Rhoades, E. (1992). Acute effects of cocaine on plasma adrenocorticotropic hormone, luteinizing hormone and prolactin levels in cocaine-dependent men. *Journal of Pharmacology and Experimental Therapeutics, 263(2),* 505–509.

Merab, J. (1988). Acute dystonic reaction to cocaine. *American Journal of Medicine, 84,* 564.

Merigian, K. S. and Roberts, J. R. (1987). Cocaine intoxication: Hyperpyrexia, rhabdomyolysis, and acute renal failure. *Journal of Toxicological and Clinical Toxicology, 25,* 135–148.

Metzger, D., Woody, G., De Philippis, D., McLellan, A. T., O'Brien, C. P., and Platt, J. J. (1991). Risk factors for needle sharing among methadone-treated patients. *American Journal of Psychiatry, 148(5),* 636–640.

Meyer, R. E. (1992). New pharmacotherapies for cocaine dependence . . . revisited. *Archives of General Psychiatry, 49,* 900–904.

Michalec, E., Zwick, W. R., Monti, P. M., Rohsenow, D. J., Varney, S., Niaura, R. S., and Abrams, D. B. (1992). A cocaine high-risk situations questionnaire: Development and psychometric properties. *Journal of Substance Abuse, 4,* 377–391.

Milburn, N. G. and Booth, J. A. (1992). Illicit drug and alcohol use among homeless black adults in shelters. *Ethnic and Multicultural Drug Abuse,* 115–155.

Milkman, H. and Frosch, W. A. (1973). On the preferential abuse of heroin and amphetamine. *Journal of Nervous and Mental Disease, 156,* 242–248.

Miller, B. L., Chiang, F., McGill, L., Sadow, T., Goldberg, M. A., and Mena, I. (1993). Cerebrovascular complications from cocaine: Possible long-term sequelae. In H. Sorer (Ed.), *Acute cocaine intoxication: Current methods of treatment* (NIDA Research Monograph No. 123). Rockville, Md.: NIDA, pp. 129–146.

——— Mena, I., Giombetti, R., Villanueva-Meyer, J., and Djenderedjian, A. H. (1992). Neuropsychiatric effects of cocaine: SPECT measurements. *Cocaine: Physiological and Physiopathological Effects,* 47–58.

Miller, F. T. and Tanenbaum, J. H. (1989). Substance abuse in schizophrenia. *Hospital and Community Psychiatry, 40,* 847–849.

Miller, N. S., Gold, M. S., and Belkin, B. M. (1990). The diagnosis of alcohol and cannabis dependence in cocaine dependence. *Advances in Alcohol and Substance Abuse, 8(3&4),* 33–42.

——— Gold, M. S., and Klahr, A. L. (1990). The diagnosis of alcohol and cannabis dependence (addiction) in cocaine dependence (addiction). *International Journal of the Addictions, 259(7),* 735–744.

——— Gold, M. S., and Mahler, J. C. (1991). Violent behaviors associated with cocaine use: Possible pharmacological mechanisms. *International Journal of the Addictions, 26(10),* 1077–88.

——— Gold, M. S., and Millman, R. B. (1989). Cocaine: General characteristics, abuse, and addiction. *New York State Journal of Medicine, 89,* 390–395.

——— Millman, R. B., and Keskinen, S. (1989). The diagnosis of alcohol, cocaine, and other drug dependence in an inpatient treatment population. *Journal of Substance Abuse Treatment, 6,* 37–40.

——— Summers, G. L., and Gold, M. S. (1993). Cocaine dependence: Alcohol and other drug dependence and withdrawal characteristics. *Journal of Addictive Diseases, 12(1),* 25–35.

——— Gold, M. S., Belkin, B. M., and Klahr, A. (1989). Family history and diagnosis of alcohol dependence in cocaine dependence. *Psychiatric Research, 29,* 113–121.

——— Klahr, A. L., Gold, M. S., Sweeney, K., Cocores, J. A., and Sweeney, D. R. (1990). Cannabis diagnosis of patients receiving treatment for cocaine dependence. *Journal of Substance Abuse Treatment, 2,* 107–111.

Miller, W. R. (1985). Motivation for treatment: A review with special emphasis on alcoholism. *Psychological Bulletin, 98,* 84–107.

——— and Hester, R. K. (1986). Inpatient alcoholism treatment: Who benefits? *American Psychologist, 41,* 794–805.

——— and Rollnick, S. (Eds.) (1991). *Motivational interviewing: Preparing people to change addictive behaviors.* New York: Guilford.

Millman, R. B. (1988). Evaluation and clinical management of cocaine abusers. *Journal of Clinical Psychiatry, 49 (suppl 2),* 27–33.

Millon, T. (1984). Interpretive guide to the Millon Clinical Multiaxial Inventory. In P. McReynolds and G. J. Chelune (Eds.), *Advances in psychological assessment.* Vol. 6. San Francisco: Jossey-Bass, pp. 1–41.

Minkoff, H. L., McCalla, S., Delke, I., Stevens, R., Salwen, M., and Feldman, J.

(1990). The relationship of cocaine use to syphilis and human immunodeficiency virus infections among inner city parturient women. *American Journal of Obstetrics and Gynecology, 163,* 521–526.

Mirchandani, H. G., Rorke, L. B., Sekula-Perlman, A., and Hood, I. C. (1994). Cocaine induced agitated delirium, forceful struggle, and minor head injury. A further definition of sudden death during restraint (review). *American Journal of Forensic Medicine and Pathology, 15(2),* 95–99.

Mittleman, R. E. and Wetli, C. V. (1984). Death caused by recreational cocaine use: An update and comment. *Journal of the American Medical Association, 26(14),* 1889–93.

Mody, C. K., Miller, B. L., McIntyre, H. B., Cobb, S. K., and Goldberg, M. A. (1988). Neurologic complications of cocaine abuse. *Neurology, 38,* 1189–93.

Moffett, C. (1911). Rx cocaine. *Hampton's Magazine, 26,* 595–606.

Moise, R., Reed, B. G., and Connell, C. (1981). Women in drug abuse treatment programs: Factors that influence retention at very early and later stages in two treatment modalities: A summary. *International Journal of the Addictions, 16,* 1295–1300.

——— Reed, B. G., and Ryan, V. (1982). Issues in the treatment of heroin-addicted women: A comparison of men and women entering two types of drug abuse programs. *International Journal of the Addictions, 17,* 109–139.

Molotsky, I. (1988, October 30). Capital's homicide rate is at a record. *New York Times,* p. 20.

Monardes (1569). *Joyful Newes out of the New-found Worlde, wherein are declared the rare and singular virtues of divers Herbs, Trees, Plants, Oyles, and Stones, with their Applications as well as to the use of Physick as of Chirurgery, &c. The Three Books of Doctor Monardes of Sevil. Englished by John Frampton, Merchant.* London, 1596; reprinted in G. F. Dowdeswell (1876). The coca leaf: Observations. *Lancet,* 632.

Moore, K. E., Ciueh, C. C., and Zeldes, G. (1977). Release of neurotransmitters from the brain in vivo by amphetamine, methylphenidate and cocaine. In E. H. Ellinwood, Jr., and M. M. Kilbey (Eds.), *Cocaine and other stimulants.* New York: Plenum, pp. 143–160.

Moore, N. (1993). Drugs in ancient populations (letter; reply). *Lancet, 341,* 1157.

Morgan, C., Kosten, T., Gawin, F., and Kleber, H. (1988). A pilot trial of amantadine for ambulatory withdrawal for cocaine dependence. In L. S. Harris (Ed.), *Problems of drug dependence, 1987* (NIDA Research Monograph No. 81). Washington, D.C.: NIDA, pp. 81–85.

Morgan, J. P. (1992). Prohibition was and is bad for the nation's health. In J. H. Lowinson, P. Ruiz, and R. B. Millman (Eds.), *Substance abuse: A comprehensive textbook.* Baltimore: Williams & Wilkins, pp. 1012–18.

Morrow, P. L. and McQuillen, J. B. (1993). Cerebral vasculitis associated with cocaine abuse. *Journal of Forensic Sciences, 38(3),* 732–738.

Moscovitz, H., Brookoff, D., and Nelson, L. (1993). A randomized trial of bromocriptine for cocaine users presenting to the emergency department. *Journal of General Internal Medicine, 8(1),* 1–4.

Mott, S. H., Packer, R. J., and Soldin, S. J. (1994). Neurologic manifestations of cocaine exposure in childhood. *Pediatrics, 93(4),* 557–560.

Muntaner, C., Kumor, K., Nagoshi, C., and Jaffe, J. (1988). Effects of nifedipine (a Ca++ modulator) pre-treatment on cardiovascular and subjective responses to intravenous cocaine administration in humans. In L. S. Harris (Ed.), *Problems of drug dependence, 1988* (NIDA Research Monogrpah No. 90). Washington, D.C.: NIDA, p. 388.

—— Kumor, K. M., Nagoshi, C., and Jaffe, J. H. (1991). Effects of nifedipine pretreatment on subjective and cardiovascular responses to intravenous cocaine in humans. *Psychopharmacology, 105(1),* 37–41.

Murphy, S. and Rosenbaum, M. (1992). Women who use cocaine too much: Smoking crack vs. snorting cocaine. *Journal of Psychoactive Drugs, 24(4),* 381–388.

Murphy, S. B., Reinarman, C., and Waldorf, D. (1989). An 11-year follow-up of a network of cocaine users. *British Journal of Addictions, 84,* 427–436.

Murray, R., Smialek, J., Golle, M., and Albin, R. (1988). Pulmonary vascular abnormalities in cocaine users. *American Review of Respiratory Disease, 137(4; suppl.),* 459.

Musto, D. F. (1992). Cocaine's history, especially the American experience. *Cocaine: Scientific and social dimensions* (Ciba Foundation Symposium No. 166). Chichester: Wiley, pp. 7–19.

Nace, E. P., Davis, C. W., and Gaspari, J. P. (1991). Axis II comorbidity in substance abusers. *American Journal of Psychiatry, 148(1),* 118–120.

Nadelmann, E. A. (1989). Drug prohibition in the United States: Costs, consequences, and alternatives. *Science, 245,* 939–947.

—— (1991a). Beyond drug prohibition: Evaluating the alternatives. In M. B. Krauss and E. P. Lazear (Eds.), *Searching for alternatives: Drug-control policy in the United States.* Palo Alto, Calif.: Hoover Institution Press, pp. 241–250.

—— (1991b). A rational approach to drug legalization. *American Journal of Ethics and Medicine (Spring),* 3–7.

—— (1992). Thinking seriously about alternatives to drug prohibition. *Daedalus, 121(3),* 85–132.

Nademanee, K., Gorelick, D. A., Josephson, M. A., Ryan, M. A., Wilkins, J. N., Robertson, H. A., Mody, F. V., and Intarachot, V. (1989). Myocardial ischemia during cocaine withdrawal. *Annals of Internal Medicine, 111,* 876–880.

Nair, P., Rothblum, S., and Hebel, R. (1994). Neonatal outcome in infants with evidence of fetal exposure to opiates, cocaine, and cannabinoids. *Clinical Pediatrics, 33(5),* 280–285.

Nakamura, G. R. and Noguchi, T. T. (1981). Fatalities from cocaine overdose in Los Angeles County. *Clinical Toxicology, 18(8),* 895–905.

Nanji, A. A. and Filipenko, J. D. (1984). Asystole and ventricular fibrillation associated with cocaine intoxiciation. *Chest, 85,* 132–133.

Naranjo, C. A., Poulos, C. X., Bremner, K. E., and Lanctot, K. L. (1994). Flouxetine attenuates alcohol intake and desire to drink. *International Clinical Psychopharmacology, 9(3),* 163–172.

National Institute of Justice (1994a). *Drug use forecasting 1993: Annual report on adult arrestees.* Washington, D.C.: U.S. Department of Justice.

—— (1994b). *Drug use forecasting 1993: Annual report on juvenile arrestees/ detainees: Drugs and crime in America's cities.* Washington, D.C.: U.S. Department of Justice.

Newcomb, M., Maddahian, E., and Bentler, P. M. (1986). Risk factors for drug use among adolescents: Concurrent and longitudinal analyses. *American Journal of Public Health, 76,* 525–531.

Newcomb, M. D., Bentler, P. M., and Fahy, B. (1987). Cocaine use and psychopathology: Associations among young adults. *International Journal of the Addictions, 22(12)*, 1167–88.

Newman, N. M., DiLoreto, D. A., Ho, J. T., Klein, J. C., and Birnbaum, N. S. (1988). Bilateral optic neuropathy and osteolytic sinusitis: Complications of cocaine abuse. *Journal of the American Medical Association, 259*, 72–74.

Newman, R. G. (1979). Detoxification treatment of narcotic addicts. In R. Dupont, A. Goldstein, J. O'Donnell, and B. S. Brown (Eds.), *Handbook on drug abuse*. Washington, D.C.: NIDA, pp. 21–29.

Nicholi, A. M. (1984). Historical perspective: The long and colorful history of erythoxylon coca. *Journal of American College Health*, 252–257.

NIDA (1992). *Annual Medical Examiner Data, 1991: Data from the Drug Abuse Warning Network (DAWN):* Series 1, No. 11-B. Washington, D.C.: Department of Health and Human Services, DHHS Pub. No. (ADM) 92–1955.

Nunes, E. V., Quitkin, F. M., and Klein, D. F. (1989). Psychiatric diagnosis in cocaine abuse. *Psychiatry Research, 28*, 105–114.

―――― McGrath, P. J., Wager, S., and Quitkin, F. M. (1990). Lithium treatment for cocaine abusers with bipolar spectrum disorders. *American Journal of Psychiatry, 147(5)*, 655–657.

Nurco, D. N., Stephenson, P. E., and Hanlon, T. E. (1990–91). Aftercare/relapse prevention and the self-help movement. *International Journal of the Addictions, 25(9A and 10A)*, 1179–1200.

―――― Stephenson, P. E., and Naesea, L. (1981). *Manual for setting up self-help groups of ex-narcotic addicts*. Washington, D.C.: U.S. Government Printing Office.

―――― Kinlock, T. W., Hanlon, T. E., and Ball, J. C. (1988). Nonnarcotic drug use over an addiction career: A study of heroin addicts in Baltimore and New York City. *Comprehensive Psychiatry, 29(5)*, 450–459.

―――― Wegner, N., Stephenson, P., Makofsky, A., and Shaffer, J. W. (1983). *Ex-addicts' self-help groups: Potentials and pitfalls*. New York: Praeger.

O'Brien, C. P., Childress, A. R., and McLellan, A. T. (1991). Conditioning factors may help to understand and prevent relapse in patients who are recovering from drug dependence. In R. W. Pickens, C. G. Leukefeld, and C. R. Schuster (Eds.), *Improving drug abuse treatment* (NIDA Research Monograph No. 106). Rockville, Md.: NIDA, pp. 293–312.

―――― Ehrman, R. N., and Ternes, J. W. (1986). Classical conditioning in human opioid dependence. In S. R. Goldberg and I. P. Stolerman (Eds.), *Behavioral analysis of drug dependence*. Orlando, Fla.: Academic Press, pp. 329–356.

―――― Childress, A. R., Arndt, I. O., McLellan, A. T., Woody, G. E., and Maany, I. (1988). Pharmacological and behavioral treatments of cocaine dependence: Controlled studies. *Journal of Clinical Psychiatry, 49 (suppl. 2)*, 17–22.

―――― Childress, A. R., McLellan, A. T., and Ehrman, R. (1990a). The use of cue exposure as an aid in the prevention of relapse to cocaine or heroin dependence. *Addictive Behaviors, 17(5)*, 491–499.

―――― Childress, A. R., McLellan, A. T., and Ehrman, R. (1990b). Integrating systematic cue exposure with standard treatment in recovering drug dependent patients. *Addictive Behaviors, 15*, 355–365.

—— Childress, A. R., McLellan, T., and Ehrman, R. (1992). A learning model of addiction. In C. P. O'Brien and J. H. Jaffe (Eds.), *Addictive states*. New York: Raven Press, pp. 157–177.

—— Childress, A. R., McLellan, A. T., and Ehrman, R. (1993). Developing treatments that address classical conditioning (review). In F. M. Tims and C. G. Leukefeld (Eds.), *Cocaine treatment: Research and clinical perspectives* (NIDA Research Monograph No. 135). Rockville, Md.: NIDA, pp. 71–91.

—— McLellan, A. T., Alterman, A., and Childress, A. R. (1992). Psychotherapy for cocaine dependence. *Ciba Foundation Symposium, 166,* 207–223.

—— O'Brien, T. J., Mintz, J., and Brady, J. P. (1975). Conditioning of narcotic abstinence symptoms in human subjects. *Drug and Alcohol Dependence, 1,* 115–123.

—— Testa, T., O'Brien, T. J., Brady, J. P., and Wells, B. (1977). Conditioned narcotic withdrawal in humans. *Science, 195,* 1000–1002.

O'Donnell, A. E., Mappin, G., Sebo, T. J., and Tazelaar, H. (1991). Interstitial pneumonitis associated with "crack" cocaine abuse. *Chest, 100(4),* 1155–57.

O'Farrell, T. J. and Langenbucher, J. (1987). Inpatient treatment of alcoholism: A behavioral approach. *Journal of Substance Abuse Treatment, 4(3–4),* 215–231.

Olshaker, J. S. (1994). Cocaine chest pain (review). *Emergency Medicine Clinics of North America, 12(2),* 391–396.

Olson, K. R., Kearney, T. E., Dyer, J. E., Benowitz, N. L., and Blanc, P. D. (1994). Seizures associated with poisoning and drug overdose. *American Journal of Emergency Medicine, 12(3),* 392–395.

O'Malley, J. E., Anderson, W. H., and Lazare, A. (1972). Failure of outpatient treatment of drug abuse. I. Heroin. *American Journal of Psychiatry, 128(7),* 865–868.

O'Malley, P. M., Johnston, L. D., and Bachman, J. G. (1985). Cocaine use among American adolescents and young adults. In H. G. Kozel and E. H. Adams (Eds.), *Cocaine use in America: Epidemiologic and clinical perspectives* (NIDA Research Monograph No. 61). Rockville, Md.: NIDA, pp. 50–75.

O'Malley, S., Adamse, M., Heaton, R. K., and Gawin, F. H. (1992). Neuropsychological impairment in chronic cocaine abusers. *American Journal of Drug and Alcohol Abuse, 18(2),* 131–144.

O'Malley, S. S. and Gawin, F. H. (1990). Abstinence symptomatology and neuropsychological impairment in chronic cocaine abusers. In J. W. Spencer and J. J. Boren (Eds.), *Residual effects of abused drugs on behavior* (NIDA Research Monograph No. 101). Rockville, Md.: NIDA, pp. 179–190.

—— Adamse, M., Heaton, R.K., and Gawin, F. H. (1988). Neuropsychological impairment in chronic cocaine abusers. Presented at the Annual Meeting of the Society of Psychologists in Addictive Behaviors, Atlanta, August.

—— Gawin, F. H., Heaton, R., and Kleber, H. D. (1989). Cognitive deficits associated with cocaine abuse. Presented at the annual meeting of the American Psychiatric Association, San Francisco, May.

Oppenheimer, E., Sheehan, M., and Taylor, C. (1988). Letting the client speak: Drug misusers and the process of help seeking. *British Journal on Addiction, 83,* 635–647.

Osol, A. and Pratt, R. (Eds.) (1973). *The United States dispensatory.* Philadelphia: Lippincott, p. 329.

Owens, W. D. (1912). Signs and symptoms presented by those addicted to cocain. *Journal of the American Medical Association, 58(5)*, 329–330.

Paly, D., Jatlow, P., Van Dyke, C., Jeri, F. R., and Byck, R. (1982). Plasma cocaine concentrations during cocaine paste smoking. *Life Sciences, 30*, 731–738.

―――― Van Dyke, C., Jatlow, P., Cabieses, F., and Byck, R. (1979). Cocaine plasma concentrations in coca chewers. *Clinical Pharmacology and Therapeutics, 25*, 240.

Parker, S. and Knoll, J. L. (1990). Partial hospitalization: An update. *American Journal of Psychiatry, 147*, 156–160.

Parr, D. (1976). Sexual aspects of drug abuse in narcotic addicts. *British Journal of Addictions, 71*, 261–268.

Parsche, F., Balabanova, S., and Pirsig, W. (1993). Drugs in ancient populations. *Lancet, 341*, 503.

Parsons, L. H., Schad, C. A., and Justice, J. B., Jr. (1993). Co-administration of the D2 antagonist pimozide inhibits up-regulation of dopamine release and uptake induced by repeated cocaine. *Journal of Neurochemistry, 60(1)*, 376–379.

Pascual-Leone, A., Dhuna, A., and Anderson, D. (1991). Cerebral atrophy in habitual cocaine abusers: A planimetric CT study. *Neurology, 41*, 34–38.

Passannante, M. R., Wells, D. V. B., Quinones, M. A., Jackson, J. F., and Rotkiewicz, L. G. (1991). AIDS education in drug user treatment programs. *International Journal of the Addictions, 26(5)*, 577–594.

Patterson, M. A. (1976). *Hooked? NET: New approach to drug cure*. London: Faber & Faber.

―――― (1984). Treatment of drug, alcohol and nicotine addiction by neuroelectric therapy: Analysis of results over 7 years. *Journal of Bioelectricity, 3*, 193–221.

―――― Firth, J., and Gardiner, R. (1984). Effects of neuroelectric therapy (NET) in drug addiction. *United Nations Bulletin on Narcotics, 28*, 55–62.

Pearlson, G. D., Jeffery, P. J., Harris, G. J., Ross, C. A., Fischman, M. W., and Camargo, E. E. (1993). Correlation of acute cocaine-induced changes in local cerebral blood flow with subjective effects. *American Journal of Psychiatry, 150(3)*, 495–497.

Pearman, K. (1979). Cocaine: A review. *Journal of Laryngology and Otology, 93*, 1191–99.

Pearsall, H. R. and Rosen, M. I. (1992). Inpatient treatment of cocaine addiction. In T. R. Kosten and H. D. Kleber (Eds.), *Clinician's guide to cocaine treatment: Theory, research, and treatment*. New York: Guilford, pp. 314–334.

Peng, S. K., French, W. J., and Pelikan, P. C. D. (1989). Direct cocaine cardiotoxicity demonstrated by endomyocardial biopsy. *Archives of Pathology and Laboratory Medicine, 113*, 842–845.

Pentel, P. R. and Thompson, T. N. (1993). Potential adverse interactions of drugs with cocaine. In H. Sorer (Ed.), *Acute cocaine intoxication: Current methods of treatment* (NIDA Research Monograph No. 123). Rockville, Md.: NIDA, pp. 156–171.

Perez-Reyes, M. (1994). The order of drug administration: Its effects on the interaction between cocaine and ethanol. *Life Sciences, 55(7)*, 541–550.

Peterson, P. K., Gekker, G., Chao, C. C., Schut, R., Molitor, T. W., and Balfour,

H. H., Jr. (1991). Cocaine potentiates HIV-1 replication in human peripheral blood mononuclear cell cocultures. Involvement of transforming growth factor-beta. *Journal of Immunology, 146(1),* 81–84.

Petty, G. W., Brust, J. C. M., Tatemichi, T. K., and Barr, M. L. (1990). Embolic stroke after smoking "crack" cocaine. *Stroke, 21,* 1632–35.

Phibbs, C. S., Bateman, D. A., and Schwartz, R. M. (1991). The neonatal costs of maternal cocaine use. *Journal of the American Medical Association, 266(11),* 1521–26.

Phillippe, M. (1983). Fetal catecholamines. *American Journal of Obstetrics and Gynecology, 146,* 840–855.

Phillips, A. G., Broekkamp, C. L. E., and Fibiger, H. C. (1983). Strategies for studying the neurochemical substrates of drug reinforcement in rodents. *Progress in Neuro-Psychopharmacology and Biological Psychiatry, 7,* 585–590.

Physician's Desk Reference [PDR] (1994). Montvale, N.J.: Medical Economics Data Production.

Pickens, R. W., Battjes, R., Svikis, D. S., and Gupman, A. E. (1993). Substance use risk factors for HIV infection. *Psychiatric Clinics of North America, 16,* 119–125.

Pickering, H. and Stimson, G. (1994). Prevalence and demographic factors of stimulant use. *Addiction, 89,* 1385–89.

Pickett, G., Kosten, T. R., Gawin, F. H., Byck, R., Fleming, J., Silverman, D., Kosten, T. A., and Jatlow, P. (1990). Concurrent effects of acute intravenous cocaine in context of chronic desipramine in humans. In L. S. Harris (Ed.), *Problems of drug dependence, 1990* (NIDA Research Monograph No. 105). Rockville, Md.: NIDA, pp. 508–509.

Pirozhkov, S. V., Watson, R. R., and Chen, G. J. (1992). Ethanol enhances immunosuppression induced by cocaine. *Alcohol, 9(6),* 489–494.

Platt, J. J. (1986). *Heroin Addiction: Theory, Research, and Treatment.* 2nd ed. Malabar, Fla.: Krieger.

——— (1995a). *Heroin Addiction.* Vol. 2. *The addict, the treatment process, and social control.* Melbourne, Fla.: Krieger.

——— (1995b). *Heroin Addiction.* Vol. 3. *Treatment advances and AIDS.* Melbourne, Fla.: Krieger.

——— and Labate, C. (1976). *Heroin addiction: Theory, research, and treatment.* New York: Wiley.

——— and Metzger, D. S. (1987). Cognitive interpersonal problem-solving skills and the maintenance of treatment success in heroin addicts. *Psychology of Addictive Behaviors, 1,* 5–13.

——— Bühringer, G., Widman, M., Kunzel, J., and Lidz, V. (1996). Uniform standards for substance abuse treatment research: An example from Germany for the United States. *Substance Use and Misuse, 31(4),* 479–492.

——— Kirby, K., Marlowe, D., Lamb, R., and Lidz, V. (1995). Effectiveness of outpatient versus day treatment for cocaine users. Abstract submitted for 1995 annual College on Problems of Drug Dependence meeting, Palm Beach, Fla., June.

——— Steer, R. A., Ranieri, W. F., and Metzger, D. S. (1989). Differences in the Symptom Check List-90 profiles of black and white methadone patients. *Journal of Clinical Psychology, 45(2),* 342–345.

Plessinger, M. A. and Woods, J. R. (1993). Maternal, placental, and fetal patho-physiology of cocaine exposure during pregnancy. *Clinical Obstetrics and Gynecology, 36(2)*, 267–278.

Pohl, R., Balon, R., and Yergani, V. K. (1987). More on cocaine and panic dis-order (letter). *American Journal of Psychiatry, 144,* 1363.

———— Yeragani, V. K., Balon, R., and Lycaki, H. (1988). The jitteriness syndrome in panic disorder patients treated with antidepressants. *Journal of Clinical Psychiatry, 49,* 100–104.

Pollack, M. H. and Rosenbaum, J. F. (1991). Fluoxetine treatment of cocaine abuse in heroin addicts. *Journal of Clinical Psychiatry, 52(1),* 31–33.

———— Brotman, A. W., and Rosenbaum, J. F. (1989). Cocaine abuse and treat-ment. *Comprehensive Psychiatry, 30,* 31–44.

Pollock, D. A., Holmgreen, P., Lui, K. J., and Kirk, M. L. (1991). Discrepancies in the reported frequency of cocaine-related deaths, United States, 1983 through 1988. *Journal of the American Medical Association, 266(16),* 2233–37.

Pope, H. G., Keck, P. E., and McElroy, S. L. (1986). Frequency and presentation of neuroleptic malignant syndrome in a large psychiatric hospital. *American Journal of Psychiatry, 143(10),* 1227–32.

Popkin, S. J., Johnson, W. A., Clatts, M. C., Wiebel, W. W., and Deren, S. (1993). Homelessness and risk behaviors among intravenous drug users in Chicago and New York City. In B. S. Brown and G. M. Beschner (Eds.), *Handbook on risk of AIDS: Injection drug users and sexual partners.* Westport, Conn.: Greenwood Press, pp. 313–327.

Post, R. M. (1975). Cocaine psychosis: A continuum model. *American Journal of Psychiatry, 132(3),* 225–231.

———— and Kopanda, R. T. (1976). Cocaine, kindling and psychosis. *American Journal of Psychiatry, 133(6),* 627–634.

———— and Rose, H. (1976). Increasing effects of repetitive cocaine administra-tion in the rat. *Nature, 260,* 731–732.

———— and Weiss, S. R. (1988). Psychomotor stimulant vs. local anesthetic ef-fects of cocaine: Role of behavioral sensitization and kindling. In D. Clouet, K. Ashgar, and R. Brown (Eds.), *Mechanisms of cocaine abuse and toxicity* (NIDA Research Monograph No. 88). Rockville, Md.: NIDA, pp. 217–238.

———— and Weiss, S. R. (1989). Sensitization, kindling, and anticonvulsants in mania. *Journal of Clinical Psychiatry, 50 (suppl.),* 23–30.

———— Kopanda, R. T., and Black, K. E. (1976). Progressive effects of cocaine on behavior and central amine metabolism in the rhesus monkey: Relationship to kindling and psychosis. *Biological Psychiatry, 11,* 403–419.

———— Weiss, S. R. and Pert, A. (1984). Differential effects of carbamazepine and lithium on sensitization and kindling. *Progress in Neuropsychopharmacology and Biological Psychiatry, 8,* 425–434.

———— Lockfeld, A., Squillace, K. M., and Contel, N. R. (1981). Drug-environ-ment interaction: Context dependency of cocaine-induced behavioral sen-sitization. *Life Sciences, 28,* 755–760.

———— Weiss, S. R., Pert, A., and Uhde, T. W. (1987). Chronic cocaine adminis-tration: Sensitization and kindling effects. In S. Fisher, A. Raskin, and E. H. Uhlenhuth (Eds.), *Cocaine: Clinical and behavioral aspects.* New York: Oxford University Press, pp. 109–173.

Pottieger, A. E., Tressell, P. A., Inciardi, J. A., and Rosales, T. A. (1992). Cocaine use patterns and overdose. *Journal of Psychoactive Drugs, 24(4)*, 399–410.

Powell, B. J., Penick, E. C., Othmer, E., Bingham, S. F., and Rice, A. S. (1982). Prevalence of additional psychiatric syndromes among male alcoholics. *Journal of Clinical Psychiatry, 43*, 404–407.

Preston, K. L., Sullivan, J. T., Berger, P., and Bigelow, G. E. (1993). Effects of cocaine alone and in combination with mazindol in human cocaine abusers. *Journal of Pharmacology and Experimental Therapeutics, 267(1)*, 296–307.

Prochaska, J. O. and DiClemente, C. C. (1986). Toward a comprehensive model of change. In W. R. Miller and N. Heather (Eds.), *Treating addictive behaviors: Processes of change*. New York: Plenum, pp. 3–27.

——— and DiClemente, C. C. (1992). Stages of change in the modification of problem behaviors. In M. Hersen, R. M. Eisler, and P. M. Miller (Eds.), *Progress in behavior modification*. Sycamore, Ill.: Sycamore Press, pp. 184–214.

Pulvirenti, L. and Koob, G. F. (1993). Lisuride reduces intravenous cocaine self-administration in rats. *Neuropsychopharmacology, 8*, 213–218.

——— Swerdlow, N. R., Hubner, C. B., and Koob, C. F. (1991). The role of limbic-accumbens-pallidal circuitry in the activating properties of psychostimulant drugs. In P. Willner and J. Kruger (Eds.), *The dopamine system: From motivation to action*. London: John Wiley, pp. 131–140.

Racine, A., Joyce, T., and Anderson, R. (1993). The association between prenatal care and birth weight among women exposed to cocaine in New York City. *Journal of the American Medical Association, 270(13)*, 1581–86.

Radó, S. (1933). The psychoanalysis of pharmacothymia. *Psychoanalytic Quarterly, 2*, 1–23.

Rafla, R. L. and Epstein, R. L. (1979). Identification of cocaine and its metabolites in human urine in the presence of ethyl alcohol. *Journal of Anal Toxicology, 3*, 59–63.

Ramsey, N. F. and van Ree, J. M. (1991). Intracerebroventricular naltrexone treatment attenuates acquisition of intravenous cocaine self-administration in rats. *Pharmacology, Biochemistry and Behavior, 40(4)*, 807–810.

Rapoport, J. L., Buchsbaum, M. S., Zahn, T. P., Weingartner, H., Ludlow, C., and Mikkelsen, E. J. (1978). Dextroamphetamine: Cognitive and behavioral effects in normal prepubertal boys. *Sciences, 199(4328)*, 560–563.

Rappolt, R. T., Gay, G. R., and Inaba, D. S. (1977). Propranolol: A specific antagonistic to cocaine. *Clinical Toxicology, 10*, 265–271.

Ratner, M. S. (Ed.) (1993). *Crack pipe as pimp*. New York: Lexington Books.

Ravin, J. G. and Ravin, L. G. (1979). Blindness due to illicit use of topical cocaine. *Annals of Ophthalmology, 11*, 863–864.

Rawson, R. (1990). Cut the crack: The policymaker's guide to cocaine treatment. *Policy Review (Winter)*, 10–19.

Rawson, R. A. (1989). *Cocaine recovery issues: The neurobehavioral model of cocaine treatment*. Beverly Hills, Calif.: Matrix Institute on Addictions.

——— Obert, J. L., McCann, M. J., and Ling, W. (1991). Psychological approaches for the treatment of cocaine dependence: A neurobehavioral approach. *Journal of Addictive Diseases, 11(2)*, 97–120.

——— Obert, J. L., McCann, M. J., and Ling, W. (1993). Neurobehavioral treatment for cocaine dependence: A preliminary evaluation. In F. M. Tims and

C. G. Leukefeld (Eds.), *Cocaine treatment: Research and clinical perspectives* (NIDA Research Monograph No. 135). Rockville, Md.: NIDA, pp. 92–115.

—— Obert, J. L., McCann, M. J., and Mann, A. J. (1986). Cocaine treatment outcome: Cocaine use following inpatient, outpatient, and no treatment. In L. S. Harris (Ed.), *Problems of drug dependence, 1985* (NIDA Research Monograph No. 67). Washington, D.C.: NIDA, pp. 271–277.

—— Obert, J. L., McCann, M. J., Smith, D. P., and Ling, W. (1990). Neurobehavioral treatment for cocaine dependency. *Journal of Psychoactive Drugs, 22(2),* 159–171.

Ray, O. (1978). *Drugs, society, and human behavior.* 2nd ed. St. Louis: C. V. Mosby.

Reed, R. J. and Grant, I. (1990). The long-term neurobehavioral consequences of substance abuse: Conceptual and methodological challenges for future research. In J. W. Spencer and J. J. Boren (Eds.), *Residual effects of abused drugs on behavior* (NIDA Research Monograph No. 101). Rockville, Md.: NIDA, pp. 10–56.

Reid, R. W., O'Connor, F. L., and Crayton, J. W. (1994). The in vitro differential binding of benzoylecgonine to pigmented human hair samples. *Journal of Toxicology–Clinical Toxicology, 32(4),* 405–410.

Reinarman, C. and Levine, H. G. (1989). Crack in context: Politics and media in the making of a drug scare. *Contemporary Drug Problems, 16,* 535–577.

Resnick, R. (1983). Methadone detoxification from illicit opiates and methadone maintenance. In J. R. Cooper, F. Altman, B. S. Brown, and D. Czechowicz (Eds.), *Research on the treatment of narcotic addiction: State of the art* (NIDA Treatment Research Monograph). Rockville, Md.: NIDA, pp. 160–167.

Resnick, R. B. and Resnick, E. (1984). Cocaine abuse and its treatment. *Psychiatric Clinics of North America, 7,* 713–728.

—— and Resnick, E. (1985). Psychological issues in the treatment of cocaine abuse. In L. S. Harris (Ed.), *Problems of drug dependence, 1985* (NIDA Research Monograph Series No. 67). Rockville, Md.: NIDA, pp. 290–294.

—— Kestenbaum, R. S., and Schwartz, L. K. (1977). Acute systemic effects of cocaine in man: A controlled study by intranasal and intravenous routes. *Science, 195,* 696–698.

—— Kestenbaum, R. S., and Schwartz, L. K. (1980). Acute systemic effects for cocaine in man: A controlled study by intranasal and intravenous routes. In F. R. Jeri (Ed.), *Cocaine, 1980.* Lima, Peru: Pacific Press, pp. 17–20.

Reuband, K.-H. (1992). The epidemiology of drug use in Germany: Basic data and trends. In G. Bühringer and J. J. Platt (Eds.), *Drug addiction treatment research: German and American perspectives.* Malabar, Fla.: Krieger, pp. 3–16.

Rhodes, W. (1993). Synthetic estimation applied to the prevalence of drug use. *Journal of Drug Issues, 23(2),* 297–321.

Ricci, J. M., Fojaco, R. M., and O'Sullivan, M. J. (1989). Congenital syphilis: The University of Miami/Jackson Memorial Medical Center experience, 1986–1988. *Obstetrics and Gynecology, 74,* 687–693.

Richard, M. L., Liskow, B. I., and Perry, P. J. (1985). Recent psychostimulant use in hospitalized schizophrenics. *Journal of Clinical Psychiatry, 46(3),* 79–83.

Riffee, W. H., Wanek, E., and Wilcox, R. E. (1987). Prevention of amphetamine-induced hypersensitivity by concomitant treatment with microgram doses of apomorphine. *European Journal of Pharmacology, 135,* 255–258.

—— Wanek, E., and Wilcox, R. E. (1988). Apomorphine fails to inhibit cocaine-induced behavioral hypersensitivity. *Pharmacology, Biochemistry and Behavior, 29,* 239–242.

Ritchie, J. M. and Cohen, P. J. (1975). *The pharmacological basis of therapeutics.* In L. S. Goodman and A. Gilman (Eds.), New York: Macmillan, p. 379.

———— and Greene, N. M. (1990). Local anesthetics. In A. G. Gilman, T. W. Rall, A. S. Nies, and P. Taylor (Eds.), *Goodman and Gilman's The pharmacological basis of therapeutics.* 8th ed. Elmsford, N.Y.: Pergamon, pp. 311–313.

Ritz, M. C., Lamb, R. J., Goldberg, S. R., and Kuhar, M. J. (1987). Cocaine receptors on dopamine transporters are related to self-administration of cocaine. *Science, 237,* 1219–23.

Robbins, L. N., Helzer, J. I., Croughan, J., and Ratcliff, K. S. (1981). National Institute of Mental Health Diagnostic Interview Schedule. *Archives of General Psychiatry, 38,* 381–389.

Robbins, S. J., Ehrman, R. N., Childress, A. R., and O'Brien, C. P. (1992). Using cue reactivity to screen medications for cocaine abuse: A test of amantadine hydrocholoride. *Addictive Behaviors, 17,* 491–499.

Roberts, D. C. S., Corcoran, M. E., and Fibiger, H. C. (1977). On the role of ascending catecholaminergic systems in intravenous self-administration of cocaine. *Pharmacology, Biochemistry and Behavior, 6,* 615–620.

Roberts, J. R., Quattrocchi, E., and Howland, M. A. (1984). Severe hyperthermia secondary to intravenous drug abuse (letter). *American Journal of Emergency Medicine, 2,* 373.

Roberts, L. A. and Bauer, L. O. (1993). Reaction time during cocaine versus alcohol withdrawal: Longitudinal measures of visual and auditory suppression. *Psychiatry Research, 46(3),* 229–237.

Robins, L. N., Helzer, J. E., and Davis, D. H. (1975). Narcotic use in southeast Asia and afterward: An interview study of 898 Vietnam returnees. *Archives of General Psychiatry, 32,* 955–961.

Rockhold, R. W. (1991). Excitatory amino acid receptor antagonists: Potential implications for cardiovascular therapy and cocaine intoxication. *Medical Hypothesis, 35,* 342–348.

Rod, J. and Zucker, R. (1987). Acute myocardial infarction shortly after cocaine inhalation. *American Journal of Cardiology, 59,* 161.

Rodriguez, M.-E. (1989). Treatment of cocaine abuse: Medical and psychiatric consequences. In K. K. Redda, C. A. Walker, and G. Barnett (Eds.), *Cocaine, marijuana, designer drugs: Chemistry, pharmacology, and behavior.* Boca Raton, Fla.: CRC Press, pp. 97–112.

Roehrich, H. and Gold, M. S. (1991). Cocaine. In D. A. Ciraulo and R. I. Shader (Eds.), *Clinical manual of chemical dependence.* Washington, D.C.: American Psychiatric Press, pp. 195–231.

Rohsenow, D. J., Niaura, R. S., Childress, A. R., Abrams, D. B., and Monti, P. M. (1990–91). Cue reactivity in addictive behaviors: Theoretical and treatment implications. *International Journal of the Addictions, 25,* 957–993.

Rolfs, R. T., Goldberg, M., and Sharrar, R. G. (1990). Risk factors for syphilis: Cocaine use and prostitution. *American Journal of Public Health, 80,* 853–857.

Rosecan, J. S. (1983). The treatment of cocaine abuse with imipramine, L-tyrosine and L-tryptophan. Presented at the VII World Congress on Psychiatry, Vienna, Austria.

Rosen, H., Flemenbaum, A., and Slater, V. L. (1986). Clinical trial of carbidopa-

L-dopa combination for cocaine abuse. *American Journal of Psychiatry, 143(11),* 1493.

Rosen, M. I, Pearsall, H. R., McDougle, C. J., Price, L. H., Woods, S. W., and Kosten, T. R. (1993). Effects of acute buprenorphine on responses to intranasal cocaine: A pilot study. *American Journal of Drug and Alcohol Abuse, 19(4),* 451–464.

Rosenbaum, M. (1982). Getting on methadone: The experience of the woman addict. *Contemporary Drug Problems, 11,* 113–143.

Rosenberg, N. M., Meert, K. L., Knazik, S. R., Yee, H., and Kauffman, R. E. (1991). Occult cocaine exposure in children. *American Journal of Diseases of Children, 145(12),* 1430–32.

Ross, H. E., Glaser, F. B., and Germanson, T. (1988). The prevalence of psychiatric disorders in patients with alcohol and other drug problems. *Archives of General Psychiatry, 45,* 1023–31.

Ross, S. B. and Renyi, A. L. (1966). Uptake of some tritiated sympathomimetic amines by mouse brain cortex in vitro. *Acta Pharmacologia et Toxicologia, 24,* 297–309.

Rosse, R. B., Fay-McCarthy, M., Alim, T. N., and Deutsch, S. I. (1994). Saccadic distractibility in cocaine dependent patients: A preliminary laboratory exploration of the cocaine-OCD hypothesis. *Drug and Alcohol Dependence, 35,* 25–30.

—— Fay-McCarthy, M., Collins, J. P., Risher-Flowers, D., Alim, T. N., and Deutsch, S. I. (1993). Transient compulsive foraging behavior associated with crack cocaine use. *American Journal of Psychiatry, 150(1),* 155–156.

Roth, D., Alarcon, F. J., Fernandez, J. A., Preston, R. A., and Bourgoignie, J. J. (1988). Acute rhabdomyolysis associated with cocaine intoxication. *New England Journal of Medicine, 319,* 673–677.

Rounsaville, B. J. and Carroll, K. (1993). Interpersonal psychotherapy for patients who abuse drugs. In G. L. Klerman and M.M.Weissman (Eds.), *New application of interpersonal psychotherapy.* Washington, D.C.: American Psychiatric Press, pp. 319–352.

—— and Kleber, H. D. (1984). Psychiatric disorders and the course of opiate addictions: Preliminary findings on predictive significance and diagnostic stability. In S. M. Mirin (Ed.), *Substance abuse and psychopathology.* Washington, D.C.: American Psychiatric Press, pp. 133–151.

—— Gawin, F. H., and Kleber, H. D. (1985). Interpersonal psychotherapy adapted for ambulatory cocaine abusers. *American Journal of Drug and Alcohol Abuse, 11(3&4),* 171–191.

—— Anton, S. F., Carroll, K., Budde, D., Prusoff, B. A., and Gawin, F. (1991). Psychiatric diagnoses of treatment-seeking cocaine abusers. *Archives of General Psychiatry, 48,* 43–51.

—— Dolinsky, Z. S., Babor, T. F., and Meyer, R. E. (1987). Psychopathology as a predictor of treatment outcome in alcoholics. *Archives of General Psychiatry, 44,* 505–513.

—— Glazer, W., Wilber, C. H., Weissman, M. M., and Kleber, H. D. (1983). Short-term interpersonal psychotherapy in methadone-maintained opiate addicts. *Archives of General Psychiatry, 40,* 629–636.

—— Kleber, H. D., Wilber, C., Rosenberger, D., and Rosenberger, P. (1981). Comparison of opiate addicts' reports of psychiatric history with reports of significant-other informants. *American Journal of Drug and Alcohol Abuse, 8(1),* 51–69.

—— Kosten, T. R., Weissman, M. M., and Kleber, H. D. (1986). Prognostic significance of psychopathology in treated opiate addicts. *Archives of General Psychiatry, 43,* 739–745.

—— Kosten, T. R., Weissman, M. M., Prusoff, B., Pauls, D., Foley, S., and Merikangas, K. (1991). Psychiatric disorders in relatives of probands with opiate addiction. *Archives of General Psychiatry, 48,* 33–42.

—— Tierney, T., Crits-Chistoph, K., Weissman, M. M., and Kleber, H. D. (1982). Predictors of outcome in treatment of opiate addicts: Evidence for the multidimensional nature of addicts' problems. *Comprehensive Psychiatry, 23,* 462–478.

—— Weissman, M. M., Crits-Cristoph, K., Wilber, C., and Kleber, H. (1982a). Diagnosis and symptoms of depression in opiate addicts: Course and relationship to treatment outcome. *Archives of General Psychiatry, 39,* 151–156.

—— Weissman, M. M., Kleber, H. D., and Wilber, C. (1982b). Heterogeneity of psychiatric diagnosis in treated opiate addicts. *Archives of General Psychiatry, 39,* 161–166.

—— Wilber, C. H., Rosenberger, D., and Kleber, H. D. (1981). Comparison of opiate addicts' reports of psychiatric history with reports of significant other informants. *American Journal of Drug and Alcohol Abuse, 8,* 51–69.

Rowbotham, M. C. and Lowenstein, D. H. (1990). Neurologic consequences of cocaine use. *Annual Review of Medicine, 41,* 417–422.

—— Jones, R. T., Benowitz, N. L., and Jacob, P. (1984). Trazodone-oral cocaine interactions. *Archives of General Psychiatry, 41,* 895–899.

Ruiz, P., Cleary, T., Nassiri, M., and Steele, B. (1994). Human t-lymphocyte subpopulation and NK cell alterations in persons exposed to cocaine. *Clinical Immunology and Immunopathology, 70(3),* 245–250.

Ryan, L., Ehrlich, S., and Finnegan, L. (1987). Cocaine abuse in pregnancy: Effects on the fetus and newborn. *Neurotoxicology Teratology, 9,* 295–299.

Sabbag, R. (1976). *Snowblind.* New York: Avon.

Sachs, R., Zagelbaum, B. M., and Hersh, P. S. (1993). Corneal complications associated with the use of crack cocaine. *Opthamology, 100(2),* 187–191.

Sannerud, C. A. and Griffiths, R. R. (1988). Amantadine: Evaluation of reinforcing properties and effect on cocaine self-injection in baboons. *Drug and Alcohol Dependence, 21,* 195–202.

Santos, E. F. (1986). Naltrexone: Useful tool in the treatment of heroin users: A review of the literature. *Bulletin of the Association of Medicine of Puerto Rico, 78(3),* 95–98.

Satel, S. L. and Edell, W. S. (1991). Cocaine-induced paranoia and psychosis proneness. *American Journal of Psychiatry, 148(12),* 1708–11.

—— and Gawin, F. H. (1989). Migrainelike headaches and cocaine use. *Journal of the American Medical Association, 261(20),* 2995–96.

—— Southwick, S. M. and Gawin, F. H. (1991). Clinical features of cocaine-induced paranoia. *American Journal of Psychiatry, 148(4),* 495–498.

—— Price, L. H., Palumbo, J. M., McDougle, C. J., Krystal, J. H., Gawin, F., Charney, D. S., Heninger, G. R., and Kleber, H. D. (1991). Clinical phenomenology and neurobiology of cocaine abstinence: A prospective inpatient study. *American Journal of Psychiatry, 148(12),* 1712–16.

Schatzman, M., Sabbadini, A., and Forti, L. (1976). Coca and cocaine: A bibli-ography. *Journal of Psychoactive Drugs, 8(2),* 95–128.

Schechter, M. D. and Glennon, R. A. (1985). Cathinone, cocaine and metham-phetamine: Similarity of behavioral effects. *Pharmacology, Biochemistry and Behavior, 22,* 913–916.

Schiffer, F. (1988). Psychotherapy of nine successfully treated cocaine abusers: Techniques and dynamics. *Journal of Substance Abuse Treatment, 5,* 131–137.

Schiorring, E. (1981). Psychopathology induced by "speed drugs." *Pharmacology, Biochemistry and Behavior, 14(1),* 109–122.

Schneier, F. R. and Siris, S. G. (1987). A review of psychoactive substance use and abuse in schizophrenia: Patterns of drug choice. *Journal of Nervous and Mental Disease, 175(11),* 641–652.

Schnoll, S. H., Daghestani, A. N., and Hansen, T. R. (1984). Cocaine dependence. *Resident and Staff Physician, 30(11),* 24–31.

—— Karrigan, J., Kitchen, S. B., Daghestani, A., and Hansen, T. (1985). Characteristics of cocaine users presenting for treatment. In E. H. Adams and N. J. Kozel (Eds.), *Cocaine use in America: Epidemiologic and clinical per-spectives* (NIDA Research Monograph No. 61). Rockville, Md.: NIDA, pp. 171–181.

Schoenbaum, E. E., Hartel, D., and Friedland, G. H. (1990). Crack use predicts incident HIV seroconversion. Presented at the Sixth International Conference on AIDS. San Francisco, June 20–24.

—— Hartel, D., Selwyn, P. A., Klein, R. S., Davenny, K., Rogers, M., Feiner, C., and Friedland, G. (1989). Risk factors for human immunodeficiency virus infection in intravenous drug users. *New England Journal of Medicine, 321(13),* 874–879.

Schottenfeld, R., Carroll, K., and Rounsaville, B. (1993). Comorbid psychiatric disorders and cocaine abusers. In F. M. Tims and C. G. Leukefeld (Eds.), *Cocaine treatment: Research and clinical perspectives* (NIDA Research Monograph No. 135). Rockville, Md.: NIDA, pp. 31–47.

Schottenfeld, R. S., Kosten, T. R., Pakes, J., Ziedonis, D., and Oliveto, A. (1994). Buprenorphine vs. methadone maintenance for combined cocaine and opi-oid dependence. In L. S. Harris (Ed.), *Problems of drug dependence, 1993.* (NIDA Research Monograph No. 141). Rockville, Md.: NIDA, p. 142.

—— Pakes, J., Ziedonis, D., and Kosten, T. R. (1993). Buprenorphine: Dose-re-lated effects on cocaine and opioid use in cocaine-abusing opioid-dependent humans. *Biological Psychiatry, 34(1–2),* 66–74.

Schrank, K. S. (1993). Cocaine-related emergency department presentations. In H. Sorer (Ed.), *Acute cocaine intoxication: Current methods of treatment* (NIDA Research Monograph No. 123). Rockville, Md.: NIDA, pp. 110–128.

Schuckit, M. A. (1985). The clinical implications of primary diagnostic groups among alcoholics. *Archives of General Psychiatry, 42,* 1043–49.

—— (1994). The treatment of stimulant dependence. *Addiction, 89,* 1559–63.

Schuster, C. R. (1991). Monitoring the impact of cocaine. *Journal of the American Medical Association, 266,* 2273.

Schwartz, K. A. and Cohen, J. A. (1984). Subarachnoid hemorrhage precipitated by cocaine snorting. *Archives of Neurology, 41,* 705.

Schwartz, R. H., Luxenberg, M. G., and Hoffmann, N. G. (1991). "Crack" use by American middle-class adolescent polydrug abusers. *Journal of Pediatrics, 118(1),* 150–155.

—— Estroff, T., Fairbanks, D. N. F., and Hoffman, N. G. (1989). Nasal symptoms associated with cocaine abuse during adolescence. *Archives of Otolaryngology: Head and Neck Surgery, 115*, 63–64.

Science (1988). The biological tangle of drug addiction. In Research news. *Science, 23 (July)*, 415–417.

Seecof, R. and Tennant, F. S., Jr. (1986). Subjective perceptions of the intravenous "rush" of heroin and cocaine in opioid addicts. *American Journal of Drug and Alcohol Abuse, 12*, 79–97.

Segal, D. S. and Mandell, A. J. (1974). Long-term administration of *d*-amohetamine: Progressive augmentation of motor activity and stereotypy. *Pharmacology, Biochemistry and Behavior, 2*, 249–254.

Seibyl, J. P., Satel, S. L., Anthony, D., Southwick, S. M., Krystal, J. H., and Charney, D. S. (1993). Effects of cocaine on hospital course in schizophrenia. *Journal of Nervous and Mental Disease, 181(1)*, 31–37.

Seiden, L. S., Fischman, M. W., and Schuster, C. R. (1975). Long-term methamphetamine induced changes in brain catecholamines in tolerant rhesus monkeys. *Drug and Alcohol Dependence, 1*, 215–219.

Sellers, E. M., Naranjo, C. A., and Harrison, M. (1983). Diazepam loading simplified treatment of alcohol withdrawal. *Clinical Pharmacology and Therapeutics, 34*, 822–826.

Selwyn, P. A., Feiner, C., Cox, C. P., Lipshetz, C., and Cohen, R. L. (1987). Knowledge about AIDS and high-risk behavior among intravenous drug users in New York City. *AIDS, 1*, 247–254.

Sevy, S., Kay, S., Opler, L., and van Praag, H. (1990). Significance of cocaine history in schizophrenia. *Journal of Nervous and Mental Disease, 178(10)*, 642–648.

Shaffer, J. W., Nurco, D. N., Ball, J. C., and Kinlock, T. W. (1985). The frequency of nonnarcotic drug use and its relationship to criminal activity among narcotic addicts. *Comprehensive Psychiatry, 26(6)*, 558–566.

Shah, N. S., May, D. A., and Yates, J. D. (1980). Disposition of *levo-[^{3}H]* cocaine in pregnant and nonpregnant mice. *Toxicology and Applied Pharmacology, 53*, 279–284.

Shannon, M. (1988). Clinical toxicity of cocaine adulterants. *Annals of Emergency Medicine, 17*, 1243–47.

Shapshak, P., McCoy, C., Mash, D., Goodkin, K., Baum, M., Yoshioka, M., Sun, N., Nelson, S., Stewart, R., Srivastava, A., Shah, S., Arguello, J., Petkov, V., Wood, C., Berger, J., Bradley, W., Weatherby, N., Chitwood, D., Rivers, J., Page, B., Pardo, V., Pert, C., and Tourtellotte, W. W. (1993). The brain as an HIV-1 reservoir: Factors affecting HIV-1 infectivity. In L. S. Harris (Ed.), *Problems of drug dependence, 1992* (NIDA Research Monograph 132). Rockville, Md.: NIDA, pp. 73.

Shedlin, M. G. (1990). An ethnographic approach to understanding HIV high-risk behaviors: Prostitution and drug abuse (NIDA Research Monograph No. 93). Rockville, Md.: NIDA, pp. 134–149.

Shepherd, G. M. (1988). *Neurobiology.* 2nd ed. New York: Oxford University Press.

Sherer, M. A., Kumor, K., and Jaffe, J. H. (1989). Effects of intravenous cocaine are partially attenuated by haloperidol. *Psychiatry Research, 27*, 117–125.

—— Kumor, K. M., and Mapou, R. L. (1990). A case in which carbamazepine attenuated cocaine "rush" (letter). *American Journal of Psychiatry, 147(7)*, 950.

—— Kumor, K. M., Cone, E. J., and Jaffe, J. H. (1988). Suspiciousness induced by four-hour intravenous infusions of cocaine: Preliminary findings. *Archives of General Psychiatry*, 45, 637–677.

Sheridan, E., Patterson, H. R., and Gustafson, E. A. (1985). The problem of drug abuse. In E. Sheridan, H. R. Patterson, and E. A. Gustafson (Eds.), *Falcomer's The Drug, the Nurse, the Patient*. 7th ed. Philadelphia: W. B. Saunders.

Shesser, R., Davis, C., and Edelstein, S. (1981). Pneumomediastinum and pneumothorax after inhaling alkaloidal cocaine. *Annals of Emergency Medicine, 10*, 213–215.

Shukla, V. K., Goldfrank, L. R., Turndorf, H., and Bansinath, M. (1991). Antagonism of acute cocaine toxicity by buprenorphine. *Life Sciences, 49(25)*, 1887–93.

Siddall, J. W. and Conway, G. L. (1988). Interactional variables associated with retention and success in residential drug treatment. *International Journal of the Addictions, 23(12)*, 1241–54.

Siddiqui, N. S., Brown, L. S., Jr., and Makuch, R. W. (1993). Short-term declines in CD4 levels associated with cocaine use in HIV-1 seropositive, minority injecting drug users. *Journal of the National Medical Association, 85(4)*, 293–296.

Siegal, H. A., Carlson, R. G., and Falck, R. S. (1993). HIV infection/serostatus—outside epicenters human immunodeficiency virus (HIV-1) infection: A comparison among injection drug users in high and low seroprevalence areas. In B. S. Brown and G. M. Beschner (Eds.), *Handbook on risk of AIDS: Injection drug users and sexual partners*. Westport, Conn.: Greenwood Press, pp. 38–71.

——— Carlson, R. G., Falck, F., Reece, R. D., and Perlin, T. (1993). Conducting HIV outreach and research among incarcerated drug abusers: A case study of ethical concerns and dilemmas. *Journal of Substance Abuse Treatment, 10*, 71–75.

——— Falck, R. S., Carlson, R. G., and Li, L. (1991). Changes in needle risk behaviors: A preliminary comparative analysis of the Dayton-Columbus NADR program's standard and enhanced intervention tracks at six months. *Research in Progress*. Bethesda, Md.: Nova Research Co., pp. 12–16.

Siegel, R. K. (1978). Cocaine hallucinations. *American Journal of Psychiatry, 135(3)*, 309–314.

——— (1979). Cocaine smoking. *New England Journal of Medicine, 300(7)*, 373.

——— (1980). Cocaine: Recreational use and intoxication. In R. C. Petersen and R. C. Stillman (Eds.), *Cocaine: 1977*. (NIDA Research Monograph No. 13). Rockville, Md.: NIDA, pp. 137–152.

——— (1982a). Cocaine smoking. *Journal of Psychoactive Drugs, 14*, 271–359.

——— (1982b). Cocaine and sexual dysfunction: The curse of mama coca. *Journal of Psychoactive Drugs, 14*, 71–74.

——— (1984). Cocaine smoking disorders: Diagnosis and treatment. *Psychiatric Annals, 14(10)*, 728–732.

Silverman, K., Brooner, R. K., Montoya, I. D., Schuster, C. R., and Preston, K. L. (1994). Differential reinforcement of sustained cocaine abstinence in intravenous polydrug abusers. Poster presentation at the Fifty-Sixth Annual Scientific Meeting of the College on Problems of Drug Dependence. Palm Beach, June.

Silvestrini, B., Cioli, V., Burberi, S., and Catanese, B. (1968). Pharmacological properties of AF 1161, a new psychotropic drug. *Neuropharmacology, 7*, 587–599.

Simpson, D. D. (1979). The relation of time spent in drug abuse treatment to posttreatment outcome. *American Journal of Psychiatry, 136(11)*, 1449–53.

—— (1981). Treatment for drug abuse: Follow-up outcomes and length of time spent. *Archives of General Psychiatry, 38*, 875–880.

—— and Marsh, K. L. (1986). Relapse and recovery among opioid addicts 12 years after treatment. In F. M. Tims and C. G. Leukefeld (Eds.), *Relapse and recovery in drug abuse*. (NIDA Research Monograph No. 72). Washington, D.C.: NIDA, pp. 86–103.

—— and Sells, S. B. (1982). Effectiveness of treatment for drug abuse: An overview of the DARP research program. *Advances in Alcohol and Substance Abuse, 2*, 7–29.

—— and Sells, S. B. (Eds.) (1990). *Opioid addiction and treatment: A 12-year follow-up*. Malabar, Fla.: Krieger.

—— Savage, L. J., and Lloyd, M. R. (1979). Follow-up evaluation of treatment of drug abuse during 1969–1972. *Archives of General Psychiatry, 36*, 772–780.

Simpson, R. W. and Edwards, W. D. (1986). Pathogenesis of cocaine-induced ischemic heart disease. *Archives of Pathology and Laboratory Medicine, 110*, 479–484.

Singer, L., Arendt, R., Song, L. Y., Warshawsky, E., and Kliegman, R. (1994). Direct and indirect interactions of cocaine with childbirth outcomes. *Archives of Pediatrics and Adolescent Medicine, 148(9)*, 959–964.

Singer, L. T., Yamashita, T. S., Hawkins, S., Cairns, D., Baley, J., and Kliegman, R. (1994). Increased incidence of intraventricular hemorrhage and developmental delay in cocaine-exposed, very low birth weight infants. *Journal of Pediatrics, 124(5, pt.1)*, 765–771.

Siris, S. G. (1990). Pharmacological treatment of substance-abusing schizophrenic patients. *Schizophrenia Bulletin, 16*, 111–122.

—— Kane, J. M., Frechen, K., Sellew, A. P., Mandelli, J., and Fasano-Dube, B. (1988). Histories of substance abuse in patients with post-psychotic depressions. *Comprehensive Psychiatry, 29*, 550–557.

Sisson, R. W. and Azrin, N. H. (1989). The community reinforcement approach. In R. K. Hester and W. R. Miller (Eds.), *Handbook of alcoholism treatment approaches: Effective alternatives*. New York: Peregamon.

Small, G. W. and Purcell, J. J. (1985). Trazodone and cocaine abuse. *Archives of General Psychiatry, 42*, 524.

Smart, R. G. and Anglin, L. (1987). Do we know the lethal dose of cocaine? *Journal of Forensic Sciences, 32(2)*, 303–312.

Smith, D. E., Schwartz, R. H., and Martin, D. M. (1989). Heavy cocaine use by adolescents. *Pediatrics, 83(4)*, 539–542.

—— Wesson, D. R., and Apter-Marsh, M. (1984). Cocaine and alcohol-induced sexual dysfunctions in patients with addictive disease. *Journal of Psychoactive Drugs, 16(4)*, 359–361.

Smith, I. E., Dent, D. Z., Coles, C. D., and Falek, A. (1992). A comparison study of treated and untreated pregnant and postpartum cocaine-abusing women. *Journal of Substance Abuse Treatment, 9*, 343–348.

Snyder, C. A., Wood, R. W., Graefe, J. F., Bowers, A., and Magar, K. (1988). "Crack smoke" is a respirable aerosol of cocaine base. *Pharmacology, Biochemistry, and Behavior, 29*, 93–95.

Sobell, L. C., Maisto, S. A., Sobell, M. B., and Cooper, A. M. (1979). Reliability of alcohol abusers' self-reports of drinking behavior. *Behavior Research and Therapy, 17,* 157–160.

Soetens, E., D'Hooge, R., and Hueting, J. E. (1993). Amphetamine enhances human-memory consolidation. *Neuroscience Letters, 161(1),* 9–12.

Sorensen, J. L. Constantini, M. F., Wall, T. L., and Gibson, D. R. (1993). Coupons attract high-risk untreated heroin users into detoxification. *Drug and Alcohol Dependence, 31,* 247–252.

Sorer, H. (1993). The medications development program: A new initiative of the National Institute on Drug Abuse. In H. Sorer (Ed.), *Acute cocaine intoxication: Current methods of treatment* (NIDA Research Monograph No. 123). Rockville, Md.: NIDA, pp. 1–19.

Spencer, J. W. (1990). Why evaluate for residual drug effects. In J. W. Spencer and J. J. Boren (Eds.), *Residual effects of abused drugs on behavior* (NIDA Research Monograph No. 101). Rockville, Md.: NIDA, pp. 1–9.

Spotts, J. V. and Shontz, F. C. (1976). *The life styles of nine American cocaine users: Trips to the land of Cockaigne* (NIDA Research Monograph No. 16). Washington, D.C.: Government Printing Office.

────── and Shontz, F. C. (1980). *Cocaine users: A representative case approach.* New York: Free Press.

────── and Shontz, F. C. (1984). Drug-induced ego states. I. Cocaine: Phenomenology and implications. *International Journal of the Addictions, 19(2),* 119–151.

Stafford, J. R., Jr., Rosen, T. S., Zaider, M., and Merriam, J. C. (1994). Prenatal cocaine exposure and the development of the human eye. *Ophthalmology, 101(2),* 301–308.

Stark, M. J., Campbell, B. K., and Brinkerhoff, C. V. (1990). "Hello, may we help you?" A study of attrition prevention at the time of the first phone contact with substance-abusing clients. *American Journal of Drug and Alcohol Abuse, 16(1–2),* 67–76.

Steer, R. A., Platt, J. J., Ranieri, W. F., and Metzger, D. S. (1989). Relationships of SCL-90 profiles to methadone patients' psychosocial characteristics and treatment response. *Multivariate Experimental Clinical Research, 9(2),* 45–54.

Steinberg, M. A., Kosten, T. A., and Rounsaville, B. J. (1992). Cocaine abuse and pathological gambling. *American Journal on Addictions, 1,* 121–132.

Stephens, R. C., Feucht, T. E., and Gibbs, B. H. (1993). Needle use behavior. In B. S. Brown and G. M. Beschner (Eds.), *Handbook of risk on AIDS: Injection drug users and sexual partners.* Westport, Conn.: Greenwood Press, pp. 116–136.

Sterk, C. (1988). Cocaine and HIV seropositivity. *Lancet, 1,* 1052–53.

Stevens, V. J. and Hollis, J. F. (1989). Preventing smoking relapse, using an individually tailored skills-training technique. *Journal of Consulting and Clinical Psychology, 57(3),* 420–424.

Stewart, D. J., Inaba, T., Lucassen, M., and Kalow, W. (1979). Cocaine metabolism: Cocaine and norcocaine hydrolysis by liver and serum esterases. *Clinical Pharmcology and Therapeutics, 25,* 464–468.

────── Inaba, T., Tang, B. K., and Kalow, W. (1977). Hydrolysis of cocaine in human plasma by cholinesterase. *Life Sciences, 20,* 1557–64.

Stimmel, B. (1991). Buprenorphine and cocaine addiction: The need for caution (editorial). *Journal of Addictive Diseases, 10(3),* 1–4.

Stitzer, M. L., and Kirby, K. C. (1991). Reducing illicit drug use among methadone patients. In R. W. Pickens, C. G. Leukefeld, and C. R. Schuster (Eds.), *Improving drug abuse treatment* (NIDA Research Monograph No. 106). Rockville, Md.: NIDA, pp. 178–203.

—— Bigelow, G. E., and Liebson, I. A. (1980). Reducing drug use among methadone maintenance clients: Contingent reinforcement for morphine free urines. *Addictive Behaviors, 5,* 333–340.

—— Bigelow, G. E., and McCaul, M. E. (1983). Behavioral approaches to drug abuse. In M. Hersen and L. Eisler (Eds.), *Progress in behavior modification.* Vol. 14. New York: Acadermic Press, pp. 49–124.

—— Bickel, W. K., Bigelow, G. E., and Liebson, L. A. (1986). Effect of methadone dose contingencies on urinalysis test results of polydrug abusing methadone maintenance patients. *Drug and Alcohol Dependence, 18,1,* 341–348.

—— Bigelow, G. E., Liebson, I. A., and McCaul, M. E. (1984). Contingency management of supplemental drug use during methadone maintenance. In J. Grabowski, M. L. Stitzer, and J. E. Henningfield (Eds.), *Behavioral intervention techniques in drug abuse treatment* (NIDA Research Monograph No. 46). Rockville, Md.: NIDA, pp. 84–103.

Stone, A. M., Greenstein, R. A., Gamble, G., and McLellan, A. T. (1993). Cocaine use by schizophrenic outpatients who receive depot neuroleptic medication. *Hospital and Community Psychiatry, 44(2),* 176–177.

Strain, E. C., Stitzer, M. L., Liebson, I. A., and Bigelow, G. E. (1994). An outpatient trial of methadone versus buprenorphine in the treatment of combined opioid and cocaine dependence. In L. S. Harris (Ed.), *Problems of drug dependence, 1993* (NIDA Research Monograph No. 141). Rockville, Md.: NIDA, p. 141.

Strang, J., Johns, A., and Caan, W. (1993). Cocaine in the UK, 1991. *British Journal of Psychiatry, 162,* 1–13.

Streissguth, A. P. and Finnegan, L. P. (1996). Effects of prenatal alcohol and drugs. In J. Kinney (Ed.). *Clinical manual of substance abuse, second edition.* St. Louis: Mosby,pp. 254–270.

Strickland, T. L., Mena, I., Villanueva-Meyer, J., Miller, B. L., Cummings, J., Mehringer, C. M., Satz, P., and Myers, H. (1993). Cerebral perfusion and neuropsychological consequences of chronic cocaine use. *Journal of Neuropsychiatry and Clinical Neurosciences, 5(4),* 419–427.

Stripling, J. S. and Ellinwood, E. H., Jr. (1977). In R. H. Ellinwood and M. M. Kilbey (Eds.), *Cocaine and other stimulants.* New York: Plenum, pp. 327–351.

Strominger, M. B., Sachs, R., and Hersh, P. S. (1990). Microbial keratitis with crack cocaine (letter). *Archives of Ophthalmology, 108,* 1672.

Strug, D. L., Hunt, D. E., Goldsmith, D. S., Lipton, D. S., and Spunt, B. (1985). Patterns of cocaine use among methadone clients. *International Journal of the Addictions, 20(8),* 1163–75.

Substance Abuse and Mental Health Services Administration [SAMHSA] (1994a). *Annual Emergency Room Data, 1992* (Series I, 12-A). Rockville, Md.: DHHS.

—— (1994b). *Annual Medical Examiner Data* (Series I, 12-B). Rockville, Md.: DHHS.

—— (1994c). *Preliminary estimates from the Drug Abuse Warning Network, 1994* (Advance Report No. 8). Rockville, Md.: DHHS.

Substance Abuse and Mental Health Services Administration (1991). *National household survey on drug abuse, 1991.* Rockville, Md.: DHHS.

Sullivan, J. B., Rumack, B. H., and Peterson, R. G. (1981). Acute carbamazepine toxicity resulting from overdose. *Neurology, 31,* 621–624.

Suzuki, T., Shiozaki, Y., Masukawa, Y., Misawa, M., and Nagase, H. (1992). The role of mu- and kappa-opioid receptors in cocaine-induced conditioned place preference. *Japan Journal of Pharmacology, 58,* 435–442.

Tames, S. M. and Goldenring, J. M. (1986). Madarosis from cocaine use. *New England Journal of Medicine, 314,* 1324.

Tanenbaum, J. H. and Miller, F. (1992). Electro-cardiographic evidence of myocardial injury in psychiatrically hospitalized cocaine abusers. *General Hospital Psychiatry, 14,* 201–203.

Tardiff, K., Gross, E. M., Wu, J., Stajic, M., and Millman, R. (1989). Analysis of cocaine positive fatalities. *Journal of Forensic Science, 34,* 53–63.

———— Marzuk, P. M., Leon, A. C., Hirsch, C. S., Stajic, M., Portera, L., and Hartwell, N. (1994). Homicide in New York City: Cocaine use and firearms. *Journal of the American Medical Association, 272(1),* 43–46.

Tashkin, D. P., Gorelick, D., Khalsa, M. E., Simmons, M., and Chang, P. (1992). Respiratory effects of cocaine freebasing among habitual cocaine users. *Journal of Addictive Diseases, 11(4),* 59–70.

———— Simmons, M. S., Coulson, A. H., Clark, V. A., and Gong, H., Jr. (1987). Respiratory effects of cocaine "freebasing" among habitual users of marijuana with or without tobacco. *Chest, 92,* 638–644.

Tatum, A. L., Atkinson, A. J., and Collins, K. H. (1925). Acute cocain poisoning: Preliminary report of an experimental study. *Journal of the American Medical Association, 84(16),* 1177.

Taylor, A. T., Wagner, P. J., Pritchard, D. C., and Tollison, J. W. (1994). Fluoxetine in family practice patients. *Journal of Family Practice, 39(1),* 45–49.

Taylor, D. and Ho, B. T. (1978). Comparison of inhibition of monoamine uptake by cocaine, methylphenidate, and amphetamines. *Research Communications in Chemical Pathology and Pharmacology, 21,* 67–75.

Taylor, D. L., Ho, B. T., and Fagan, J. D. (1979). Increased dopamine receptor binding in rat brain by repeated cocaine injections. *Communications in Psychopharmacology, 3,* 137–142.

Taylor, D. P., Hyslop, D. K., and Riblet, L. A. (1980). Trazodone, a new nontricyclic antidepressant without anticholinergic activity. *Biochemical Pharmacology, 29,* 2149–50.

Teller, D. W. and Devenyi, P. (1988). Bromocriptine in cocaine withdrawal: Does it work? *International Journal of the Addictions, 23(11),* 1197–1205.

Tennant, F. S. and Sagherian, A. H. (1987). Double-blind comparison of amantadine and bromocriptine for ambulatory withdrawal from cocaine dependence. *Archives of Internal Medicine, 147,* 109–112.

Tennant, F. S., Tarver, A., and Seecof, R. (1986). Cocaine plasma concentrations in persons admitted to outpatient treatment: Relationship to treatment outcome. *Journal of Substance Abuse Treatment, 3,* 27–32.

Tennant, F. S., Jr. (1985). Effect of cocaine dependence on plasma phenylalanine and tyrosine levels and on urinary MHPG excretion. *American Journal of Psychiatry, 142,* 1200–1201.

———— and Rawson, R. A. (1983). Cocaine and amphetamine dependence treated with desipramine. In L. S. Harris (Ed.), *Problems of drug dependence, 1982* (NIDA Research Monograph No. 43). Rockville, Md.: NIDA, pp. 351–355.

Teoh, S. K., Mello, N. K., Mendelson, J. H., Kuehnle, J., Gastfriend, D. R., Rhoades, E., and Sholar, W. (1994). Buprenorphine effects on morphine- and cocaine-induced subjective responses by drug-dependent men. *Journal of Clinical Psychopharmacology, 14(1),* 15–27.

—— Mendelson, J. H., Mello, N. K., Kuehnle, J., Sintavanarong, P., and Rhoades, E. M. (1993). Acute interactions of buprenorphine with intravenous cocaine and morphine: An investigational new drug phase I safety evaluation. *Journal of Clinical Pharmacology, 13(2),* 87–99.

—— Sarnyai, Z., Mendelson, J. H., Mello, N. K., Springer, S. A., Sholar, J. W., Wapler, M., Kuehnle, J. C., and Gelles, H. (1994). Cocaine effects on pulsatile secretion of ACTH in men. *Journal of Pharmacology and Experimental Therapeutics, 270(3),* 1134–38.

Thompson, W. L. (1978). Management of alcohol withdrawal syndromes. *Archives of Internal Medicine, 138,* 278–283.

Tollefson, G. D., Birkett, M., Koran, L., and Genduso, L. (1994). Continuation treatment of OCD: Double-blind and open-label experience with fluoxetine. *Journal of Clinical Psychiatry, 55,* 69–76.

—— Rampey, A. H., Jr., Potvin, J. H., Jenike, M. A., Rush, A. J., Kominguez, R. A., Koran, L. M., Shear, M. K., Goodman, W., and Genduson, L. A. (1994). A multicenter investigation of fixed-dose fluoxetine in the treatment of obsessive-compulsive disorder. *Archives of General Psychiatry, 51(7),* 559–567.

Triffleman, E., Delucchi, K., Tunis, S., Banys, P., and Hall, S. (1993). Desipramine in the treatment of "crack" cocaine dependence: Preliminary results. In L. S. Harris (Ed.), *Problems of drug dependence, 1992* (NIDA Research Monograph No. 132). Rockville, Md.: NIDA, p. 317.

Truelson, M. E., Babb, S., Joe, J. E., and Raese, J. D. (1986). Chronic cocaine administration depletes tyrosine hydroxylase immunoreactivity in the rat brain nigral striatal system: Quantative light microscope studies. *Experimental Neurology, 94,* 744–756.

Tumeh, S. S., Nagel, J. S., English, R. J., Moore, M., and Holman, B. L. (1990). Cerebral abnormalities in cocaine abusers: Demonstration by SPECT perfusion brain scintigraphy. *Radiology, 176,* 821–824.

Tuomisto, J. and Mannisto, P. (1985). Neurotransmitter regulation of anterior pituitary hormones. *Pharmacological Reviews, 37(3),* 249–332.

Turbat-Herrera, E. A. (1994). Myoglobinuric acute renal failure associated with cocaine use. *Ultrastructural Pathology, 18(1–2),* 127–131.

U.S. Bureau of the Census (1993). *Statistical abstract of the United States: 113th edition.* Washington, D.C.: Government Printing Office.

—— (1994). *Statistrical abstract of the United States, 1993: The national data book.* Washington, D.C.: Government Printing Office.

U.S. General Accounting Office (1990). *Methadone maintenance: Some treatment programs are not effective; greater federal oversight needed* (GAO/HRD-90–104). Washington, D.C.: General Accounting Office.

Vaillant, G. E. (1973). A twenty-year follow-up of New York narcotic addicts. *Archives of General Psychiatry, 29,* 237–241.

—— (1985). *The natural history of alcoholism: Causes, patterns, and paths of recovery.* Cambridge, Mass.: Harvard University Press.

Van Dyke, C. and Byck, R. (1982). Cocaine. *Scientific American, 246,* 128–141.

—— and Byck, R. (1983). Cocaine use in man. *Advances in Substance Abuse, 3,* 1–24.

—— Barash, P. G., Jatlow, P., and Byck, R. (1976). Cocaine: Plasma concentrations after intranasal applications in man. *Science, 191,* 859–861.

—— Jatlow, P., Ungerer, J., Barash, P. G., and Byck, R. (1978). Oral cocaine: Plasma concentrations and central effects. *Science, 200,* 211–213.

—— Ungerer, J., Jatlow, P., Barash, P., and Byck, R. (1982). Intranasal cocaine dose: Relationship of psychological effects and plasma levels. *Psychiatry in Medicine, 12(1),* 1–13.

van Kammen, D. P. and Murphy, D. L. (1975). Attenuation of the euphoriant and activating effects of *d*- and *l*-amphetamine by lithium carbonate treatment. *Psychopharmacologia, 44,* 215–224.

—— Bunney, W. E., Docherty, J. P., Marder, S. R., Ebert, M. H., Rosenblatt, J. E., and Rayner, J. N. (1982). *D*-amphetamine induced heterogeneous changes in psychotic behavior in schizophrenia. *American Journal of Psychiatry, 139,* 991–997.

Vaz, A., Lefkowitz, S. S., and Lefkowitz, D. L. (1993). Effects of cocaine on the respiratory burst of murine macrophages. *Advances in Experimental Medicine and Biology, 335,* 135–142.

Verebey, K. (1987). Cocaine abuse detection by laboratory methods. In A. M. Washton, and M. S. Gold (Eds.), *Cocaine: A clinician's handbook.* New York: Guilford, pp. 214–226.

—— and Gold, M. S. (1985). Psychopharmacology of cocaine: Behavior, neurophysiology, neurochemistry and proposed treatment. In D. W. Morgan (Ed.), *Psychopharmacology: Impact on clinical psychiatry.* St. Louis: Ishiyaku EuroAmerica, pp. 219–241.

—— and Gold, M. S. (1988). From coca leaves to crack: The effects of dose and routes of administration in abuse liability. *Psychiatric Annals, 18,* 513–520.

Volkow, N. D., Fowler, J. S., Wolf, A. P., Schlyer, D., Shiue, C.-Y., Alpert, R., Dewey, S. L., Logan, J., Bendriem, B., Christman, D., Hitzemann, R., and Henn, F. (1990). Effects of chronic cocaine abuse on postsynaptic dopamine receptors. *American Journal of Psychiatry, 147(6),* 719–724.

—— Mullani, N., Gould, K. L., Adler, S., and Krajewski, K. (1988). Cerebral blood flow in chronic cocaine users: A study with positron emission tomography. *British Journal of Psychiatry, 152,* 641–648.

Voris, J., Elder, I., and Sebastian, P. (1991). A simple test of cocaine craving and related responses. *Journal of Clinical Psychology, 47,* 320–323.

Wagner, G. C., Seiden, L. S., and Schuster, C. R. (1979). Methamphetamine-induced changes in brain catecholamines in rats and guinea pigs. *Drug and Alcohol Dependence, 4,* 435–438.

Wald, D., Ebstein, R. P., and Belmaker, R. H. (1978). Haloperidol and lithium blocking of the mood response to intravenous methylphenidate. *Psychopharmacology, 57,* 83–87.

Wallace, B. C. (1987). Cocaine dependence treatment on an inpatient detoxification unit. *Journal of Substance Abuse Treatment, 4,* 85–92.

—— (1989). Psychological and enviomental determinants of relapse in crack cocaine smokers. *Journal of Substance Abuse Treatment, 6(2),* 95–106.

—— (1990a). Crack addiction: Treatment and recovery issues. *Contemporary Drug Problems 17(1),* 79–119.

——— (1990b). Treating crack cocaine dependence: The critical role of relapse prevention. *Journal of Psychoactive Drugs, 22(2)*, 149–158.

Wallach, S. J. (1989). Medical complications of the use of cocaine. *Hawaii Medical Journal, 48(11)*, 461–462.

Walsh, B. T. (1991). Psychopharmacologic treatment of bulimia nervosa (review). *Journal of Clinical Psychiatry, 52*, 34–38.

Wang, R. I. H., Cho, J.-K., Roh, B., and Salstorm, D. (1992). Bromocriptine: Anticraving and other effects in patients abusing cocaine. In L. S. Harris (Ed.), *Problems of drug dependence, 1991* (NIDA Research Monograph No. 119). Rockville, Md.: NIDA, p. 464.

——— Kalbfleisch, J., Cho, J. K., and Forbes, M. (1994). Bromocriptine, desipramine, and trazodone alone and in combination to cocaine dependent patients. In L. S. Harris (Ed.), *Problems of drug dependence, 1993* (NIDA Research Monograph No. 141). Rockville, Md.: NIDA, p. 437.

Washburn, A. M., Batki, S. L., Delucchi, K., Murphy, J., Jones, T. A., and Nanda, N. (1994). Predictors of outcome in a clinical trial of fluoxetine treatment of primary cocaine dependence. In L. S. Harris (Ed.), *Problems of drug dependence, 1993* (NIDA Research Monograph No. 141). Rockville, Md.: NIDA, p. 139.

Washton, A. M. (1987). Nonpharmacologic treatment of cocaine abuse. *Psychiatric Clinics of North America, 9*, 563–571.

——— (1989a). Cocaine abuse and compulsive sexuality. *Medical Aspects of Human Sexuality, 23*, 32–39.

——— (1989b). Outpatient treatment works, too. *US Journal of Drug and Alcohol Dependence, 13(2)*, 14.

——— and Gold, M. S. (1984). Chronic cocaine abuse: Evidence for adverse efects on health and functioning. *Psychiatric Annals, 14*, 733–743.

——— and Stone-Washton, N. (1990). Abstinence and relapse in outpatient cocaine addicts. *Journal of Psychoactive Drugs, 22(2)*, 135–147.

——— and Stone-Washton, N. (1993). Outpatient treatment of cocaine and crack addiction: A clinical perspective. In F. M. Tims and C. G. Leukefeld (Eds.), *Cocaine treatment: Research and clinical perspectives* (NIDA Research Monograph No. 135). Rockville, Md.: NIDA, pp. 15–30.

——— Gold, M. S., and Pottash, A. C. (1984). Survey of 500 callers to a national cocaine helpline. *Psychosomatics, 25(10)*, 771–775.

——— Gold, M. S., and Pottash, A. C. (1985). Treatment outcome in cocaine abusers. In L. S. Harris (Ed.), *Problems of drug dependence, 1986* (NIDA Research Monograph Series No. 67), 381–384.

——— Gold, M. S., and Pottash, A. C. (1987). Cocaine abuse: Techniques of assessment, diagnosis and treatment. *Psychiatric Medicine, 3*, 185–195.

Watson, R., Bakos, L., Compton, P., Byck, R., and Gawin, F. (1989). Cocaine use and withdrawal: The effect on sleep and mood. *Sleep Research, 8*, 83.

Watters, J. K., Reinarmen, C., and Fagan, J. (1985). Causality, context and contingency relationships between drug abuse and deliquency. *Contemporary Drug Problems, 14*, 351–373.

——— Needle, R., Brown, B. S., Weatherby, N., Booth, R., and Williams, M. (1992). The self-reporting of cocaine use (letter; comment). *Journal of the American Medical Association, 268(17)*, 2374–75.

Weatherby, N. L., Shultz, J. M., Chitwood, D. D., McCoy, H. V., McCoy, C. B.,

Ludwig, D. D., and Edlin, B. R. (1992). Crack cocaine use and sexual activity in Miami, Florida. *Journal of Psychoactive Drugs, 24(4),* 373–380.

Webber, M. P. and Hauser, W. A. (1993). Secular trends in New York City hospital discharge diagnoses of congenital syphilis and cocaine dependence, 1982–88. *Public Health Reports—Hyattsville, 108(3),* 279–284.

Webster, W. S., Brown-Woodman, P. D., and Lipson, A. H. (1990). Teratogenic properties of cocaine in rats. *Teratology, 41,* 689–697.

Weddington, W. W. (1990). Use of unproven and unapproved drugs to treat cocaine addiction. *American Journal of Psychiatry, 147(11),* 1576.

Weddington, W. W., Brown, B. S., Haertzen, C. A., Cone, E. J., Dax, E. M., Herning, R. I., and Michaelson, B. S. (1990). Changes in mood, craving, and sleep during short-term abstinence reported by male cocaine addicts. *Archives of General Psychiatry, 47,* 861–868.

——— Brown, B. S., Haertzen, C. A., Hess, J. M., Mahaffey, J. R., Kolar, A. F., and Jaffe, J. H. (1991). Comparison of amantadine and desipramine combined with psychotherapy for treatment of cocaine dependence. *American Journal of Drug and Alcohol Abuse, 17(2),* 137–152.

——— Haertzen, C. A., Hess, J. M., and Brown, B. S. (1991). Psychological reactions and retention by cocaine addicts during treatment according to HIV-serostatus: A matched-control study. *American Journal of Drug and Alcohol Abuse, 17(3),* 355–368.

Weiss, B. and Laties, V. G. (1962). Enhancement of human performance by caffeine and the amphetamines. *Pharmacological Review, 14,* 1–36.

Weiss, R. D. (1986). Recurrent myocardial infarction caused by cocaine abuse. *American Heart Journal, 111,* 793.

——— (1988). Relapse to cocaine abuse after initiating desipramine treatment. *Journal of the American Medical Association, 260(17),* 2545–46.

——— and Gawin, F. H. (1988). Protracted elimination of cocaine metabolites in long-term high-dose cocaine abusers. *American Journal of Medicine, 85,* 879–880.

——— and Mirin, S. M. (1986). Subtypes of cocaine abusers. *Psychiatric Clinics of North America, 9(3),* 491–501.

——— and Mirin, S. M. (1987). *Cocaine.* Washington, D.C.: American Psychiatric Press.

——— and Mirin, S. M. (1990). Psychological and pharmacological treatment strategies in cocaine dependence. *Annals of Clinical Psychiatry, 2,* 239–243.

——— Griffin, M. L., and Mirin, S. M. (1992). Drug abuse as self-medication for depression: An empirical study. *American Journal of Drug and Alcohol Abuse, 18(2),* 121–129.

——— Mirin, S. M., and Bartel, R. L. (1994). *Cocaine.* 2nd ed. Washington, D.C.: American Psychiatric Press.

——— Pope, H. G., and Mirin, S. M. (1985). Treatment of chronic cocaine abuse and attention deficit disorder, residual type, with magnesium pemoline. *Drug and Alcohol Dependence, 15,* 69–72.

——— Goldenheim, P. D., Mirin, S. M., Hales, C. A., and Mendelson, J. H. (1981). Pulmonary dysfunction in cocaine smokers. *American Journal of Psychiatry, 138,* 1110–12.

——— Mirin, S. M., Griffin, M. L., Gunderson, J. G., and Hufford, C. (1993). Personality disorders in cocaine dependence. *Comprehensive Psychiatry, 34(3),* 145–149.

—— Mirin, S. M., Griffin, M. L., and Michael, J. L. (1988). Psychopathology in cocaine abusers: Changing trends. *Journal of Nervous and Mental Disease, 176(12)*, 719–725.

—— Mirin, S. M., Michael, J. L., and Sollogub, A. C. (1986). Psychopathology in chronic cocaine abusers. *American Journal of Drug and Alcohol Abuse, 12(1&2)*, 17–29.

Weiss, S. R. B., Post, R. M., Costello, M., Nutt, D. J., and Tandeciarz, S. (1990). Carbamazepine prevents the development of cocaine-kindled seizures but not sensitization to cocaine's effects on hyperactivity. *Neuropsychopharmacology, 3*, 273–281.

—— Post, R. M., Pert, A., Woodward, R., and Murman, D. (1989). Context-dependent cocaine sensitization: Differential effect of haloperidol on development versus expression. *Pharmacology, Biochemistry and Behavior, 34*, 655–661.

—— Post, R. M., Szele, F., Woodward, R., and Nierenberg, J. (1989). Chronic carbamazepine inhibits the development of local anesthetic seizures kindled by cocaine and lidocaine. *Brain Research, 497*, 72–79.

Weissman, M. M., Slobetz, F., Prusoff, B., Mezritz, M., and Howard, P. (1976). Clinical depression among narcotic addicts maintained on methadone in the community. *American Journal of Psychiatry, 133(12)*, 1434–38.

Welch, M. J., Sniegoski, L. T., and Allgood, C. C. (1993). Interlaboratory comparison studies on the analysis of hair for drugs of abuse. *Forensic Science International, 63(1–3)*, 295–303.

Welch, R. D., Todd, K., and Krause, G. S. (1991). Incidence of cocaine-associated rhabdomyolysis. *Annals of Emergency Medicine, 20(2)*, 154–157.

Weller, M. P., Ang, P. C., Latimer-Sayer, D. T., and Zachary, A. (1988). Drug abuse and mental illness (letter). *Lancet, 1*, 997.

Wells, E. A., Calsyn, D. A., Saxon, A. J., and Greenberg, D. M. (1993). Using drugs to facilitate sexual behavior is associated with sexual variety among injection drug users. *Journal of Nervous and Mental Disease, 181(10)*, 626–631.

—— Peterson, P. L., Gainey, R. R., Hawkins, J. D., and Catalano, R. F. (1994). Outpatient treatment for cocaine abuse: A controlled comparison of relapse prevention and twelve step approaches. *American Journal of Drug and Alcohol Abuse, 20(1)*, 1–17.

Wells, S. R. and Carré, L. J. G. (1895). Theoretical and practical considerations of whooping-cough: With an inquiry into the therapeutic value of cocaine in upwards of 300 cases. *Lancet*, 1429–32.

Wen, H. L. and Cheung, S. Y. C. (1973). Treatment of drug addiction by acupuncture and electrical stimulation. *Asian Journal of Medicine, 9*, 138–141.

Wender, P. H. (1979). The concept of minimal brain dysfunction (MBD). In L. Bellak (Ed.), *Psychiatric aspects of minimal brian dysfunction in adults*. New York: Grune & Stratton, pp. 1–13.

Wesson, D. R. (1982). Cocaine use by masseuses. *Journal of Psychoactive Drugs, 14(1–2)*, 75–76.

—— and Smith, D. E. (1985). Cocaine treatment perspectives. In N. J. Kozel and E. H. Adams (Eds.)., *Cocaine use in America: Epidemiologic and clinical perspectives* (NIDA Research Monograph No. 61). Rockville, Md.: NIDA, pp. 193–203.

Wetli, C. V. (1993). The pathology of cocaine: Perspectives from the autopsy table. In H. Sorer (Ed.), *Acute cocaine intoxication: Current methods of treat-*

ment (NIDA Research Monograph No. 123). Rockville, Md.: NIDA, pp. 172–182.

—— and Fishbain, D. A. (1985). Cocaine-induced psychosis and sudden death in recreational cocaine users. *Journal of Forensic Science, 30,* 873–880.

—— and Wright, R. K. (1979). Death caused by recreational cocaine use. *Journal of the American Medical Association, 241(23),* 2519–22.

Wiebel, W. W. and Lampinen, T. M. (1991). Primary prevention of HIV-1 infection among intravenous drug users. *Journal of Primary Prevention, 12(1),* 35–48.

Wieder, H. and Kaplan, E. H. (1969). Drug use in adolescents: Psychodynamic meaning and pharmacogenic effect. *Psychoanalitic Study of the Child, 24,* 399–431.

Wikler, A. (1965). Conditioning factors in opiate addiction and relapse. In D. M. Wilner and G. G. Kasselbaum (Eds.), *Narcotics.* New York: McGraw-Hill, pp. 85–100.

—— (1973). Dynamics of drug dependence. Implicaitons of a conditioning theory for research and treatment. *Archives of General Psychiatry, 28,* 611–616.

Wilkinson, P., Van Dyke, C., Jatlow, P., Barash, P., and Byck, R. (1980). Intranasal and oral cocaine kinetics. *Clinical Pharmacology and Therapeutics, 27(3),* 386–394.

Williams, A. F., Peat, M. A., Crouch, D. J., Wells, J. K., and Finkle, B. S. (1985). Drugs in fatally injured young male drivers. *Public Health Report, 100,* 19–25.

Wise, R. A. (1984). Neural mechanisms of the reinforcing action of cocaine. In J. Graboski (Ed.), *Cocaine: Effects and treatment of abuse* (NIDA Research Monograph No. 50). Washington, D.C.: NIDA, pp. 15–33.

Witkin, J. M. and Katz, J. L. (1993). Preclinical assessment of cocaine toxicity: Mechanisms and pharmacotherapy. In H. Sorer (Ed.), *Acute cocaine intoxication: Current methods of treatment* (NIDA Research Monograph No. 123). Rockville, Md.: NIDA, pp. 44–69.

—— and Tortella, F. C. (1991). Modulators of N-methyl-D-aspartate protect against diazepam- or phenobarbital-resistant cocaine convulsions. *Life Science, 48,* PL51–PL56.

—— Johnson, R. E., Jaffe, J. H., Goldberg, S. R., Grayson, N. A., Rice, K. C., and Katz, J. L. (1991). The mixed opioid agonist-antagonist, buprenorphine, protects against lethal effects of cocaine. *Drug and Alcohol Dependence, 27,* 177–184.

Wojak, J. C. and Flamm, E. S. (1987). Intracranial hemorrhage and cocaine use. *Stroke, 18,* 712–715.

Wolfe, H., Vranizan, K. M., Gorter, R. G., Cohen, R., and Moss, A. R. (1990). Crack use and related risk factors in IVDUs in San Francisco. Presented at the Sixth International Conference on AIDS. San Francisco, June 20–24.

Wolff, C. (1988, December 16). Against drug tide, police holding action. *New York Times,* pp. A1, B4.

Wolfsohn, R., Sanfilipo, M., and Angrist, B. (1993). A placebo-controlled trial of L-dopa/carbidopa in early cocaine abstinence. *Neuropsychopharmacology, 9(1),* 49–53.

Wolpe, J. (1973). *The practice of behavior therapy.* New York: Pergamon.

Wood, A. (1993). Pharmacotherapy of bulimia nervosa—experience with fluoxetine. *International Clinical Psychopharmacology, 8(4),* 295–299.

Woods, N. S., Eyler, F. D., Behnke, M., and Conlon, M. (1993). Cocaine use during pregnancy: Maternal depressive symptoms and infant neurobehavior over the first month. *Infant Behavior and Development, 16,* 83–98.

Woody, G. E., McLellan, A. T., and O'Brien, C. P. (1990). Clinical-behavioral observations of the long-term effects of drug abuse. In J. W. Spencer and J. J. Boren (Eds.), *Residual effects of abused drugs on behavior* (NIDA Research Monograph No. 101). Rockville, Md.: NIDA, pp. 71–85.

―――― O'Brien, C. P., and Rickels, K. (1975). Depression and anxiety in heroin addicts: A placebo-controlled study of doxepin in combination with methadone. *American Journal of Psychiatry, 132(4),* 447–450.

―――― Luborsky, L., McLellan, A. T., O'Brien, C. P., Beck, A. T., Blaine, J., Herman, I., and Hole, A. (1983). Psychotherapy for opiate addicts. *Archives of General Psychiatry, 40,* 639–645.

―――― McLellan, A. T., Luborsky, L., and O'Brien, C. P. (1985). Sociopathy and psychotherapy outcome. *Archives of General Psychiatry, 42,* 1081–86.

―――― McLellan, A. T., Luborsky, L., O'Brien, C. P., Blaine, J., Fox, S., Herman, I., and Beck, A. T. (1984). Severity of psychiatric symptoms as a predictor of benefits from psychotherapy: The Veterans Administration–Penn Study. *American Journal of Psychiatry, 141(10),* 1172–77.

Woolverton, W. L. (1986). Effects of a D1 and a D2 dopamine antagonist on the self-administration of cocaine and piribedil by rhesus monkeys. *Pharmacology, Biochemistry and Behavior, 24,* 531–535.

―――― (1991). Discriminative stimulus effects of cocaine. In R. A. Glennon, T. U. C. Järbe, and J. Frankenheim (Eds.), *Drug discrimination: Applications to drug abuse research* (NIDA Research Monograph No. 116). Rockville, Md.: NIDA, pp. 61–74.

Wurmser, L. (1974). Psychoanalytic considerations of the etiology of compulsive drug use. *Journal of the American Psychoanalytic Association, 22,* 820–843.

Yamaguchi, K. and Kandel, D. B. (1984). Patterns of drug use from adolescence to early adulthood: III. Predictors of progression. *American Journal of Public Health, 74,* 673–681.

Yates, W. Y., Fulton, A. I., Gabel, J. E., and Brass, C. T. (1989). Personality risk factors for cocaine abuse. *American Journal of Public Health, 79,* 891–892.

Yawn, B. P., Thompson, L. R., Lupo, V. R., Googins, M. K., and Yawn, R. A. (1994). Prenatal drug use in Minneapolis–St. Paul, Minn.: A 4-year trend. *Archives of Family Medicine, 3(6),* 520–527.

Yelian, F. D., Sacco, A. G., Ginsburg, K. A., Doerr, P. A., and Armant, D. R. (1994). The effects of in vitro cocaine exposure on human sperm motility, intracellular calcium, and oocyte penetration. *Fertility and Sterility, 61(5),* 915–921.

Yokel, R. A. and Wise, R. A. (1975). Increased lever pressing for amphetamine after pimozide in rats: Implications for a dopamine theory of reward. *Science, 187,* 547–549.

Young, T. J. (1987). Illicit cocaine use in clinical perspective. *International Journal of Offender Therapy and Comparative Criminology, 3,* 179–187.

Young, T. W. and Pollock, D. A. (1993). Misclassification of deaths caused by cocaine: An assessment by survey. *American Journal of Forensic Medicine and Pathology, 14(1),* 43–47.

Yu, P. H. (1994). Pharmacological and clinical implications of MAO-B inhibitors. *General Pharmacology, 25(8),* 1527–39.

Zackon, F., McAuliffe, W. E., and Ch'ien, J. M. N. (1985). *Addict aftercare: Recovery training and self-help* (NIDA Treatment Research Monograph). Rockville, Md.: NIDA.

Zagelbaum, B. M., Tannenbaum, M. H., and Hersh, P. S. (1991). *Candida albicans* corneal ulcer associated with crack cocaine (letter). *American Journal of Ophthalmology, 111(2),* 248–249.

Zeiter, J. H., McHenry, J. G., and McDermott, M. L. (1990). Unilateral pharmacologic mydriasis secondary to crack cocaine. *American Journal of Emergency Medicine, 8(6),* 568–569.

Ziedonis, D. M. and Kosten, T. R. (1991). Depression as a prognostic factor for pharmacological treatment of cocaine dependence. *Psychopharmacology Bulletin, 27(3),* 337–343.

—— Rayford, B. S., Bryant, K. J., and Rounsaville, B. J. (1994). Psychiatric comorbidity in white and African-American cocaine addicts seeking substance abuse treatment. *Hospital and Community Psychiatry, 45(1),* 43–49.

Zucker, K. (1933). Nature of functional disturbance in cocaine hallucinations. *Lancet,* 1479–80.

Zuckerman, B. and Bresnahan, K. (1991). Developmental and behavioral consequences of prenatal drug and alcohol exposure. *Pediatric Clinics of North America, 38(6),* 1387–1406.

—— Frank, D. A., Hingson, R., Amaro, H., Levenson, S. M., Kayne, H., Parker, S., Vinci, R., Aboagye, K., Fried, L. E., Cabral, H., Timperi, R., and Bauchner, H. (1989). Effects of maternal marijuana and cocaine use on fetal growth. *New England Journal of Medicine, 320,* 762–768.

Zweben, J. E. (1987). Recovery-oriented psychotherapy: Facilitating the use of 12-step programs. *Journal of Psychoactive Drugs, 19(3),* 243–251.

—— (1989). Recovery-oriented psychotherapy: Patient resistances and therapist dilemmas. *Journal of Substance Abuse Treatment, 6,* 123–132.

Author Index

Subject Index